Latest Findings in Family Medicine

Latest Findings in Family Medicine

Editor: Nora Ortega

www.fosteracademics.com

www.fosteracademics.com

Cataloging-in-Publication Data

Latest findings in family medicine / edited by Nora Ortega.
   p. cm.
Includes bibliographical references and index.
ISBN 978-1-63242-877-6
1. Family medicine. 2. Medicine. 3. Families--Health and hygiene. I. Ortega, Nora.
RC46 .L38 2020
610--dc23

Foster Academics,
118-35 Queens Blvd., Suite 400,
Forest Hills, NY 11375, USA

ISBN 978-1-63242-877-6 (Hardback)

Contents

Preface

In my initial years as a student, I used to run to the library at every possible instance to grab a book and learn something new. Books were my primary source of knowledge and I would not have come such a long way without all that I learnt from them. Thus, when I was approached to edit this book; I became understandably nostalgic. It was an absolute honor to be considered worthy of guiding the current generation as well as those to come. I put all my knowledge and hard work into making this book most beneficial for its readers.

Family medicine is a specialization in medicine, which is concerned with the provision of comprehensive healthcare to individuals and families. Unlike other medical specialties, which are limited to the treatment of a particular disease or management of a specific organ, this field integrates care for patients across all ages, genders and diseases. This field deals with a range of diverse acute and chronic healthcare concerns. Besides the diagnosis and treatment of illness, health-risk assessments, preventive care, routine checkups, personalized counseling, and immunization and screening tests, are essential aspects of family medicine. Family physicians participate in integrated outpatient and inpatient learning in obstetrics and gynecology, pediatrics, psychiatry and neurology, internal medicine, community medicine and surgery. This book elucidates the concepts and innovative models around prospective developments with respect to family medicine. While understanding the long-term perspectives of the topics, the book makes an effort in highlighting their impact as a modern tool for the growth of the discipline. It attempts to assist those with a goal of delving into this field.

I wish to thank my publisher for supporting me at every step. I would also like to thank all the authors who have contributed their researches in this book. I hope this book will be a valuable contribution to the progress of the field.

Editor

General practitioners' perspectives on management of early-stage chronic kidney disease

Carola van Dipten[1]*[iD], Saskia van Berkel[1], Wim J. C. de Grauw[1], Nynke D. Scherpbier-de Haan[1], Bouke Brongers[1], Karel van Spaendonck[1], Jack F. M. Wetzels[2], Willem J. J. Assendelft[1] and Marianne K. Dees[1]

Abstract

Background: Guideline adherence in chronic kidney disease management is low, despite guideline implementation initiatives. Knowing general practitioners' (GPs') perspectives of management of early-stage chronic kidney disease (CKD) and the applicability of the national interdisciplinary guideline could support strategies to improve quality of care.

Method: Qualitative focus group study with 27 GPs in the Netherlands. Three analysts open-coded and comparatively analysed the data. Mind-mapping sessions were performed after data-saturation.

Results: Five themes emerged: defining CKD, knowledge and awareness, patient-physician interaction, organisation of CKD care and value of the guideline. A key finding was the abstractness of the CKD concept. The GPs expressed various perspectives about defining CKD and interpreting estimated glomerular filtration rates. Views about clinical relevance influenced the decision-making, although factual knowledge seems lacking. Striving to inform well enough without creating anxiety and to explain suitably for the intellectual ability of the patient caused tension in the patient-physician interaction. Integration with cardiovascular disease-management programmes was mentioned as a way of implementing CKD care in the future. The guideline was perceived as a rough guide rather than a leading document.

Conclusion: CKD is perceived as an abstract rather than a clinical concept. Abstractness plays a role in all formulated themes. Management of CKD patients in primary care is complex and is influenced by physician-bound considerations related to individual knowledge and perception of the importance of CKD. Strategies are needed to improve GPs' understanding of the concept of CKD by education, a holistic approach to guidelines, and integration of CKD care into cardiovascular programmes.

Keywords: Chronic kidney disease, Guidelines, Primary care, Qualitative research, Quality of care

Background

Chronic kidney disease (CKD) is an important healthcare problem. The estimated prevalence in the Netherlands is 12% [1], which is similar to the prevalence in the US and the UK (13%) [2, 3]. CKD causes substantial morbidity and mortality, mainly related to increased cardiovascular risk [4–6]. It is expected that the number of CKD patients will increase due to aging of the population and increased prevalence of diabetes and hypertension [5, 7].

Most early-stage CKD patients receive care from general practitioners (GPs). Several international guidelines have been developed to improve the quality of care in primary care [8, 9]. In the Netherlands GPs function as gatekeepers and are supported by nurse practitioners in the area of chronic diseases. The Dutch interdisciplinary guideline for CKD (DIG-CKD) [10] for family practice and nephrology provides recommendations for GPs

* Correspondence: Carola.vanDipten@radboudumc.nl
[1]Department of Primary and Community Care, Radboud University Medical Center, PO Box 9101, 6500 HBPostal Route 117, Nijmegen, The Netherlands
Full list of author information is available at the end of the article

about the identification and management of CKD and serves as a guide for shared care with nephrologists [10]. This guideline was introduced in 2009. It is very similar to the NICE guideline for CKD, is distributed by the Dutch College of General Practitioners and freely available, in print and online.

Despite guideline recommendations, a number of quantitative studies indicate substantial deficiencies in the quality of care delivered, including CKD recognition and monitoring as well as reaching blood pressure targets [11–13]. Several barriers for implementation of CKD management have already been described; objections to the label CKD because of fear, stigmatisation and physiological decrease of kidney function; lack of time; low expectations of management; and guideline familiarity [14–16]. A commonly mentioned solution is education, but GPs who participated in a recent Dutch CKD trial in which they received extra education on CKD management, had difficulties implementing the guideline recommendations [17]. In order to improve the implementation of CKD care, it is important to know GPs' underlying thoughts and beliefs about CKD and the implementation of the guideline. The present study therefore aims to explore the perspectives of GPs who were familiar with the guideline on CKD management in daily practice. We also examined the applicability of the national interdisciplinary guideline.

Methods

Study design

Given the explorative character of the research aim, we considered a qualitative approach to be the most appropriate. We selected a focus group design because perspectives are more likely to be revealed by interaction and discussion with peers. Grounded theory was used as a theoretical framework [18]. We used the consolidated criteria for reporting qualitative health research (COREQ) as a reporting structure [19]. Besides adjustment of the topic list, we made no further modifications of the methods during the study.

Selection of participants

Four focus group interviews were conducted with 27 Dutch GPs. We recruited (by phone and e-mail) from practices that had participated in the CONTACT study (Consultation Of Nephrology by Telenephrology Allows optimal Chronic kidney disease Treatment in primary care) [20]. These GPs were definitely informed about the guideline. We assumed they used the guide in daily practice, thus being able to provide knowledge about the perspectives of implementation of CKD management. In the Netherlands, GPs are responsible for providing and implementing CKD care. Although Dutch nurse practitioners (NPs) are involved in care programmes for diabetes and

cardiovascular disease, their involvement in CKD care is minor. We therefore recruited only GPs. Two GPs were not involved in the CONTACT trial study. They participated because two participants in focus group 4 cancelled at the last minute. They were involved in scientific research and familiar with the guideline.

A purposive stepwise sampling strategy [21] was applied to ensure heterogeneity for gender, age, urbanization, and experience in general practice (Table 1). Sampling, data collection and analysis occurred iteratively. Practice and personal data were collected prior to the interviews. All GPs consented to participation, and they were assured that anonymity and confidentially was guaranteed. No patient data were used.

Data collection

Before starting, a topic list (Additional file 1) was created by reviewing relevant literature and in consultation with the research team and two CKD-patients of the Dutch

Table 1 Participant characteristics

Sex n (%)	
Male	13 (48.1%)
Female	14 (51.9%)
Age in years	
Mean	50
Range	30–62
Working experience in Years	
Mean	19
Range	1–33
Familiarity with DIG-CKD n (%)[a]	
Scarce	3 (11.1%)
Reasonable	13 (48.1%)
Good	8 (29.6%)
Very good	3 (11.1%)
Frequency of DIG-CKD usage n (%)[b]	
Weekly	3 (11.1%)
Monthly	11(40.7%)
< than once a month	8 (29.6%)
Rarely	4 (14.8%)
Never	1 (3.7%)
Usage of telenephrology	21 (77.8%)
Practice urbanization n (%)	
Rural	11 (40.7%)
Urban	16 (59.3%)
Active as practice holder n (%)	26 (96.3%)
Presence of a nurse practitioner n (%)	27 (100%)

DIG-CKD: Dutch Interdisciplinary Guideline for Chronic Kidney Disease
[a]Subjective perception of the participating GPs
[b]Defined as the minimal use of the guideline

Kidney Foundation. A senior psychologist (KvS) with extensive experience in medical healthcare and chairing focus group studies moderated the focus groups. Either one of the two investigators (CD or SB), both GP trainees, PhD students and trained in qualitative research, and a research intern (BB) observed the focus groups and noted non-verbal communication and details about group interaction. The sessions lasted 120 min each. After each focus group, the investigator and Chair discussed observations made during the sessions and adjusted the topic list for each following focus group, in discussion with the research team. All focus group discussions were audio-taped and transcribed verbatim. In the analysis of the fourth focus group, no new codes or concepts were found. We decided that saturation had been reached at that moment.

Data analysis

The transcripts were analysed with the constant comparative analysis method [21] and with the aid of a computer program (Atlas.ti version: 7.1.5). Analyses started after the first focus group interview. The analysts (SB and BB) independently used open and inductive coding. They discussed and merged codes after each focus group. In the case of disagreement, members of the peer group (MD and WG) were consulted. A consensus code list arose, which was used to code the second transcript. New codes were added and discussed as described after each next coded transcript. After three focus group sessions, another researcher (CD) became involved as SB left the research project. This researcher coded all transcripts as a third coder. The research intern (BB) and the second researcher (CD) independently coded the fourth session. After saturation was reached, the codes were sorted into categories and themes. It took five consensus meetings in which members of the research group (CD, SB, BB, MD, NS, and WG) participated to construct the final thematic map. For a detailed description of the analysis process, see Additional file 2. A native-English speaker translated the illustrative quotes.

Results

Participants

Four focus group interviews were conducted between November 2014 and March 2016. A total of 147 GPs were invited to participate, of whom 71 responded. Forty-one GPs were interested in participating, while 30 GPs declined, mostly due to lack of time. Altogether, 27 GPs were included by purposive sampling, and 5 to 8 GPs participated in each session. Table 1 presents the characteristics of the participants.

Overview

Five main themes emerged: 1) defining CKD, 2) knowledge and awareness, 3) patient-physician interaction, 4) organisation of CKD care, and 5) value of the guideline. For a detailed description of codes, categories and themes, see Additional file 3.

Defining CKD

CKD was experienced as a difficult and abstract concept. CKD seems intangible. The diagnosis is not a clinical one, but is merely based upon laboratory findings without patient complaints and- in the view of participants- in some cases without clinical consequences. The participants struggled to interpret the eGFR values due to eGFR fluctuations and strict cut-off points. Age and physiology were considered relevant to interpret eGFR values, but also whether to label patients with the CKD diagnosis. Participants felt that there was no fixed definition of CKD. Furthermore, whether CKD is a disease on its own or a risk factor for cardiovascular disease, like hypertension, was discussed.

"The initial question was what is your picture of chronic kidney damage, and honestly, that picture is just a check mark in a row of risk factors." (FG1, man, 60-70y)

Knowledge and awareness
Professional competence

Educational gaps in the contents of the guideline and about proteinuria were reported. Nevertheless, there was a shared feeling that awareness of CKD has improved due to increased monitoring of diabetes and cardiovascular disease and the introduction of the DIG-CKD. The recurrent use of the guideline appeared to facilitate a learning curve so that managing CKD patients became easier. This reduced the urge to consult or refer to a nephrologist.

"Yes, at a certain point you know what the nephrologist will say. If I have heard it a few times, then I think: ok, that's the next step that I can take with this patient." (FG2, woman, 50-60y)

Perception of the importance of CKD

Due to insufficient knowledge about the clinical consequences of CKD, treatment and adherence to the guideline were trivialised. There was scepticism concerning health profit for patients if GPs would fully adhered to the guideline. GPs' decision making was influenced by expectations about poor prognosis and quality of life.

"I think it's a difficult problem ... a lot of medication, that influences kidney function. But then I think I'd rather have poor kidney function than be a patient who is extremely short of breath." (FG4, woman, 50-60y)

Patient-physician interaction
Informing patients
It appeared difficult to find the best approach for informing patients. The major concern was to inform enough without creating anxiety. Both straightforward communication and metaphors were used to explain the CKD diagnosis.

"...That there is a kind of rinsing machine in your body that keeps your blood clean, I say then. And if that machine doesn't work well, then your blood gets poisoned." (FG1, man, 60-70y)

Striving to adequately inform patients without creating unnecessary anxiety and to ensure the explanations and education was tailored to the patients educational level was found difficult. The right moment to inform patients and a lack of information material were also discussed.

Patient empowerment
The GPs felt the urge to empower patients in managing their CKD, but struggled to provide methods to increase patients health literacy. GPs felt that patients should especially take preventive measures, but they also had doubts about the efficacy of self-management. They felt that gaining patients' compliance would require time-consuming explanations. Especially in the case of co-morbidity, the balance between energy spent on self-management and the return it would generate worked out negatively.

"Yes, but that is in the whole of chronic care, it is certainly very difficult because people with kidney function disorders, even not considering age, so often have other problems with smoking, blood pressure, weight, etc." (FG4, man, 40-50y)

Organisation of CKD care
Primary care
There was not always consensus regarding GPs' policies within the practices, though the participants agreed about the importance of congruence of CKD care. The presence of alignments about task delegation to the nurse practitioner varied. There was discussion about the future implementation of CKD care.

"They usually come into the picture through the annual blood test in chronic-disease management programmes, so that you have already checked them in connection with other disorders." (FG1, man, 40-50y)

Primary-secondary care interface
The accessibility of nephrologists and the transfer of medical information needs improvement. The participants found it instructive to consult a nephrologist. The preferred method of contacting nephrologists (teleconsultation or by phone) differed.

"Formerly, specialist were easy to reach, now you get lost in the logistics of the hospital." (FG3, man 50-60y)

Medical specialists
The views towards nephrologists varied and were mainly based on previous experiences in contact and communication with them. Some had doubts about the added value of nephrologists' involvement. Losing control over patients' treatment after referral to a specialist was difficult for the GPs. They considered that other aspects should be taken into account, influencing how aggressively patients should be treated. GPs also experienced one-way communication and held the opinion that nephrologists do not involve GPs enough.

"I always find it sad when people land at the nephrologists' and have a blood pressure that is 2 mmHg too high. Then they have to come back three times. While I think: yeah right, boys, yeah." (FG3, man, 50-60y)

Value of the guideline
Facilitators
Accepting the recommendations of the existing interdisciplinary guideline induced a sense of safety. The guideline was used by the GPs to reduce knowledge gaps, resulting in a learning curve. The shared opinion was that the guideline created more awareness for CKD and improved the quality of care for patients.

Barriers
The GPs found treatment and referral criteria in the interdisciplinary CKD guideline too strict and precise, which made following the guideline time consuming. Furthermore, a feeling of medicalization of CKD patients was mentioned.

"What is the use of medicalising someone of great age with everything?" (FG4, woman, 40-50y)

Advice for improvements

According to the GPs more attention should be paid to the context of CKD patients and to how to interpret laboratory and clinical findings, while at the same moment taking the context of the patient into account. More advice about how to enlarge patient empowerment would be helpful.

Discussion

Summary of main findings

Perception of CKD as an abstract concept is a key finding in this study. The perceived abstract CKD concept seems to play a role in all formulated themes. It influences the GPs' experienced confidence on CKD knowledge. Clinical relevance also seems to be lacking, and there is scepticism concerning treatment benefits for patients. GPs act at their own discretion, taking into account patients' age, prognosis and quality of life. The interdisciplinary guideline is therefore seen as a rough guide rather than leading. The abstractness of the CKD concept forms an obstacle in conveying the CKD concept to patients.

Comparison with existing literature

Abstractness

Previous findings like educational gaps, guideline familiarity, tensions surrounding ICPC (international classification of primary care) labeling and physiology are in line with our study results [14–16, 22–24]. However, the importance of the perceived abstractness of the CKD concept, which in our study was a key finding, has never been highlighted as a central theme, causing difficulties for GPs in managing CKD. Since our findings are based on a study of trained GPs with special interest in CKD we presume that CKD as a concept will be even more difficult for other GPs who have not been trained in CKD explicitly. We indentified several factors that contribute to the abstractness of the CKD concept. Of these factors, renal aging, a diagnosis based on eGFRs and the tension between disease and risk factors have been earlier discussed in studies of Crinson and Simmonds [14, 22]. In our study, another aspect of the abstractness of CKD appeared to be the struggle to interpret eGFRs (i.e. fluctuating eGFRs, eGFR versus severity of CKD). This is a new and fascinating insight, which raises the question of how the interpretation of an eGFR value differs from the interpretation of a blood glucose level. Both a CKD diagnosis and a diabetes diagnosis are laboratory based, have strict cut-off points, and have no symptoms in an early stage. Despite these similarities, diabetes management is well integrated in daily practice in primary care while CKD management is not. In the knowledge that CKD provides as much risk of cardiovascular disease as diabetes does [25], this is a remarkable difference.

Education

We have seen that extra education for the GPs in our previous study did not meet their needs in interpreting and managing CKD [20]. We hypothesise that educational interventions should be even more intense, as Pang found in a study in which GPs perceived an increase in knowledge after interventions during which they were personally mentored by nephrologists [26].

Patient empowerment

GPs prefer to make CKD patients partners in care, but they encounter several barriers. Patient empowerment is time-consuming, and GPs have doubts about the efficacy of self-management. If patient empowerment is recommended in guidelines, attention should be paid to these barriers.

Strengths and limitations

The heterogeneity of the participants supported the generalisability of the findings. Internal validity was established through independent coding in triplicate, the use of Atlas.ti and the mind-mapping sessions with the research team in which additional perspectives and interpretation of analysis and findings were discussed. Analysis by three analysts and similar findings from previous other studies helped to triangulate the findings. The rigor of the data is supported by the iterative approach of the focus group and the interim data analysis. Some limitations should be considered. The focus groups were performed in Dutch, so that representative quotations needed translation. This may have caused loss of nuance, which we tried to limit through translation by a native-English speaker. The moderator was a psychologist, which could be a restriction regarding in-depth interviewing in the medical field. Another possible limitation is that most recruited GPs were previous participants in the CONTACT study. This might be related to a special interest in the research theme, possibly influenced their knowledge of and commitment to the subject. However, GPs who are not familiar with the subject may have even more difficulties with CKD care while they have insufficient knowledge about the guideline to provide answers to the research question. In order to avoid analysis bias as much as possible, the research team members differed in profession, age, experience regarding CKD care, and experience as a GP. Some had been involved in previous research on CKD (including the trial), but others had no specific experience in CKD research when the focus group study was performed. All researchers were GPs (in training). These background factors may have influenced our findings, but we can't indicate the direction of a possible bias.

Implications for practice

Our study provides insight into the perspectives of GPs concerning early-stage CKD management and could give input for future quality-improvement interventions. A major direction should be to improve GPs' understanding of the clinical concept of CKD. This could be done by education, which should also focus on clinical relevance, prognostic value of CKD, proteinuria and the interpretation of eGFRs in relation to age and comorbidity. Instructions on how to give a suitable explanation of the CKD diagnosis to patients might as well be part of GPs' education.

Our opinion is that embedding CKD care in an integrated care programme of all cardiovascular risk factors, including CKD, hypertension and diabetes, may support GPs and patients to maintain an overview. For those who were not diagnosed with diabetes or cardiovascular disease, a comparable care program provides the best chance of creating awareness and improving the quality of care for CKD patients. The tension between disease-specific guidelines and the holistic care preferred by GPs is - besides the abstract concept of CKD - perhaps the most important implementation barrier. GPs wish to maintain a patient-centred approach in providing high-quality CKD care, deviating from guideline recommendations when necessary.

Conclusions

This paper shows that care for patients with chronic kidney disease in primary care is a complex interplay of an abstract concept and physician-bound considerations. Difficulty interpreting the concept of CKD and doubts about the clinical relevance of CKD in the light of the patient's personal situation are the main reasons for deviating from guideline recommendations. Quality improvement strategies should focus on education of GPs in CKD-specific knowledge, especially in judging CKD relevance and GP-patient communication. Guidelines should include more guidance in eGFR interpretation, clinical consequences, and suggestions for tailoring interventions to the personal context of the individual patient. GPs feel there is tension between personalised healthcare and CKD-specific guidelines.

Abbreviations

CKD: Chronic kidney disease; CONTACT: Consultation of nephrology by telenephrology allows optimal chronic kidney disease Treatment in primary care; COREQ: COnsolidated criteria for REporting Qualitative health research; DIG-CKD: Dutch interdisciplinary guideline for chronic kidney disease; eGFR: Estimated glomerular filtration rate; FG: Focus group; GPs: General practitioners; KDIGO: Kidney disease: improving global outcomes; UK: United Kingdom; US: United States

Acknowledgements

Participating general practitioners.
Lea Peters, research assistant.
Dutch kidney foundation for financial support.

Funding

The Dutch Kidney Foundation funded the study. Grant no. 13A4D302. The funder agreed with the researchers' study design, but had no direct influence on the data collection, analysis, interpretation and reporting of the project.

Authors' contributions

All authors read and approved the final manuscript. CD: organised focus groups, coded, analysed and wrote the article. SB: organised focus groups, coded and analysed. WG: was consulted in case of disagreement (between CD, SB, BB), participated in the mind map sessions and in the writing process. NS: submitted an application, participated in the mind map sessions and in the writing process. BB: transcribed, coded and analysed. KS: chaired the focus groups and participated in the writing process. JW: involved in the design of the study, involved in the supervision of the PhD and participated in the writing process. WA: involved in the design of the study, involved in the supervision of the PhD and participated in the writing process. MD: was consulted in case of disagreement (between CD, SB, BB), participated in the mind map sessions and in the writing process.

Competing interests

The authors declare that they have no financial or non-financial competing interests.

Author details

[1]Department of Primary and Community Care, Radboud University Medical Center, PO Box 9101, 6500 HBPostal Route 117, Nijmegen, The Netherlands. [2]Department of Nephrology, Radboud University Medical Center, PO Box 9101, 6500 HBPostal Route 464, Nijmegen, The Netherlands.

References

1. de Zeeuw D, Hillege HL, de Jong PE. The kidney, a cardiovascular risk marker, and a new target for therapy. Kidney Int Suppl. 2005;(98):S25–9.
2. Roderick PRM, Mindell J. Prevalence of chronic kidney disease in England: findings from the 2009 health survey for England. J Epidemiol Commun H. 2011;65(Suppl I):A12.
3. Coresh J, Selvin E, Stevens LA, Manzi J, Kusek JW, Eggers P, et al. Prevalence of chronic kidney disease in the United States. JAMA. 2007;298(17):2038–47.
4. Go AS, Chertow GM, Fan D, McCulloch CE, Hsu CY. Chronic kidney disease and the risks of death, cardiovascular events, and hospitalization. N Engl J Med. 2004;351(13):1296–305.
5. Fox CS, Matsushita K, Woodward M, Bilo HJG, Chalmers J, Lambers Heerspink HJ, et al. Associations of kidney disease measures with mortality and end-stage renal disease in individuals with and without diabetes: a meta-analysis. Lancet. 2012;380(9854):1662–73.
6. Matsushita K, van der Velde M, Astor BC, Woodward M, Levey AS, de Jong PE, et al. Association of estimated glomerular filtration rate and albuminuria with all-cause and cardiovascular mortality in general population cohorts: a collaborative meta-analysis. Lancet. 2010;375(9731):2073–81.
7. Mahmoodi BK, Matsushita K, Woodward M, Blankestijn PJ, Cirillo M, Ohkubo T, et al. Associations of kidney disease measures with mortality and end-stage renal disease in individuals with and without hypertension: a meta-analysis. Lancet. 2012;380(9854):1649–61.
8. Kidney Disease: Improving Global Outcomes (KDIGO) CKD Work Group. KDIGO 2012 Clinical Practice Guideline for the Evaluation and Management of Chronic Kidney Disease. Kidney Inter Suppl. 2013;3:1–150.
9. NICE Clinical guideline: Chronic kidney disease. Early identification and management of chronic kidney disease in adults in primary and secondary care. London: National Collaborating Centre and National Institute for health and care excellence; 2008. September (last modified 2014)

10. De Grauw WJC, Kaasjager HAH, Bilo HJG, Faber EF, Flikweert S, Gaillard CAJM. Landelijke transmurale afspraak chronische nierschade. Huisarts Wetenschap. 2009;52:586–97.

11. Allen AS, Forman JP, Orav EJ, Bates DW, Denker BM, Sequist TD. Primary care management of chronic kidney disease. J Gen Intern Med. 2011;26(4):386–92.

12. Lenz O, Mekala DP, Patel DV, Fornoni A, Metz D, Roth D. Barriers to successful care for chronic kidney disease. BMC Nephrol. 2005;6:11.

13. Van Gelder VA, Scherpbier-De Haan ND, De Grauw WJ, Vervoort GM, Van Weel C, Biermans MC, et al. Quality of chronic kidney disease management in primary care: a retrospective study. Scand J Prim Health Care. 2016;34(1): 73–80.

14. Crinson I, Gallagher H, Thomas N, de Lusignan S. How ready is general practice to improve quality in chronic kidney disease? A diagnostic analysis. Br J Gen Pract. 2010;60(575):403–9.

15. Blakeman T, Protheroe J, Chew-Graham C, Rogers A, Kennedy A. Understanding the management of early-stage chronic kidney disease in primary care: a qualitative study. Br J Gen Pract. 2012;62(597):e233–42.

16. Abdel-Kader K, Greer RC, Boulware LE, Unruh ML. Primary care physicians' familiarity, beliefs, and perceived barriers to practice guidelines in non-diabetic CKD: a survey study. BMC Nephrol. 2014;15:64.

17. van Dipten C, van Berkel S, van Gelder VA, Wetzels JF, Akkermans RP, de Grauw WJ, et al. Adherence to chronic kidney disease guidelines in primary care patients is associated with comorbidity. Fam Pract. 2017;34(4):459–66.

18. Walker D, Myrick F. Grounded theory: an exploration of process and procedure. Qual Health Res. 2006;16(4):547–59.

19. Tong A, Sainsbury P, Craig J. Consolidated criteria for reporting qualitative research (COREQ): a 32-item checklist for interviews and focus groups. Int J Qual Health Care. 2007;19(6):349–57.

20. van Gelder VA, Scherpbier ND, van Berkel S, Akkermans RP, De Grauw IS, Adang EM, et al. Web-based consultation between general practitioners and nephrologists, a cluster randomized controlled trial. Fam Pract. 2017; 34(4):430–6.

21. Marshall MN. Sampling for qualitative research. Fam Pract. 1996;13(6):522–5.

22. Simmonds R, Evans J, Feder G, Blakeman T, Lasserson D, Murray E, et al. Understanding tensions and identifying clinician agreement on improvements to early-stage chronic kidney disease monitoring in primary care: a qualitative study. BMJ Open. 2016;6(3):e010337.

23. Vest BM, York TR, Sand J, Fox CH, Kahn LS. Chronic kidney disease guideline implementation in primary care: a qualitative report from the TRANSLATE CKD study. J Am Board Fam Med. 2015;28(5):624–31.

24. Lo C, Teede H, Ilic D, Russell G, Murphy K, Usherwood T, et al. Identifying health service barriers in the management of co-morbid diabetes and chronic kidney disease in primary care: a mixed-methods exploration. Fam Pract. 2016;33(5):492–7.

25. Matsushita K, Coresh J, Sang Y, Chalmers J, Fox C, Guallar E, et al. Estimated glomerular filtration rate and albuminuria for prediction of cardiovascular outcomes: a collaborative meta-analysis of individual participant data. Lancet Diabetes Endocrinol. 2015;3(7):514–25.

26. Pang J, Grill A, Bhatt M, Woodward GL, Brimble S. Evaluation of a mentorship program to support chronic kidney disease care. Can Fam Physician. 2016;62(8):e441–7.

2

Formative evaluation and adaptation of pre-and early implementation of diabetes shared medical appointments to maximize sustainability and adoption

Christine P. Kowalski[1]*(iD), Miranda Veeser[1] and Michele Heisler[1,2]

Abstract

Background: Understanding the many factors that influence implementation of new programs, in addition to their success or failure, is extraordinarily complex. This qualitative study examines the implementation and adaptation process of two linked clinical programs within Primary Care, diabetes shared medical appointments (SMAs) and a reciprocal Peer-to-Peer (P2P) support program for patients with poorly controlled diabetes, through the lens of the Consolidated Framework for Implementation Research (CFIR). We illustrate the role and importance of pre-implementation interviews for guiding ongoing adaptations to improve implementation of a clinical program, achieve optimal change, and avoid type III errors.

Methods: We conducted 28 semi-structured phone interviews between September of 2013 and May of 2016, four to seven interviewees at each site. The interviewees were physician champions, chiefs of primary care, pharmacists, dieticians, nurses, health psychologists, peer facilitators, and research coordinators. Modifiable barriers and facilitators to implementation were identified and adaptations documented. Data analysis started with immersion in the data to obtain a sense of the whole and then by cataloging principal themes per CFIR constructs. An iterative consensus-building process was used to code. CFIR constructs were then ranked and compared by the researchers.

Results: We identified a subset of CFIR constructs that are most likely to play a role in the effectiveness of the diabetes SMAs and P2P program based on our work with the participating sites to date. Through the identification of barriers and facilitators, a subset of CFIR constructs arose, including evidence strength and quality, relative advantage, adaptability, complexity, patient needs and resources, compatibility, leadership engagement, available resources, knowledge and beliefs, and champions.

Conclusions: We described our method for identification of contextual factors that influenced implementation of complex diabetes clinical programs - SMAs and P2P. The qualitative phone interviews aided implementation through the identification of modifiable barriers or conversely, actionable findings. Implementation projects, and certainly clinical programs, do not have unlimited resources and these interviews allowed us to determine which facets to target and act on for each site. As the study progresses, these findings will be compared and correlated to outcome measures. This comprehensive adaptation data collection will also facilitate and enhance understanding of the future success or lack of success of implementation and inform potential for translation and public health impact. The approach of using the CFIR to guide us to actionable findings and help us better understand barriers and facilitators has broad applicability and can be used by other projects to guide, adapt, and improve implementation of research into practice.

(Continued on next page)

* Correspondence: Christine.Kowalski@va.gov
[1]Center for Clinical Management Research (CCMR- VA), VA Ann Arbor Healthcare System, 2800 Plymouth Road Bld. 16, Ann Arbor, MI 48109, USA
Full list of author information is available at the end of the article

(Continued from previous page)

Keywords: Formative evaluation, Implementation, Diabetes, Shared medical appointments, Qualitative research, Facilitation, CFIR, Adaptation

Background

Understanding the many factors that influence implementation of new programs, in addition to their success or failure, is extraordinarily complex. Formative evaluation, defined as a rigorous assessment process designed to identify potential and actual influences on the progress and effectiveness of implementation efforts, is an essential means to systematically approach this complexity [1].

Many implementation studies rely exclusively on summative data– or data outputs, products, and outcomes— to determine program success or failure. While summative data is useful, it is not adequate to understand critically important implementation processes [1, 2]. When used in isolation, summative data often leads to the term "implementation black box" [3]: there is no way to understand the specific reasons the intervention succeeded or failed, how it was actually implemented, and how local contextual factors affected implementation. This is where formative evaluation comes in, to fill in these gaps and to systematically examine key features of the local implementation setting, detect and monitor unanticipated events and adjust if necessary in real-time, optimize implementation to improve potential for success, and avoid type III errors—the failure to detect differences between the original intervention plan and the ultimate manner of implementation that lead to failure to achieve outcomes [1, 4]. This understanding is essential for efforts to sustain, scale up, and disseminate any new program–otherwise there is potential for failure to account for specific contextual issues in program implementation.

Adaptations have been found to be necessary for sustainable implementation [5] and are considered part of the traditional translation pipeline (adaptations as required) [6]. Progress has been made in advancing the science of implementation, but too often the complexity of translating research into practice is overlooked or follows an overly simplistic model [7]. In the words of implementation experts Dr. Chambers and Dr. Norton, "Rather than assuming that adaptation of a manualized intervention is at odds with good implementation, the field can systematically collect information on the impact of adaptation to individuals, organizations, and communities and use this information to extend the knowledge base of implementation of evidence-based practices as well as ongoing improvement of the evidence-based practices themselves" [8]. Indeed other efforts in implementation have been described where adaptations are catalogued on an ongoing basis. [9] While the static view of adaptation has been that it is bad or to be avoided and/or eliminated, the dynamic sustainability model believes adaptation to be "inevitable and encouraged." [7] Likewise, simplified intervention implementation overlooks the complexities of translating research to practice and relies on a set of assumptions that limits enhancement of fit between evidence-based interventions and delivery setting. [10]

Additionally, while the evidence-to-practice gap for interventions is receiving attention, it tends to be understudied in primary care. [11] A recent study highlighted the importance of paying attention to context, which was noted as frequently failing to be acknowledged, described, or taken into account during implementation in primary care. [11]

Accordingly, to fill this gap in the literature, we sought to illustrate the role and importance of pre-implementation (early) interviews for guiding ongoing adaptations to improve implementation of a clinical program, achieve optimal change, and avoid type III errors. We gathered detailed pre-implementation data across five health system sites, within primary care settings, that had each committed to institute Shared Medical Appointments (SMAs) and in some SMA cohorts an additional offered mutual peer support program (P2P) for adult patients with poorly controlled diabetes. In particular, we examined modifiable barriers and facilitators to implementation. We then documented the adaptations that were made in real-time to attempt to improve implementation. This comprehensive data will also facilitate and enhance understanding of the future success or lack of success of implementation of new innovative clinical programs such as SMAs and inform potential for translation and public health impact of these [2].

Methods

This qualitative study is part of a larger implementation study, "The Shared Health Appointments and Reciprocal Enhanced Support (SHARES) study" [12]. The SHARES study is a multi-site cluster randomized trial of five geographically diverse Veterans Affairs (VA) health systems evaluating the effectiveness and implementation of diabetes Shared Medical Appointments (SMAs) with and without an additional reciprocal Peer-to-Peer (P2P) support program, when compared to usual care.

SMAs bring patients with the same chronic condition together with an interdisciplinary team of providers to provide shared education and support. The diabetes SMAs consist of a series of 1–2 h sessions of 8–10 patients led by a team of health professionals. At each site, participants have a total of approximately 8 h of sessions, and the sessions are intended to be interactive and focus on key diabetes self-management topics (e.g., diet, medications, physical activity, self-monitoring). The P2P program comprises periodic peer support, [13, 14] group sessions, and telephone contact between SMA participant pairs to promote more effective diabetes self-management and sustain gains achieved through the SMAs after completion of these sessions. Outcomes will be examined across three different treatment groups: (1) SMAs; (2) SMAs plus P2P; and 3) usual care.

We undertook a type of formative evaluation (FE), labeled implementation-focused evaluation, of the SMAs and of P2P [1]. This type of FE occurs throughout implementation of the project plan: before, during, and after implementation. This manuscript focuses on the real-time FE that took place during the early stages of implementation and pre-implementation.

The overarching framework for the SHARES qualitative discovery– including the interviews, formative evaluation, implementation, and analysis– was the Consolidated Framework for Implementation Research (CFIR) [15]. The CFIR provides a framework of 39 constructs from across published implementation frameworks that describe the organizational and contextual setting and are believed to influence implementation. We are tracking the CFIR constructs across the sites throughout the project and will ascertain how they influence implementation success during future program evaluation.

Institutional Review Board (IRB) approval was obtained from the Central IRB.

Data collection and analysis

A brief phone survey was conducted with key informants from each site to identify potential key CFIR constructs. We then conducted 28 semi-structured phone interviews with participants at five VA health systems, four to seven interviewees at each site (see Table 1). Interviews were conducted between September of 2013 and May of 2016 and lasted between 22 and 56 min (mean of 34 min). Two interviewers participated in all interviews; detailed notes were taken by both, while most of the questions were asked by the first interviewer. The interviewees were physician champions, chiefs of primary care, pharmacists, dieticians, nurses, health psychologists, P2P facilitators, and research coordinators from the local sites. After each initial interview, the interviewee was then asked to recommend other informants. This type of recruitment, called snowball sampling, means that rather than determining individuals to

interview ahead of time, we asked everyone that we interviewed to recommend other potential participants, including key clinical opinion leaders. Interviewees from each site were continually recruited until the research team felt that qualitative data discovery had reached saturation—the point at which new data only confirmed the themes and conclusions already achieved [16].

Phone interviews were qualitative and, unlike a survey, all questions were open-ended; interviewees were encouraged to share their experiences in detail to enable a thorough understanding of the implementation experience from their varying perspectives. Conducting multiple interviews at each site enabled us to understand how perspectives compared from staff in different positions.

Our interview guide included questions about the interviewee's role in the diabetes SMAs and P2P groups, aspects of the program they would like to change, barriers and facilitators with regards to implementing/ expanding the diabetes SMAs and P2P programs, what kinds of resources or tools they would need for implementation, need for and awareness of evidence for the P2P program in addition to SMAs, existence of a clinical champion or local opinion leader, and types of feedback they would like to receive as the study progressed. Although CFIR-relevant questions were asked, there were opportunities to explore non-CFIR issues in that the interviewees could discuss anything related to their implementation experience, which was described by the participants in detail. After each interview, we developed a list of barriers, facilitators, and tasks that we needed to accomplish or follow up on with key staff at each of the local sites as part of the implementation process.

The initial lists of barriers and facilitators were developed from the detailed interview notes with a quick turnaround time to implement an immediate feedback loop to the sites because the primary consideration was not collecting data for "research," but rather to implement adaptations to overcome barriers and improve the implementation process. After these barriers were reviewed, the implementation team worked with the local staff from each site to make adaptations as necessary. Of note, some of the adaptations were driven by local clinical staff (see Table 2 for these details). We shared feedback with each local site continually while the phone interviews progressed so that suggestions could be incorporated in a timely manner. Each of these items was addressed to the extent that it could be prior to a mid-implementation site visit. For any barriers that we had not been able to address before each site visit, a detailed summary packet was written by the project qualitative analyst (CPK) and distributed to the implementation team members attending the site visit, with background information and a list of questions and tasks that still needed to be addressed. In addition, conference

Table 1 Qualitative interviewee titles

Job title of interviewee	Site 1001 $n = 6$	Site 1002 $n = 6$	Site 1003 $n = 5$	Site 1004 $n = 7$	Site 1005 $n = 4$	$n = 28$
Clinical pharmacist (PharmD)	1	1	1	3		6
Primary Care physician	1	1	1		2	5
Nurse Manager	1	1				2
Health Psychologist (PhD)	2		1			3
Research Coordinator	1			1		2
P2P group facilitator			1	1		2
Chief of Cardiology				1		1
Chief of Primary Care				1		1
Dietician			1		1	2
Associate Chief of Staff					1	1
Chief of Ambulatory Care		1				1
Nurse		2				2

calls with individual sites occurred throughout this study period and detailed notes about important issues were documented and included in analysis.

Subsequent data analysis started with immersion in the data to obtain a sense of the whole and then by cataloging principal themes that emerged according to the CFIR framework constructs [17, 18]. This is a type of qualitative directed-content analysis [19] (directed initially by the CFIR constructs). Given the CFIR has 39 broad constructs related to implementation, although we analyzed, we did not discover any strong themes outside of the organizational parameters outlined in the framework.

Two authors (CK and MV) used an iterative consensus-building process to code; first each team member independently coded transcripts, and then met as a group to discuss and reconcile codes, identify emergent themes, and resolve discrepancies through consensus. Each of the CFIR constructs was ranked on a scale of − 2 to + 2 (Table 3) independently by CK and MV for each site and then were discussed until consensus ranking was reached, taking all of the qualitative data into account. The valence of each construct reflects the impact on implementation (negative or positive); the numbers provide a reference for the impact on implementation as weak or strong, with 2 being the strongest. [20]

Results

Key constructs or areas of focus varied across sites. Table 2 is organized by site and CFIR construct and within that row, highlights how the findings (barrier column) informed our actions to improve or facilitate implementation (facilitator column) and what actions were taken (adaptations).

Based on our work with the participating sites to date, we identified a subset of CFIR constructs that are most likely to play a role in the implementation and possibly

effectiveness of the diabetes SMAs and the P2P program, including evidence strength and quality, relative advantage, adaptability, complexity, patient needs and resources, compatibility, leadership engagement, available resources, knowledge and beliefs, and champions (Table 4). Although data from any organizational aspect mentioned by interviewees, and all CFIR constructs, were coded (see Table 2), these specific constructs formed the basis of primary qualitative analyses due to the depth and frequency of the construct throughout the interviews and qualitative analysis. A definition of each CFIR construct is included in Table 2.

Evidence strength and quality
Diabetes SMA

The evidence strength and quality construct constitutes stakeholders' perceptions of the quality and validity of evidence supporting the belief that the innovation will have desired outcomes. This construct was rated positively for all sites except 1002 (see Table 2), where every interviewee mentioned that the diabetes SMAs were seen as extra work without added value or belief that the innovation will have the desired outcomes. 1002 nurse summarized these thoughts: *"I've got to tell you, it's a hard sell with physicians. Even now, I don't have a champion for the diabetes SMA. They see it as extra work. They don't see the added value. It troubles me a lot that it's so hard to get the docs involved."* After this barrier was discovered, our facilitation team made a visit to present evidence and met with the local primary care team to help educate and influence the physicians.

Diabetes SMA and P2P

The remaining four sites' interviews demonstrated local staff belief in the positive evidence quality for both the diabetes SMAs and P2P. A leader from site 1004 stated,

Table 2 Detailed adaptations made in real-time by site and CFIR construct

Construct	Barrier	Facilitator or Adaptation
INTERVENTION CHARACTERISTICS		
Intervention Source Definition: Perception of key stakeholders about whether the innovation is externally or internally developed.		1001: Internal
		1002: External
		1003: Internal
		1004: External
		1005: Internal
Evidence Strength & Quality Definition: Stakeholders' perceptions of the quality and validity of evidence supporting the belief that the innovation will have desired outcomes.		1001: • Interviewees see benefit in social support that SMA and P2P programs would provide. This was also shown in their trial program. • See also, Trialability. • See also, Knowledge and Beliefs.
	1002: • Repeated throughout all the interviews, that the SMAs and P2P programs are seen as extra work and staff do not see any added value – overall negative mindset to this implementation. • Diabetes SMAs have been a hard sell with physicians; they are not on board – they do not see an added value.	1002: • Our team presented evidence during the site visit and during a local primary care team meeting to help educate and influence the physicians.
		1003: • "Buddy system" (similar to P2P) has been effective in other settings in the facility, which has in turn increased support for P2P program. • HBC believes evidence behind SMAs is good and they were already looking for opportunities to improve their diabetic population outcomes. Believes the SMA and P2P will be very "fruitful and helpful." • Physicians involved believe they have seen evidence that having a peer or buddy for support will help the diabetic population.
		1004: • Leadership is on board and thinks there is good evidence for the positive effect of being part of a group for the SMAs and the P2P components. • See also, Knowledge and Beliefs. • See also, Leadership Support.
		1005: • The ACOS for Ambulatory Care believes strongly in the evidence for SMAs. • SMA PCP feels there is evidence that the SMA and P2P will engage the patients (participants); feels they are more motivated by hearing from peers than from a clinician- belief of local evidence that the group portion of the SMA and the P2P group will be beneficial. • See also, Knowledge and Beliefs. • See also, Leadership Support.
Relative advantage Definition: Stakeholders' perception of the advantage of implementing the innovation versus an alternative solution.	1001: • According to some interviewees, staff were not encouraging their patients to attend the SMAs because they did not see an advantage of the SMAs compared to usual care.	1001: • We had local staff present information about the SMA program and the value of it to the PCPs.

Table 2 Detailed adaptations made in real-time by site and CFIR construct *(Continued)*

Construct	Barrier	Facilitator or Adaptation
	1002:	• Our team presented evidence during the site visit and during a local primary care team meeting to help educate and influence the physicians.
		• "Don't see how it could hurt" attitude.
	• Physicians see the diabetes SMAs as extra work; do not see the added value. • See also, Evidence Strength & Quality.	1002: • Our team presented evidence during the site visit and during a local primary care team meeting to help educate and influence the physicians.
		• Nursing staff seems to be on board – believe in peer support aspect to improve diabetes care/outcomes for Vets. Believe Veterans listen to peers more than clinicians.
		1003:
		• Have had other diabetes studies at site, but group support was not formalized, "no mechanism for patients who have been-there-done-that providing support to others."
		• Health psychologist and other staff saw SMAs as an advantage to their already mandated diabetes education classes because they had not translated into any action.
		1004: • Staff see a need for peer mentoring program in Veterans especially because they are deployed in a unit and relate to their Veteran peers.
		• A physician leader thinks that there may be a financial benefit to the SMA group and P2P component.
		• See also, Cost. 1005: • The Associate Chief of Staff sees the advantage of the diabetes SMAs because he thinks it will help with access, efficiency, and help Veterans to learn from each other. • Currently, the ACOS says there are 5–6 separate patients meeting with the clinical pharmacist specialist for 30 min each going over the same information with some tweaking for their condition. • Some PCPs talked about how they could see the relative advantage of doing group visits vs. one on one patient visits. • See also, Cost.
	1005: • Possible added work for clinicians due to number of patients needing clinical notes following SMAs; described as: *"It is a little bit of extra work because I have to write you know, 8 to 12 notes rather than just the four that I would write in two hours, but it potentially helps, but, as a doc, that['s] the biggest detriment I see to it."* • While PCP SMA lead is excited about the prospect of group visits, there was only a 50/50 excitement from other PCPS at this site for expansions of SMAs. Levels of enthusiasm varied because some PCPs simply like the idea of group appointments and some do not.	
Adaptability	1001:	1001:

Table 2 Detailed adaptations made in real-time by site and CFIR construct *(Continued)*

Construct	Barrier	Facilitator or Adaptation
Definition: The degree to which an innovation can be adapted, tailored, refined, or reinvented to meet local needs.	• Concern from staff if the program was not adaptable and patients may not want to work with their assigned partner and this may cause them to leave the study. • Several staff were concerned that the locally designed recruitment plan was too ambitious. • Nurses originally going to take charge of SMAs, varying levels of comfort and would need to train too many facilitators. 1002: • Staff here were concerned with the standardization that they perceived was required of their local SMAs. This site did not feel the program was very adaptable initially.	• We worked with the site to come up with an adapted plan whereby a patient who does not work well with his/her partner can be re-paired or put into a group of 3. We also worked with the nurses and PCPs for their recommendation on patients that will work well together. The site appreciated us working with them to make the peer pairing adaptable. • During a pre-implementation local site visit our project staff discussed recruitment; the site did change their recruitment strategy to be more realistic. • HBC or psychology fellow to fill role of nurses as leaders of SMAs. 1002: • We were able to work with the local team through meetings and calls to ensure that the SMAs could be adapted as each site saw fit. Each sub-site was able to come up with its own SMA plan. 1004: • Site has tailored current SMA visits according to Veteran feedback so they can get what they want out of sessions.
Trialability Definition: The ability to test the innovation on a small scale in the organization, and to be able to reverse course (undo implementation) if warranted.		1001: • Pilot SMA was conducted before our clinical program began. Local staff involved decided it was too difficult for patients to absorb all the information in a one-day SMA. Also, because they were making meta-adjustments/medication changes, they felt the sessions needed to be longitudinal to titrate. *"We feel we can't fix all of that in just one visit."* 1002: • Piloted SMAs locally prior to implementation. 1005: • Piloted SMAs locally prior to implementation.
Complexity = 4 Definition: Perceived difficulty of the innovation, reflected by duration, scope, radicalness, disruptiveness, centrality, and intricacy and number of steps required to implement.	1002: • Staff are "busy and stretched thin;" it is difficult to do anything additional. • Contrary to all our other sites we were told that the amount of training for the peer facilitator needed to be minimal. They had trouble finding a P2P facilitator because of their perception of the work required. • Originally staff felt this project was only supposed to be adding on the P2P component. "Yet, somehow it has ended up to be a lot more work for the SMA people." Staff feel they had to make multiple changes to the SMAs that they were not anticipating. • Staff expressed annoyance about the work involved and administrative tasks: "very frustrating," "just more stress." The timeline getting pushed back "just became unnerving." They did not anticipate that this project "would be so much work." 1003: • Staff told us their largest barrier is always funding and finding time in staff schedules to devote to this project. 1004: • Very busy staff and many competing initiatives; not only diabetes, but overall information overload.	1001: • Interestingly, this is the only site where we did not hear about staff being overly busy, stretched thin. 1002, 1003, 1004, 1005: • Facilitation team worked with the sites through team meetings and phone meetings to streamline documentation, shared diabetes SMA clinical note templates across the sites, worked to better integrate into existing workflow with input from staff.

Table 2 Detailed adaptations made in real-time by site and CFIR construct *(Continued)*

Construct	Barrier	Facilitator or Adaptation
	1005: • Although the ACOS is very supportive of the SMAs he did say that it cannot add extra work to his employees. • Clinical pharmacist notes are a large barrier. Generally, clinical pharmacist notes are very comprehensive and they are the SMA documenters for this site. ACOS is concerned about the amount of time the documentation of the diabetes SMAs will take for the clinical pharmacists. He wants someone to make sure that we build thoughtful templates that capture what is taking place, but for the most part are standard curriculum.	
Design Quality and Packaging Definition: Perceived excellence in how the innovation is bundled, presented, and assembled.	All sites: We added this because of the comments from all sites that clinical staff was not always aware of what was happening and what the intervention actually was –many of the staff did not understand what P2P was and we spent a good portion of the interviews explaining P2P. This was not really the intention of the interviews going in, but we spent a lot of time on clarifications and answering questions.	
Cost Definition: Costs of the innovation and costs associated with implementing the innovation including investment, supply, and opportunity costs.	1002: • Nursing leadership has suggested cost, in terms of staff time for the P2P facilitators, as a barrier to implementation of this program.	1004: • A physician leader thinks that there may be a financial benefit to the SMA group and P2P component. 1005: • The ACOS feel that SMAs should improve efficiency of care and access.
Outer setting		
Patient Needs & Resources Definition: The extent to which the needs of those served by the organization (e.g., patients), as well as barriers and facilitators to meet those needs, are accurately known and prioritized by the organization.	1001: • Patients have pre-paid phones, run out of minutes and are not able to make calls at the end of the month. • Patients are "guarded" and may not want to share phone numbers with their peer. • Clinicians stated top barrier would be "convincing the patients to show up." • Patients not motivated in general to come to appointments or sessions unless compensated financially. • Lack of patient motivation or follow-though. • Low patient attendance to SMAs and P2P drop-ins. • Concern that copay could contribute to poor attendance. • Concern about early morning start – some Veterans come in without eating before, which leads to very low blood sugars. • Delays to the start of the diabetes SMAs; knowing when the patients arrive and where to take vitals (time). • Plan for post-SMA continuation of care. 1002: • Difficulties with patient recruitment for SMAs; believe they will experience the same problem for the P2P groups. Lack of motivation among patients to attend. • Local patients are elderly and very private. May not want to work with a peer; concern about potential mis-matches alienating patients from participating.	1001: • The local RA facilitated patient attendance through reminder calls and letters. • We worked with the local nurses to determine how to ensure staff are better aware of when the patients arrive for SMAs to ensure a timely start. • Moved SMA start time to early in morning to resolve parking issue and in hopes to increase attendance. • Studied barriers to attendance – poor attendance correlated with adherence issues. • Adapted so that the SMA is no longer one full day. This was done to allow time for medication adjustments, which could not be done when the SMA as only 1 day. • We consulted with staff from the site to take into account their perspective on matching peers together and who would work best together allowing for adaptability and patient re-pairing. • We also worked with site to ensure whenever possible that these facilitators would be sustainable across time when the research team would no longer be involved (transference of some of these tasks in time to local clinical and administrative staff). • Worked to guarantee eligibility for travel pay for SMAs. 1002: • The local RA facilitated patient attendance through reminder calls and letters.

Table 2 Detailed adaptations made in real-time by site and CFIR construct *(Continued)*

Construct	Barrier	Facilitator or Adaptation
	• Concern about distance – many Veterans live far from this VA. • Concern Veterans may not want to stay after the SMA for P2P. 1003: • Patient attendance/compliance is low—particularly among patients with A1cs over 9. Elderly population with less financial means; many do not have phones or access to the internet. • Patients resistant to change. • Concerns from multiple staff about "passive patient population" through experience with SMAs patients tend to be passive and expect you to do something rather than making a change for themselves. • Some patients prefer not coming to clinic unless they will receive travel pay. • Concerns about attendance due to ongoing construction. 1004: • All interviewees mentioned that it is difficult to get buy-in from patients to participate in groups. • In their experience with recruiting for the diabetes SMAs you need to recruit 3 patients for every 1 who attends. • VA does not reimburse patients for travel to research visits. Sometimes patients would like to join the groups but cannot afford to travel without compensation. • Many patients at this site use disposable phones so their phone numbers frequently change. Nurses have this experience when they try to call patients for reminders. • Some Veterans work and take classes, making timing/attendance difficult.	• Presentations were given at staff meetings to increase patient attendance/ referrals. • We worked with staff from the site to consider their perspective on matching peers together and which would work best together (taking into account disease state, gender, age). • Worked to guarantee eligibility for travel pay for SMAs. • As above worked with site to ensure sustainability of facilitators. 1003: • The local RA facilitated patient attendance through reminder calls and letters. • Word of mouth support from Veterans who have participated in the diabetes SMAs to other Veterans has helped. This has been mostly serendipitous rather than organized. We discussed this with the local site PI and she presented information on P2P to a Veteran-run wellness group to help with the word-of-mouth support. • We instituted a way to distribute reminders for the P2P groups. • We worked to make sure the initial group script is very dynamic. • Worked to guarantee eligibility for travel pay for SMAs. • SMAs have been modified to better fit patient needs (number of sessions, etc.) • Veterans appreciate having an interdisciplinary team to guide them. • Social support will increase patient accountability/attendance. • As above worked with site to ensure sustainability of facilitators. 1004: • The local RA facilitated patient attendance through reminder calls and letters. • One facilitator staff has noticed is having 2 health psychologists participate in the SMAs to make sure that patients' needs and wants are addressed in the class and moving the sessions to more of a conversation rather than a didactic session—has already been successful. • Vets will benefit from added social support and "hearing from 'equals' rather than somebody else." • Worked to guarantee eligibility for travel pay for SMAs. • As above worked with site to ensure sustainability of facilitators. 1005: • The importance of goal setting, as a patient need, was discussed in regards to prior SMAs and how that was needed to improve outcomes – being held accountable helps to improve patient outcomes. • The local RA facilitated patient attendance through reminder calls and letters. • Social support is seen as a patient need and the SMA and P2P groups will fill a gap in patient needs. • PCPs here view the well-controlled patients attending the SMAs as a facilitator. • Worked to guarantee eligibility for travel pay for SMAs.

Table 2 Detailed adaptations made in real-time by site and CFIR construct *(Continued)*

Construct	Barrier	Facilitator or Adaptation
Structural Characteristics Definition: The social architecture, age, maturity, and size of an organization.		1005: • There is a new patient education room with the exam room attached. This site was getting ready to ramp up the SMA model. *"We are well situated to make this work."*
Networks /Communications Definition: The nature and quality of webs of social networks, and the nature and quality of formal and informal communications within an organization.	1002: • Concern that there would be a communication gap between the SMA coordinator and the P2P facilitators. • Very large project and having 3 local sites makes it even more complicated because each site has some differing challenges. • Communication between main study site and 1002 cited as problematic. • Staff can be difficult to reach and get in contact with. • Concern word still needs to be spread about project. • The overall project site staff has ongoing difficulties in communicating with this site.	1001: • Nurse that managed previous SMAs has well established relationships with key stakeholders. • PharmD & health psychology fellow offered and gave more information to physicians at staff meetings. • Keeping project on MDs minds will help with referrals to program, so staff ensure this was done. • Champion is also chief – runs primary care meetings and encourages support from physicians. 1002: • We worked with this site and held team conference calls and developed a plan to address communication. • A staff member who knows the patient panels well is working to communicate with and enlist her providers.
Culture Definition: Norms, values, and basic assumptions of a given organization.	1001: • Multiple staff describe this site as a culture of Veterans not wanting to participate in group settings. • Veterans here are very "guarded" and have culture of not being very motivated to make their own changes, do not bring back homework, do not bring in things asked to bring. 1002: • Culturally have great difficulty getting staff to commit a few hours a week to any type of project, even though this site has more financial resources than others. The site is still very cautious to commit staff; they will not commit to having a pharmacist attend the SMAs unlike all other sites. There is also a reluctance to write down responsibilities because of a fear they will become an expectation.	
Tension for change Definition: The degree to which stakeholders perceive the current situation as intolerable or needing change.	1003: • Diabetes education classes have been mandated, but have not "translated into action."	1001: • This site has a lack of group appointments, interviewees see need for program that will provide extra social support. 1003: • SMAs seen as potential solution to lack of action/improvement in diabetes management. • Staff see need for innovation at their facility. 1004: • "Benefit to hearing from 'equals' rather than somebody else – someone lateral as opposed to top down…" • Always looking for new programs to help their "frequent flyers."
Compatibility Definition: The degree of tangible fit between meaning and values attached to the innovation by involved individuals, how those align with individuals' own norms, values, and perceived risks and needs, and how the innovation fits with existing workflows and systems.	1002: • Had mixed drop-in sessions which they now cannot do with diabetes SMAs. 1004: • According to the chief of primary care, it is very important that this process fit into the existing workflow for implementation to succeed.	1001: • Local staff have confidence that research implementation will be smooth at facility because it will fit within existing programs. • This innovation is considered by staff to be good compliment to what is already going on in patient care. • Not a lot of diabetes programming, fits need.

Table 2 Detailed adaptations made in real-time by site and CFIR construct *(Continued)*

Construct	Barrier	Facilitator or Adaptation
	• It is very important that we foster buy-in from frontline providers and they need to see this [P2P] as integrated and not imposed or there will be pushback. We need to coordinate our work into the suite of already existing programs.	1002: • SMAs were already in place at this site and P2P perceived as easy to add on. 1003: • Intervention fits within existing structure, some minor changes able to be made with information provided by innovation staff. 1004: • Chief of primary care presented information about P2P at a monthly staff meeting. • We spoke with several front-line staff about how to best integrate this with their already existing work. • The Director of primary care sent emails about the project. Coming from him will help elevate the status of the project. • The Director of primary care will present information at the bi-weekly meetings with team leaders. • Diabetes groups already running, innovation will be able to fit within context of ongoing groups.
Relative Priority Definition: Individuals' shared perception of the importance of the implementation within the organization.	1002: • Intervention not on leadership radar – voluntary, so can be first of things to go. 1004: • The top barrier was stated to be infringement on their previous initiatives. During the interviews, we determined that if the staff already involved in diabetes management feel their work is being challenged or re-directed by P2P it will "put their backs up." • Very busy staff and many competing initiatives; not only diabetes, but overall information overload. They	1001: • Leadership thinks the SMA expansion will easily fit in because already had SMAs ongoing. 1002: • Nurses want program to be success – trying to enlist more people/rally support. 1004: • The qualitative interviews with front line nurses and physicians helped determine how to integrate P2P with their existing workflow and programs. We also asked for their suggestions for modifications to enable local success and gain buy-in. • Chief of primary care circulated info to those involved in a strategic planning initiative to let them know what will be happening and how to incorporate it. • To overcome sense of infringement the chief of primary care suggested 3 people as potential champions and said it was very important for us to get them on board: 1) a diabetes management nurse, who is the "epicenter of things" and the "clearing point" for diabetes management, 2) the acting chief of pharmacy, who oversees the clinical pharmacists in primary care, and 3) a highly-engaged dietician. We interviewed all three to get their perspective and pull them into the study. • We sent the Chief of primary care a summary to circulate to those involved in the strategic planning initiative so all can be on same page, let them know what's coming and how to incorporate it. He pulled together a distribution list.
Readiness for implementation Definition: Tangible and immediate indicators of organizational commitment to its decision to implement an innovation.		1001: • This site is ready for implementation: the plan for when study related SMAs will begin is in place – recruitment strategies, SMAs already running and have been through trial and error period.
Leadership Engagement	1002: • Leadership engagement is lacking compared to the other 4 sites. Physicians are not	1001: • We were impressed with Chief of primary care as are local staff. Helped to convince providers

Table 2 Detailed adaptations made in real-time by site and CFIR construct *(Continued)*

Construct	Barrier	Facilitator or Adaptation
Definition: Commitment, involvement, and accountability of leaders and managers with the implementation of the innovation.	engaged or supportive of SMAs and the P2P groups. The leader who is the chief for one site and our local PI was mentioned as not being influential by several local staff. This could be complicated by the fact that there are 3 local sites. • Also, there was a barrier discussed confidentially by multiple staff about a high level leader being a barrier for this project, specifically, as well as other projects. This person is not supportive and has blocked nurses from being involved in this as well as other projects. Solving this issue was beyond the scope of our project.	to enroll patients, blocked out time for clinicians to be at groups, guaranteed space, and made sure the project ran smoothly overall. • At this site we have support from leaders across disciplines. • General support for SMAs from staff. 1002: • Multiple interviewees said staff and clinicians are aware these programs. 1003: • Interviewees suggest leadership engagement is present and they have leadership support for the SMAs and P2P. This came from multiple staff including physicians. 1004: • Very impressive chief of primary care. Was very thoughtful in his remarks and what will need to be done on his behalf for this program to succeed. Several other staff also mentioned his as a very supportive leader who is engaged in this study. • Chief of primary care offered to help us to make sure staff see P2P as a benefit, leading from a high level, tell others why we are implementing P2P and that this is important work. • Director of primary care said data feedback is important for his staff to stand behind this and he offered to disseminate data to the strategic initiative quad and everyone involved in diabetes care. 1005: • We were very impressed with the ACOS for Ambulatory Care. He is extremely supportive of the diabetes SMAs and pushing them forward and making sure PharmDs are able to participate despite time constraints. He sees an advantage to having the SMAs in terms of efficiency. • See also, Relative Advantage and Knowledge and Beliefs.
Available resources Definition: The level of resources organizational dedicated for implementation and on-going operations including physical space and time.	1001: • Space constraints for group visits. • Rooms have been scheduled for SMAs, but when patients arrive that space is occupied. • Patient parking is often not available. • Psychologist who was the P2P facilitator and SMA facilitator was not renewed and now they must find someone new and re-train. • Not all resources are available for getting patients checked in and vitals taken prior to SMAs. For example, need their own scale. 1002: • Space is so limited that groups here are scheduled based on room availability rather than staff availability. • Facility covers a large geographic area; some Veterans live 200 miles away from their facility. • Cost concerns have meant that they use volunteers for the P2P facilitator position. This caused concern that they may not be here at the right time or not have the right skills to serve as the P2P facilitator. Indeed there was P2P facilitator turnover and re-training required.	All sites: • Worked to find a guaranteed room (applies to all except 1005). • Scheduled out all rooms for SMAs and P2P open group sessions in advance. • P2P phone access to peers is available and always a viable option for all. • We did write scripts for the P2P facilitators to ease their workload and make it easier to understand their role. We also hosted bi-monthly training and question and answer sessions for them to talk to the facilitators as well as all other site P2P facilitators. 1003: • Made sure the classroom was reserved early for next couple of years for P2P. • Likely patient parking/construction problems will be resolved by time funding comes through. 1004: • We worked with the local staff to ensure that the P2P process will fit into the existing workflow. Additionally, P2P was presented at a monthly staff meeting by study staff. • Director of primary care offered to help us to make sure staff see this as a benefit, leading

Table 2 Detailed adaptations made in real-time by site and CFIR construct *(Continued)*

Construct	Barrier	Facilitator or Adaptation
	• The amount of training for the peer facilitator really needs to be minimal. We did not hear this from the other sites. • Staff are "busy and stretched thin;" it is difficult to do anything additional. 1003: • Patient parking is lacking and there are construction projects ongoing. • Group meeting space is constrained (SMAs and P2P drop-in). • Staff told us their largest barrier is always funding and finding time in staff schedules to devote to this project. 1004: • Time demands on staff are a major issue. We were told that if a lot of time would be required for patient recruitment and screening that implementation would be very difficult. • Busy staff, competing initiatives; overall information overload. • Space constraints for group meetings. • Concern there will not be enough resources to continue program after study period ends (SUSTAINABILITY). • Parking can be issue. 1005: • There is a big issue with lack of resources at this site. This was seen in terms of clinical pharmacist leaving and they were not able to replace her and the resulting lack of time for the remaining pharmDs. This may be related to the insistence that the SMAs be kept team specific. This issue came up at local team meetings with pharmacists and dieticians. • From the ACOS, *"We are short-staffed right now and we are unable to hire people."*	from a high level, tell others why we're doing P2P, 'this is important work.' • We will send ongoing data to the director of primary care and he will disseminate to the strategic initiative quad and everyone involved in diabetes care. • RA will help to relieve time demands of staff for implementing initiative 1005: • The ACOS is very on board (see also Leadership) and did help to overcome some of these barriers, such as securing time from the PharmDs despite their initial statements that they did not have enough time. However, see his caveat at left.
Access to knowledge &information Definition: Ease of access to digestible information and knowledge about the innovation and how to incorporate it into work tasks.	1001: • Chief of Primary Care aware of study. 1002: • Extended project delays (over a year) and the roll-out keeps getting pushed back with a lot of time to not know what is happening has made staff uncomfortable. Other key stake-holders may not be aware of project because of these delays – leadership has not pushed it due to delays. • Lack of awareness of project	1001: • PharmDs speak at primary care meetings to educate MDs about SMA groups. • In general, most staff aware of the way study will be conducted. 1004: • P2P facilitator engaged and knowledgeable of her role.
CHARACTERISTICS OF INDIVIDUALS		
Knowledge & Beliefs about P2P and SMA Definition: Individuals' attitudes toward and value placed on the innovation, as well as familiarity with facts, truths, and principles related to the innovation.	1001: • Staff mentioned that they are curious to see if this P2P has an added benefit to the SMAs. Kind of a wait and see how it goes approach more than already believing in the evidence. • Unclear how much clinicians know about P2P aspect of program. • Some confusion over how patients will be communicating. • Some concern about patients sharing incorrect medical information. 1002: • Some staff were worried about the P2P group and its purpose. They thought the patients would be giving incorrect clinical advice to each other. • Some staff generally confused about the way implementation/P2P would work. 1004:	1001: • Champion (also chief) understands program well and can use his knowledge to gain more support from clinicians. • HBC PhD Psychologist sees a potential benefit to the P2P program in addition to the already ongoing SMAs. • Conference call to discuss concerns about P2P groups—the intention and the instructions that the P2P patients will be given; patients will be educated and should not be exchanging clinical advice—this will be covered in the do's and don'ts' s card and in the patient orientation. 1002: • We held a conference call with this site to go into detail about the P2P groups—the intention and the instructions that the P2P patients will be given; patients will be

Table 2 Detailed adaptations made in real-time by site and CFIR construct *(Continued)*

Construct	Barrier	Facilitator or Adaptation
	• Some staff questioned aspects of the P2P study evaluation such as the patients recalling and self-reporting the number of times they had spoken with their peer partner (for those not using the telephone system). They do not think patients will be able to accurately recall. 1005: • Concern was common at this site that the patient may give each other incorrect clinical information when paired up in peer-to-peer. • The dietician discussed a negative belief about the interaction of peers and how one could be over-bearing and change the tone. • PCP interviewee talked about his beliefs that it may be possible that the pairing might not be well thought out and patients may clash or disagree.	educated and should not be exchanging clinical advice—this will be covered in the do's and don'ts' s card and in the patient orientation. Team calls also clarified this. 1003: • Much more positive about the evidence behind P2P than the other sites. Absolutely see a need for the P2P program. Believe based on work with other Veteran groups that it will be very fruitful. Believe having a peer will help with attendance and motivate Veterans to attend. A previous local veteran-paired smoking group has been successful. 1005: • The ACOS is very supportive of SMAs. When introduced to PACT in 2009/2010, was introduced to concepts of SMAs – got education on SMAs and started reading about them and thought, *"Hey this is a fantastic way to actually create some efficiency in the way we provide care."* He is a practicing PCP and has numerous diabetic patients—he has been using the clinical pharmacists and nursing staff to help manage his diabetes patients for years. • Leadership says that clinicians recognize that this will have a good impact on patients, they understand impacts on efficiency, and they understand the concepts of peer support. • Dieticians believe P2P will work because patients really enjoy having someone check up on them.
Self-efficacy Definition: Individual belief in their own capabilities to execute courses of action to achieve implementation goals.	1005: • Physician talking about engaging other providers: *"Some Primary Care providers are better than others, and I think it's all going to have to do with their personality basically. I think some docs would be very well-suited for this where they're not preaching at them and uh, and is okay with, like I'm kind of okay with it going off-topic every now and then but I'll steer it back, uh, but I don't have to be the center of attention, do you know what I mean? I don't know, so it's more of a Socratic method."*	1002: • "Champion" confident he can organize the logistics for the startup of project. 1003: • P2P facilitator confident in ability to help Veterans make changes and reach goals.
	PROCESS	
Planning Definition: The degree to which a scheme or method of behavior and tasks for implementing an innovation are developed in advance, and the quality of those schemes or methods.	1002: • Staff unclear of roles in SMAs – not yet defined. • Lack of schedule for SMAs.	1001: • Curriculum for SMAs tested and set prior to implementation. • Roles of clinicians in SMAs well defined prior to implementation (had nurse following up with patients for lab work, appointments, health psychologist working on goals with Vets, etc.) • Educational materials are prepared for patient use. • Nurse involved in SMAs willing to help/seek help in pairing Vets for P2P – can have group of three if pairing doesn't work well. • Recruitment strategies thought out in terms of available patient pools. 1002: • Did SMA trial period prior to implementation. • Ready for implementation due to planning – gotten buy in at sub-site A, have organized RA. 1003: • Self-initiated local planning. The Site PI thought about ways to get buy-in from providers and planned for ways to spread the word to

Table 2 Detailed adaptations made in real-time by site and CFIR construct *(Continued)*

Construct	Barrier	Facilitator or Adaptation
		patients by presenting information at other groups. • P2P facilitator in place and has been attending SMAs to plan/learn more. 1004: • A lot of local planning was done. The Chief of primary care was very involved in making sure this was presented to involved staff multiple times and that buy-in from providers was obtained. 1005: • MD SMA group 2, talks about how the month interval is a good plan to follow because of the timing for when changes in behavior occur. See also knowledge and beliefs.
Opinion Leaders Definition: Individuals in an organization that have formal or informal influence on the attitudes and beliefs of their colleagues with respect to implementing the innovation.	1002: • The opinion leader for primary care was named by several staff; however, he has not been formally pulled into our project – we tried, but have not been able to yet. The named opinion leader/champion does not have the necessary influence, i.e. is not really an opinion leader. 1004: • PI and the chief of primary care seem to be opinion leaders backing this project—however, as pointed out in champions, the PI has not been able to influence 1 of the 2 SMAs groups to be supportive of this project.	1001: • The Director of primary care was named as an opinion leader; he also happens to be the champion, and a good supporter of this project. 1003: • Health Behavior psychologist is more of champion, but is also somewhat of an opinion leader for the primary care staff.
Formally appointed implementation leaders Definition: Individuals from within the organization who have been formally appointed with responsibility for implementing an innovation as coordinator, project manager, team leader, or other similar role.	1001: • Need for P2P facilitator who can engage participants. 1002: • The appointed physician implementation leader has little influence over staff at 2 of the local sites and several staff mentioned this. Also, he seems to think that he has the necessary influence, which compounds the problem. • General concern over roles in project/who will be filling roles. • P2P facilitator role of concern because seen as a lot of work/time.	1001: • RA role will be huge help for implementation of program (dedicated person to perform study related tasks). 1003: • Have P2P leaders in mind prior to implementation – is extremely engaged and prioritizes innovation.
Champions Definition: "Individuals who dedicate themselves to supporting, marketing, and 'driving through' an [implementation]", overcoming indifference or resistance that the innovation may provoke in an organization.	1002: • No overall physician champion. The physicians have not bought into the diabetes SMAs. • The physicians see the diabetes SMA as extra work. They do not see the added value. • The physicians will not participate in the diabetes SMAs. Whereas, the nurses want a physician to be there for medical questions. • The named physician champion for the SMA/P2P project, does not have the influence that he needs to have (wrong champion selected) according to multiple staff.	1001: • Great champion in the director of primary care firm A. Helps with presentations, helps convince providers to enroll patients, blocks out time for providers to be at the groups, secures space, oversees local running of the project. 1002: We worked with the chief of primary care to present the study and try to gain physician buy-in for the SMAs as well as P2P groups. • Given the named champion is thought to not have adequate influence, we tried to pull in and speak with a physician who was named as being influential. 1003: • The health psychologist is a great champion for this site. He has a great deal of expertise and ideas to help with the project. He is very communicative. He is very passionate about this project and staff listen to him. 1004: • The Chief of Primary Care is a good champion for the diabetes SMAs.

Table 2 Detailed adaptations made in real-time by site and CFIR construct *(Continued)*

Construct	Barrier	Facilitator or Adaptation
		• Chief of PC also offered to send any emails to staff that we need him to. He said the material coming from him, would help. See also construct – leadership support. 1005: • The NP lead facilitator of most of the new SMAs is a champion, she started the SMAs (see also innovation sources), but she is also a champion. • Diabetes SMA has a nurse who was a big champion and really helped with the success of these groups according to the dietician and the lead MD facilitator. • The MD of the 2nd SMA group is a good champion and his group was well run and had good outcomes. See also innovation participants about how the PCP champion strategically used well-controlled patients in his groups.
Key stakeholders Definition: Individuals from within the organization that are directly impacted by the innovation, e.g., staff responsible for making referrals to a new program or using a new work process.	1002: • Hard sell for physicians – do not see benefit, takes too much time.	1001: • PharmDs speak at primary care meetings to educate MDs about SMA groups – overall support from clinicians for SMAs. • Champion also chief – engages key stakeholders (clinicians). 1002: • One interviewee cited a possible solution to engage residents in innovation. • One provider cited as enlisting physicians on her panel. 1004: • Chief of primary care will work to engage key stakeholders. 1005: • The ACOS for Ambulatory Care is a good supporter and has been working to engage key stakeholders in the SMAs.
Innovation participants Definition: Individuals served by the organization that participate in the innovation, e.g., patients in a prevention program in a hospital.	1001: • Poor attendance at group meetings – Vets at this site may not be comfortable in groups. • Success dependent upon engagement of participants. • Concern over finding enough interested participants. 1002: Participants need to see added value in SMA to get engagement. 1003: • Site SMAs began with recruitment of those with A1c's over 9, attendance/engagement was very low. 1004: • Patient engagement low, patient drop-off high.	1001: • Scheduling ahead and getting reminder calls may help Vet attendance/engagement. • Pairing aspect of P2P may increase engagement among participants – peer holding them accountable. 1002: • Voluntary program – participants more likely to be motivated/engaged. 1003: • Include Vets with A1c's under 9, which has increased attendance and engagement in program. • Having formally appointed implementation leaders (RA & P2P leader) to engage innovation participants will help. • Social support will increase engagement in SMAs. • Group setting/P2P will help to engage "passive patient population." • Because travel is an issue, one interviewee suggested a carpool setup. 1004: • To increase engagement in SMAs/P2P, pair up Veterans at first or second SMA (previous SMA was only one visit). • Psychologists have been asking Veterans what they would like to get out of sessions/for feedback to increase engagement. • Let Veterans know they can self-refer.

Table 3 CFIR construct ranking after pre-implementation phone interviews. Rating − 2 to + 2

Construct	Site #1 (1001)	Site #2 (1002)	Site #3 (1003)	Site #4 (1004)	Site #5 (1005)
Intervention characteristics					
Intervention Source	Internal	External	Internal	External	Internal
Evidence Strength & Quality	+ 1	−2	+ 1	+ 2	+ 1
Relative advantage	−1	− 2	+ 1	+ 1	Mixed
Adaptability	−1	− 1	Missing	+ 1	Neutral
Trialability	+ 1	+ 1	Missing	Missing	Neutral
Complexity	+ 1	−2	Mixed	−1	− 2
Design Quality and Packaging	−1	− 1	− 1	−1	− 1
Cost		−1		+ 1	+ 1
Outer setting					
Patient Needs & Resources	−2	−1	−2	− 1	+ 1
Inner setting					
Networks / Communications	+ 1	−2	Neutral	Neutral	Neutral
Culture	−2	−2	Neutral	Neutral	Neutral
Tension for Change	Mixed	Neutral	+ 1	+ 1	Neutral
Compatibility	+ 1	Mixed	+ 1	Neutral	Neutral
Relative Priority	+ 1	−2	Neutral	−1	Neutral
Leadership Engagement	+ 2	−2	+ 2	+ 2	+ 1
Available Resources	−1	−1	− 1	− 1	−1
Access to knowledge & info	−1	−2	−1	− 1	−1
Characteristics of individuals					
Knowledge & Beliefs about P2P	Mixed	−1	+ 2	+ 1	− 1
Self-efficacy	Missing	Neutral	+ 1	Neutral	Neutral
Process					
Planning	+ 2	Mixed	+ 1	+ 1	Neutral
Opinion Leaders	+ 1	−1	+ 1	Mixed	Neutral
Formally appointed implementation leaders	Neutral	−1	+ 1	Neutral	Neutral
Champions	+ 2	−2	+ 2	+ 2	+ 1
Key Stakeholders	+ 1	−2	Neutral	+ 1	+ 1
Innovation Participants	−1	Neutral	−1	− 1	Neutral

"*I think [SMA and P2P] is another means for providing guidance and motivation for patients with diabetes struggling with their glucose to meet goals. I think we do a lot of telling patients what to do, and I really think there's a benefit to hearing from 'equals' rather than somebody else—someone lateral as opposed to top down with the guiding and coaching.*" A Primary Care Physician (PCP) from site 1005 explained, "*No matter how much I say, 'Yeah, I know diabetes does this, diabetes does that,' I don't have to deal with it and there's one guy saying,*

Table 4 CFIR construct importance as ranked by local sites

All sites ranked very important in phone survey, and subsequent interview data confirmed this	All sites ranked very important or important in phone survey, and subsequent interview data confirmed this	Phone survey ranked as not very important; however, data came out strongly during the qualitative interviews
Complexity	Adaptability	Evidence Strength and Quality
Available Resources	Compatibility	Relative Advantage
Champions	Patient Needs and Resources	
Leadership Engagement		
Knowledge and Beliefs about P2P		

'Yeah, my blood sugar's like this, I made this little change and it dropped like, you know, dropped 20 or 30 points,' and they believe them more." Sites 1001 and 1003 also mentioned that local evidence had shown that having a peer or buddy for support, as is the case in the diabetes SMAs and the P2P pairs and group sessions, helps patients with diabetes.

Relative advantage
Diabetes SMA
Perceptions of the relative advantage of diabetes SMA programs were mixed across sites. Those sites that had an overall positive ranking for stakeholder's perception of the advantage of these programs were 1003 and 1004. As an example, a 1003 health psychologist stated, *"We do have also a diabetes education class... There's a great bit of information given. There is only a very small percentage of diabetes patients that have not taken that class because it is essentially mandated. But, we're finding that for some reason this doesn't translate into action."* The need for and potential advantages of the peer support program in this population was mentioned at site 1004: *"...especially in Veteran population because they're deployed in a unit and they come back in a unit. So the peer support would be even more effective in theory than in the general population..."*.

There were also some references from clinicians about advantages to leading group visits instead of one-on-one patient appointments and that format provided a means to hear more detailed information about patient behaviors, *"I love talking to patients but I get tired of half-hour slots, so anything that kind of breaks up my clinic, it's a slightly different format...and it's a chance to kind of listen to the more of the social stories and kind of what's going in [food] why do they eat at Coney Island every day and their diet hasn't changed, or why they're not going to change that."*

Sites 1001 and 1002 had negative ratings; staff did not see an advantage compared to usual care or likewise because they saw the SMAs as added worked, without any added value. For those sites with a negative ranking, we asked local staff to present information about the value and advantage to their local PCPs. During our site visits, we also presented evidence to the primary care staff from the literature, engaged them, and answered any questions they had.

Diabetes SMA and P2P
Another noted advantage (see Cost in Table 2) was the belief that the SMAs and P2P program will improve efficiency of care and, therefore, increase patient access and decrease cost. A physician leader from site 1004 said, *"I also think that it's a good way to cut costs from healthcare because if a peer mentor can help the patient, he* can remind him to follow his appointments, take his medications, exercise; it's much simpler than a health professional trying to do the same thing while juggling other things. I think it helps from the clinical aspect, as well as having a financial benefit..."* A site 1005 clinical leader said, *"Let that dietician go over information with 8-12 people at one time, instead of one at a time. Those kinds of efficiencies are really great and I think it will help my dieticians, my clinical pharmacists, and my psychologist a lot, and I think it will help the physicians to manage their population of patients."*

Adaptabiliy
Diabetes SMA
Sites 1001 and 1002 had concerns initially that the SMA program was not adaptable. They thought that the overseeing site would be dictating the content and manner that each of the SMA sessions would be run. We worked with both sites continually through phone calls and virtual meetings to explain that the local team had flexibility and control over the SMA sessions and that our fidelity assessment would help to account for any differences across sites.

Site 1004 had a positive rating for adaptability of SMAs because they realized the importance of flexibility and had tailored their SMA sessions to be adaptable so Veterans could get what *"they want and need out of each session."* Staff at this site also had a good understanding that we wanted the local clinical programs to be adaptable to fit local context.

P2P
Views on the potential adaptability of the peer support component of the program were mixed. Site 1001 had concerns that the program could not be adapted for patients who did not mesh well with their assigned peer. We worked with that site to come up with an adapted plan whereby a patient could be easily re-paired, even with a patient outside their cohort if need be, or assigned to a new group of 3 patients. We also implemented a way of working with the local nurses and PCPs to get their recommendations on patient pairs that would work well together. Site 1001 also had some issues surrounding their locally developed recruitment plan that the clinical and research teams thought was not feasible. During the site visit, we discussed this with the local team and they adapted their recruitment plan to be more realistic.

Complexity
Diabetes SMA and P2P
Interestingly, site 1001 staff had no concerns, even when prompted, about staff being so busy that it would be difficult to do anything additional or complex. However,

that was the only site with a positive ranking. The other four sites expressed concerns that if the programs were complex, this would make the programs much more difficult to implement. An Associate Chief of Staff at 1005 said, *"I am very supportive of this, but it can't add work to my people. It will have to be very efficient."* One specific complexity concern was in terms of the clinical notes and documentation required for each SMA visit and that the notes would be cumbersome for the clinical pharmacist, who was the documenter at one site. *"I just want the pharmacist who will be involved to write very short, patient specific changes. That is going to be VERY important to me. If it is burdensome to them, they are not going to be able to continue."* The facilitation team worked with the site through team meetings and in-person discussions with the clinical pharmacists to streamline the documentation and share diabetes SMA clinical note templates across the sites.

Sites 1002, 1003, 1004, and 1005 all expressed concern with staff being busy and that it would be difficult to add additional programs and find staff time to help facilitate the SMA and/or P2P group sessions. To impact the complexity barriers, the facilitation team worked with the local sites through team meetings and phone calls to streamline documentation and shared diabetes SMA clinical note templates across the sites. Additional efforts were made to integrate the process within existing workflow–for example, allowing the clinician who documented the diabetes SMA notes to be adaptable: in some sites a clinical pharmacist, others a nurse practitioner, or primary care physician. Likewise, the role of the P2P facilitator varied.

Patient needs and resources
Diabetes SMA and P2P
All sites except 1005 perceived the new programs as facing multiple barriers within the CFIR construct of addressing patient needs and resources. This was the most negatively ranked construct overall. There were a plethora of barriers across the sites, including staff concerns about patients being guarded and not wanting to pair up or exchange numbers, lack of motivation in patient population, low patient attendance especially without financial compensation for the P2P or SMA visits, difficulties with patient recruitment, long distance drives for patients to the hospital, patients' lack of financial resources, patient resistance to change, and lack of patient follow-through when asked to bring in or complete materials or goals. A clinical pharmacist from site 1003 expressed it this way, *"There are many obstacles to bringing the patients in... [to SMAs or P2P group sessions] Our population tends to be older and on the financial scale of things, having more difficulty. Those factors set into place some natural barriers to being compliant with appointments."*

A primary care physician at site 1001 stated, *"Definitely the top barrier will be convincing the patients to show up. We invite an average of 10 people and we usually have between 4 and 7 who come and continue to show up. I think patient buy-in is definitely a barrier."* Site 1001 health psychologist, *"I can say generally we have a hard time getting patients to come to groups here. We're trying to hold them first thing in the morning so that parking will be easier, but parking is a huge barrier. Patients don't want to come to anything that they perceive as extra a lot of the time, because they find it so challenging to actually physically get here, get parked and get to their appointment."*

Site 1004 research coordinator, *"People with diabetes don't feel well and getting them involved in something—it is difficult. And some of our patients are still working, so if we have classes during the day, that's an obstacle. And transportation. We've had that experience in the past where they'd like to join but they can't get here."*

To overcome these barriers the facilitation team worked to make sure that patients would be eligible for travel pay for attendance to the SMA clinical appointments and helped with attendance by making additional reminder calls and sending reminder letters. We worked with all sites to ensure that, when possible, appointments were scheduled at a convenient time for patients (also considering which time of day each facility has the most parking availability). We consulted with staff from the sites to consider their perspective on matching peers together and who would work best together and again, allowing for adaptability and patient re-pairing. We also worked with sites to ensure whenever possible that these facilitators would be sustainable across time when the research team would no longer be involved (transference of some of these tasks in time to local clinical and administrative staff).

Compatibility
Diabetes SMA and P2P
Perceptions of the compatibility of the SMA and P2P programs were either mixed, neutral or positive for all sites. Site 1001 and 1003 staff were confident that the implementation process would be smooth because both programs were designed in a way that they believed was compatible and fit within their existing workflow and programs. At site 1004, we heard from multiple staff that it was very important for us to make sure the programs were integrated into their suite of already existing programs or there would be push-back from staff. To do so, we spoke with several front-line staff about how to best integrate the programs with their existing work. The Chief of Primary Care at this site also worked with us to present information at their monthly staff meetings.

Other compatibility adaptations meant that we were very flexible about the type of clinicians who could facilitate the SMAs—the main facilitators varied between clinical pharmacists, nurses, dieticians, and primary care providers; as long as multiple types of clinicians were involved, the lead was adaptable to best suit their local needs and staffing considerations. Additionally, we were flexible about the role of the P2P facilitators; Veterans with and without diabetes, research associates, and volunteers.

Leadership engagement
Diabetes SMA and P2P
Leadership engagement was ranked positively at all sites except one. Leaders were considered engaged when multiple interviewees expressed that a leader did things such as: help with convincing providers to enroll patients, block out time for clinicians to facilitate the SMAs and staff to facilitate the P2P groups, guarantee space for the SMA and P2P programs to be held, garner general support from staff, help with results/outcome feedback to staff, lead from a high level, and express to staff why they feel these programs are important. At site 1002 where leadership was lacking, a named leader for the project was mentioned by local staff as not being influential. Additionally, there were some issues with general lack of high leadership support at this site (beyond the scope of this project).

Available resources
Diabetes SMA and P2P
The availability of resources was ranked the same negative value across all sites (– 1). Issues of concern included space constraints for SMA and P2P group visits, lack of patient parking, SMA and P2P facilitator staff leaving after trained, staff generally busy and stretched thin, competing initiatives, overall information overload, and being short-staffed, "We are short-staffed right now and we are unable to hire people." Space was so limited at site 1002 that SMA sessions had to be scheduled based on room availability, rather than staff availability.

The facilitation team helped to find guaranteed rooms, scheduled SMAs and P2P sessions early so rooms could be booked well in advance, wrote scripts for staff, and had monthly training for the P2P facilitators to ease their workload and make it easier to understand their role.

Knowledge and beliefs
Diabetes SMA and P2P
There were concerns from several sites stemming from beliefs that the patients in the SMAs or as part of their pairing would share incorrect clinical information. Site 1002 health psychologist explained: "And one other barrier potentially could be misinformation, people talk and sometimes myths get out there and misconceptions and what they hear by word of mouth which is not very accurate information so...the group sessions, we don't know what's going to be said between the Veterans and I think it's important to make sure proper education being shared among them but I mean that's going to be hard to control, so that's another downfall."

Site 1005 had the most concerns about the patients being paired and chatting in the SMAs, largely based on their prior experience: "There's been two people that used to call each other and kind of hold each other accountable, however, they were both very non-compliant and didn't give off the best information, so we were kind of like, 'Eh, that didn't work out very well.'" This site also had a concern about peer interaction during the SMAs, as a dietician talked about a negative belief about the interaction of peers and how one could be over-bearing and change the tone. "Then there's this other guy that was coming to diabetes SMA and he made so many good changes, [But] he kind of came off really hard to others. He was losing weight, he was improving his A1C and we first told him, 'Can you share your story, can you try to motivate these people?' and it became really aggressive... someone would say, 'No, I haven't started exercising,' and he's like, 'Why not?? Why can't you do that?' and it was really offending patients. We actually had to talk to him after...he was giving advice that more a provider should've given and it was not supportive and we had several patients call and complain about it."

At site 1001, 1002, 1005, we held separate conference calls, where we gave a detailed outline of the P2P program, we explained that patients would receive orientation materials and instruction and be advised not to exchange any clinical advice, and allowed staff to discuss any of their concerns with facilitators.

"In the group [SMA] we do try to set goals each time. We'll go over the goals that they made last month...goal-setting holds them accountable, we say, 'Mr. so and so, did you get on the treadmill like you said you were going to last month?' and if he hasn't, it's kind of like, 'Oh, I let my group down.' It might motivate them to try again this month and them kind of working off of each other and holding each other accountable, which is nice."

P2P
Site 1001 had what we termed a "wait and see" approach to observe if the peer program had any benefit. When prompting interviewees on their beliefs about the peer program, we were able to clear up some misperceptions and confusion about how the patients would be communicating.

Site 1003 was the most confident in the benefits of the peer program—they stated that they saw an absolute need for the peer program based on other local work with patient groups that were fruitful. They believed having a peer would help with attendance and motivate patients to attend. Furthering their confidence in the peer program, a previous local veteran-paired smoking group had been successful.

There was pushback at sites 1001, 1002, and 1005 stemming from beliefs that matching peers would be difficult for multiple reasons. Site 1001 nurse, *"Matching the patients up will probably be the hard part, I mean if one person doesn't like their partner, I could see them wanting to stop."*

Champions

Champions were ranked positively at all but one site (1002). Interestingly, the champions' organizational role varied across sites: Director of Primary Care (3), Clinical Health Psychologist (1), and Nurse Practitioner (1).

Positive champions were defined as those working to push through any barriers and positively advocating for the clinical programs to gain staff buy-in. The Chief of Primary Care for 1004 was deemed a good champion by staff at his site. He also said, *"I see my role as making sure that primary care, as a service, sees this [SMA and P2P] as a benefit. Leading it from a high level rather and being able to tell others why we're doing this. I can say, 'this is important work.'"* Descriptions of what the champions did included: help with presentations, help convince providers to enroll patients, block out time for providers to facilitate/attend the groups, secure space, and oversee local management of the project.

Many interviewees at site 1002 saw their site champion as non-influential. Facilitators worked with the local site to try to gain physician buy-in for the SMAs and P2P groups. In addition, we tried to pull in and speak with a physician who was named as being influential by interviewees and staff we met on site visits.

Discussion

In this article, we described our method for identification of contextual factors that influenced implementation of complex diabetes clinical programs -SMAs and P2P. The qualitative phone interviews aided implementation through the identification of modifiable barriers or conversely, actionable findings. Implementation projects, and certainly clinical programs, do not have unlimited resources and these interviews allowed us to determine which facets to target and act on for each site.

Likewise, our facilitation team used formative evaluation to understand the context and organizational issues at each of these VA health systems. Our approach used the CFIR to guide us to actionable findings and help us better understand barriers and facilitators, and variations of those, across constructs and sites. Using the CFIR to do this allowed us to improve the generalizability and efficiency of our findings by highlighting factors that prior research have identified as influencing implementation (each of the published constructs). Additionally, our

project team and the local sites benefited from the use of formative evaluation throughout the early implementation process; we identified, in an ongoing manner, problems that we had not anticipated but that needed to be addressed to optimize implementation.

The implementation of a new clinical program is very complex and the field has recognized the need to utilize theoretical bases of implementation to facilitate implementation itself and there have been more calls for researchers to utilize existing frameworks to gain insights into the mechanisms by which implementation is more likely to succeed and to achieve common terminology. [21] We believe our approach of using the CFIR to accomplish those goals has broad applicability and can be used by other projects to guide, adapt, and improve implementation of research into practice.

We have illustrated how pre- and early-implementation FE is critically important in preparing for and gaining early understanding of key factors that influence implementation processes, and future success or failure. This early formative research shaped our implementation to minimize type III failures. Our rich examples highlight areas that were challenging as well as those that facilitated implementation of both shared medical appointments, and peer-to-peer programming. It is important to note that there was no site that was universally positive or negative across constructs, as often is assumed of "laggard" or "early adopting" sites. Evidence strength and quality was a negative issue at only one site (1002), but it was very impactful there (see Table 3, 2 ranking) and important for the facilitators to be aware of and to work to overcome. As a result, our team presented evidence during the site visit and during a local primary care team meeting to help educate and influence the physicians. In contrast patient needs and resources was a negatively rated construct at 4 of the 5 sites, but at the 5th (1005) was a positively ranked construct—illustrating that implementation scientists need to be very cautious of labeling any construct as universally problematic.

Because of our intentional broad range of interviewees, CFIR constructs could be mixed within a site. When this was the case, the findings were discussed, weighed and used to come up with one overall score as per CFIR guidelines. The process is similar to consensus-based coding; "Analysts apply a summary rating, taking all the individual ratings and supporting qualitative summary and rationale into consideration, and then discuss ratings to achieve consensus" [22].

There are several limitations to this study. Constructs were assigned only one rating per site using weighted data from all respondents. Additionally, it is challenging for implementation researchers to identify when modifications create an additional intervention; however, in this case we classified these as local adaptations because the core underlying conceptual nature of the interventions was maintained in each case. Program drift is sometimes thought of as resulting in lower intervention success due to lack of fidelity [7]. However, experts in the field recognize that view is overly simplistic and encourages an unnecessarily rigid view of fidelity; "this designation decreased opportunities to learn from evidence-based intervention adaptations that result in improvements beyond what is expected" [10].

Conclusions

As the SHARES study progresses, these findings will be compared and correlated to outcome measures. This comprehensive adaptation data collection will also facilitate and enhance understanding of the future success or lack of success of implementation and inform potential for translation and public health impact. Crossing the bridge from research to practice in primary care and family practice settings is crucially important because in many ways we are not reaping the full public health benefits of our investment in research. [23] While the evidence-to-practice gap for interventions in primary care is receiving attention, it tends to be understudied. [11] We believe our approach of using the CFIR to guide us to actionable findings and help us better understand barriers and facilitators, has broad applicability and can be used by other projects to guide, adapt, and improve implementation of research into practice in primary care and other clinical settings.

Abbreviations
CFIR: Consolidated Framework for Implementation Research; FE: Formative Evaluation; IRB: Institutional Review Board; P2P: Peer-to-Peer; PCP: Primary Care Physician; SHARES: Shared Health Appointments and Reciprocal Enhanced Support; SMA: Shared Medical Appointments; VA: Veterans Affairs

Funding
The SHARES study is funded by the VA Health Services Research & Development (HSR&D) IIR 15–321. The study funder did not design the study or data collection, and did not participate in the analysis or interpretation of data.

Authors' contributions
CPK lead all the interviews, lead the coding and analysis of the qualitative data, and wrote this manuscript. MV helped in the interviewing process, participated fully in the qualitative coding and analysis of data, and editing this manuscript. MH conceived and designed the overall SHARES study and critically revised this manuscript. All authors read and approved the final manuscript. CPK, MV, and MK, all agree to be accountable for all aspects of the work and in ensuring that questions related to the accuracy or integrity of any part of the work are appropriately investigated and resolved.

Author's information
CPK was trained in epidemiology at the University of Michigan and works for the Center for Clinical Management Research (CCMR) at the Ann Arbor Veterans Affairs Healthcare System. She leads a national Implementation Research Group (IRG) of 250 members for the Center for Evaluation and Implementation

Resources (CEIR) that provides continuing education, training, and sharing of best practices in implementation science. Her expertise over the last 15 years includes formative evaluation, qualitative interviewing and analysis, adaptations and fidelity, and implementation science.
MV obtained her Bachelor of Science from the University of Michigan and currently works as the research associate on the SHARES study.
MK is a physician Research Scientist at the Ann Arbor Center for Clinical Management Research (CCMR). She is also Director of the Community Engagement and Outreach Core of the Michigan Center for Diabetes Translational Research (MCDTR), one of five DTRs funded by the National Institutes of Health to provide assistance to researchers conducting novel interventions to improve diabetes care. MK has expertise in the development and evaluation of health system and behavioral interventions to improve between-clinic visit chronic disease self-management and outcomes. She has served as PI on multiple multi-site effectiveness and implementation studies evaluating different peer support models and health team outreach programs to improve glycemic, blood pressure, and other risk factor control in diabetes. She is also PI on an AHRQ grant that developed a diabetes web-based decision aid that peer mentors and other outreach workers can use with patients to improve diabetes treatment decision-making.

Ethics approval and consent to participate
The SHARES study was approved by the Veterans Affairs Central Institutional Review Board (C-IRB) (reference number 13–21). All participants consented to participate and were informed that their participation was completely voluntary. The consent process was executed as governed by the Central IRB. Staff members were provided with a Study Information Sheet at the time of recruitment and verbal consent was obtained prior to the start of the interview. Verbal consent for staff interviews was approved by the CIRB, as the study is considered minimal risk and obtaining written consent would place an additional burden on participants.

Competing interests
The authors declare that they have no competing interests.

Author details
¹Center for Clinical Management Research (CCMR- VA), VA Ann Arbor Healthcare System, 2800 Plymouth Road Bld. 16, Ann Arbor, MI 48109, USA. ²Department of Internal Medicine, University of Michigan, 1500 East Medical Center Drive, Ann Arbor, MI 48109, USA.

References
1. Stetler CB, et al. The role of formative evaluation in implementation research and the QUERI experience. J Gen Intern Med. 2006;21 (Suppl 2):S1–8.
2. Glasgow RE, Lichtenstein E, Marcus AC. Why don't we see more translation of health promotion research to practice? Rethinking the efficacy-to-effectiveness transition. Am J Public Health. 2003;93(8):1261–7.
3. Hasson H. Systematic evaluation of implementation fidelity of complex interventions in health and social care. Implement Sci. 2010;5:67.
4. Hulscher ME, Laurant MG, Grol RP. Process evaluation on quality improvement interventions. Qual Saf Health Care. 2003;12(1):40–6.
5. Mitchell SE, et al. Implementation and adaptation of the re-engineered discharge (RED) in five California hospitals: a qualitative research study. BMC Health Serv Res. 2017;17(1):291.
6. Brown CH, et al. An overview of research and evaluation designs for dissemination and implementation. Annu Rev Public Health. 2017;38:1–22.
7. Chambers, D.A., R.E. Glasgow, and K.C. Stange, The dynamic sustainability framework: addressing the paradox of sustainment amid ongoing change. Implement Sci, 2013. 8: p. 117.
8. Chambers DA, Norton WE. The Adaptome: advancing the science of intervention adaptation. Am J Prev Med. 2016;

9. Aarons GA, et al. Dynamic adaptation process to implement an evidence-based child maltreatment intervention. Implement Sci. 2012;7:32.
10. Chambers DA, Norton WE. The Adaptome: advancing the science of intervention adaptation. Am J Prev Med. 2016;51(4 Suppl 2):S124–31.
11. Lau R, et al. Achieving change in primary care–causes of the evidence to practice gap: systematic reviews of reviews. Implement Sci. 2016;11:40.
12. Heisler M, et al. The shared health appointments and reciprocal enhanced support (SHARES) study: study protocol for a randomized trial. Trials. 2017; 18(1):239.
13. Heisler M, et al. Diabetes control with reciprocal peer support versus nurse care management: a randomized trial. Ann Intern Med. 2010;153(8):507–15.
14. Heisler M, et al. Randomized controlled effectiveness trial of reciprocal peer support in heart failure. Circ Heart Fail. 2013;6(2):246–53.
15. Damschroder LJ, et al. Fostering implementation of health services research findings into practice: a consolidated framework for advancing implementation science. Implement Sci. 2009;4:50.
16. Maxwell, J.A., *Qualitative Research Design: An Interactive Approach*. 3 ed. applied social research methods. 2013: Sage Publications. 232.
17. Mason J. Qualitative researching. Thousand Oaks: Sage Publications; 2002.
18. Patton MQ. Enhancing the quality and credibility of qualitative analysis. Health Serv Res. 1999;34(5 Pt 2):1189–208.
19. Hsieh HF, Shannon SE. Three approaches to qualitative content analysis. Qual Health Res. 2005;15(9):1277–88.
20. Damschroder LJ, et al. Implementation evaluation of the telephone lifestyle coaching (TLC) program: organizational factors associated with successful implementation. Transl Behav Med. 2017;7(2):233–41.
21. Nilsen P. Making sense of implementation theories, models and frameworks. Implement Sci. 2015;10:53.
22. CFIRguide. *Consolidated Framework for Implementation Research - Qualitative Data Analysis*. [cited 2017 April 18, 2017]; available from: http://cfirguide.org/qual.html.
23. Lenfant C, lecture S. Clinical research to clinical practice–lost in translation? N Engl J Med. 2003;349(9):868–74.

3

'The big buzz': a qualitative study of how safe care is perceived, understood and improved in general practice

Carl de Wet[1,2,3*], Paul Bowie[1,2] and Catherine O'Donnell[2]

Abstract

Background: Exploring frontline staff perceptions of patient safety is important, because they largely determine how improvement interventions are understood and implemented. However, research evidence in this area is very limited. This study therefore: explores participants' understanding of patient safety as a concept; describes the factors thought to contribute to patient safety incidents (PSIs); and identifies existing improvement actions and potential opportunities for future interventions to help mitigate risks.

Methods: A total of 34 semi-structured interviews were conducted with 11 general practitioners, 12 practice nurses and 11 practice managers in the West of Scotland. The data were thematically analysed.

Results: Patient safety was considered an important and integral part of routine practice. Participants perceived a proportion of PSIs as being inevitable and therefore not preventable. However, there was consensus that most factors contributing to PSIs are amenable to improvement efforts and acknolwedgement that the potential exists for further enhancements in care procedures and systems. Most were aware of, or already using, a wide range of safety improvement tools for this purpose. While the vast majority was able to identify specific, safety-critical areas requiring further action, this was counter-balanced by the reality that additional resources were a decisive requirment.

Conclusion: The perceptions of participants in this study are comparable with the international patient safety literature: frontline staff and clinicians are aware of and potentially able to address a wide range of safety threats. However, they require additional resources and support to do so.

Keywords: Patient safety, Patient safety incidents, General practice, Family medicine, Quality improvement

Background

In the last few decades, a growing body of evidence suggests that patient safety incidents (PSIs) commonly occur and that a substantial minority result in preventable, iatrogenic harm to patients in primary care [1–3]. Improving care quality and safety is now a priority in many modern health care systems, including the UK National Health Service (NHS). Consequently, a diverse range of improvement initiatives and interventions have been developed and implemented, ranging from small-scale, informal actions in single units, practices or care teams to formal collaborative-type large-scale programmes at regional and national levels [4–6].

The Scottish Patient Safety Program (SPSP) is an example of this approach [7]. It initially focused on specific, high-risk processes in secondary and tertiary care centres only, before being extended into primary care [4]. As a result, there are now a range of potential improvement methods, tools and interventions available that have been adapted and contextualised for the general practice setting [8–15].

Despite these initiatives and a growing research agenda, there is still limited evidence that the standards of care, including in general practice, have been significantly improved as a result of specific interventions. While there are many potential reasons for this, they typically relate to two interlinked issues. The first is the characteristics of

* Correspondence: carl.dewet@health.qld.gov.au
[1]Medical Directorate, NHS Education for Scotland, Glasgow, UK
[2]General Practice & Primary Care, Institute of Health & Wellbeing, College of Medical, Veterinary and Life Science, University of Glasgow, Glasgow, Scotland
Full list of author information is available at the end of the article

the intervention, in particular whether it is useful, acceptable, feasible and implemented as intended by those who developed and tested it. The second issue is whether the intended users of these complex health care interventions are willing and able to effectively implement them and continue to use them.

In order to fully understand these issues, it is therefore important, and possibly essential, that health care policy makers and researchers elicit and attempt to understand the perceptions of frontline staff groups (the 'on-the--ground' implementers) before attempting to implement such complex interventions, not least because these perceptions largely determine how an intervention is understood and implemented in routine practice [16]. However, to date, the perceptions of general practice team members remains, for the most part, unknown [17].

Method
Study aims
The aims of this study were threefold:

1. To describe the perceptions, understanding and experiences of safe care from a range of general practice team members in Scotland;
2. To identify and describe the issues perceived as important contributing factors to patient safety incidents (PSI); and.
3. To identify existing improvement actions and strategies and explore team perceptions about potential opportunities for future interventions.

Design
This is a qualitative study, using semi-structured interviews, conducted with general practitioners (GP), practice nurses (PN) and practice managers (PM). The decision to interview different team members was motivated by the multidisciplinary nature of general practice, its strong ethos of integrated working to explore clinical and non-clinical perceptions and experiences of how safe care is understood and delivered.

Setting and sample
The study was undertaken in Scotland in two mainland NHS Health Boards: one covering a large, urban setting with 262 general practices (designated Health Board A); the other covering a mixed urban-rural setting, with 56 practices (Health Board B). For the purposes of this study practies were considered 'semirural' if they were in outlying areas adjacent to suburbs. In April 2012, all practice managers in each Board area were sent written information via e-mail about the proposed study and an invitation for the PM, one GP and a PN to participate. Due to time and resource constraints, a convenience sample of the first 12 GP practices who responded was

constructed: 10 practices from Board A and 2 from Board B.

Data collection
An open-ended interview guide was developed based on a scan of the international patient safety and implementation science literature and from previous experience of the authors. A single, one-to-one interview was conducted in the practice premises of each participant at a time convenient to them, starting in July 2012 until June 2013. As part of the sampling process, the interviews occurred in a fluid manner between the different practices and team members. Prior to the interviews, the reasons for the research were explained to the participants and informed consent was obtained. They were assured that the research team genuinely wanted to understand their perceptions of patient safety and that this would help inform potential improvement initiatives. All interviews were conducted by the same investigator (CdW), who introduced himself as a GP and researcher. Interviews were digitally recorded and supplemented with contemporaneous fieldnotes.

Data analysis
All interviews were transcribed verbatim but were not reviewed by participants. Transcripts were anonymised and the twelve participating practices assigned a unique, double digit identifier. A thematic analysis was undertaken, which allowed the identification of emergent codes and themes. The six stages described by Braun and Clarke were followed, namely: familiarisation with data; generation of initial codes; searching for themes among codes; reviewing themes; defining and naming themes; and producing the final report [18]. The codes and themes were mapped and displayed with NVivo version 9.2.81.0. The number and nature of the themes are described in the results section.

The analysis aimed to be emergent and exploratory and was not intended to identify numeric differences in responses. The data were independently coded by CdW and COD and all authors met regularly to discuss the findings, ensure consistency and agree and verify data interpretations. There were also regular meetings with a research peer who were not directly involved in the study and who did not have a background in direct clinical care. This was considered valuable as these offered perspectives that were not shaped by personal experience of general medical practice.

Results
The demographic data of the participating practices are summarized in Table 1. A total of 34 interviews were held with 11 general practitioners, 12 practice nurses and 11 practice managers. One participant had the dual role of practice nurse and manager and one GP initially agreed to

Table 1 Demographic data of the participating practices

Practice no	Patient list size[a]	GPs (n)		Area	Training practice (Yes/No)
		Partners	Other		
1	2100	1	–	Semi-rural	No
2	4300	3	1 salaried	Urban	Yes
3	3200	1	1 salaried	Urban	No
			1 long-term locum		
4	4100	3	1 Retainer	Urban	Yes
5	11,000	8	–	Semi-rural	Yes
6	5900	4	1 Salaried	Urban	Yes
7	8200	7	–	Urban	Yes
8	6800	3	2 Salaried	Urban	Yes
9	6400	3	1 Salaried	Urban	No
10	9900	6	1 Retainer	Urban	Yes
11	3000	4	1 Retainer	Urban	Yes
12	7500	6	1 Salaried	Urban	Yes

[a]At the time of the interviews, rounded to the nearest hundred

participate but had to withdraw due to personal reasons. Although the final sample size for the study was fixed a priori, analysis eventually stopped identifying new themes and content, indicating that theoretical saturation was achieved.

Perceptions and experiences of 'patient safety'

A few participants were able or attempted to provide a 'working' definition of patient safety, but most felt that a formal definition of this notion had little value for them. However, all were able to articulate what patient safety meant to them in practical terms.

> It's about taking personal and professional responsibility for that patient... not passing the buck, taking responsibility for each patient (PN02)

The themes that emerged were that patient safety is: (i) *important*; (ii) *integral* to care; (iii) characterized by *impermanence*; and (iv) amenable to *improvement efforts*.

Patient safety is important

All participants agreed that patient safety is important; some considered it *the* most important characteristic of care. However, with other equally important priorities competing for limited time and resources, the relative importance of patient safety fluctuated over time.

> [Patient safety] is almost the 'be all and end all'. Whatever you do you have to make sure that patient safety is your highest priority (GP11)

> It's just I suppose for most practices, it's just something else to do in your already crammed up day (PM10)

Circumstances that increased its importance within the practice were after detection and reporting of a significant PSI or as a result of the practice team participating in an improvement programme promoted by the Health Boards.

Patient safety is integral to care

The vast majority of participants felt that patient safety had been an integral part of their practice for many years, even if they had not explicitly acknowledged this. According to them, external agencies had only recently started to show an interest in this area with the result that it was becoming *'fashionable', 'sexy'* (GP04) and a *'buzz word'*. As an example, some of the participants referred to the SPSP that had been launched nationally in 2008 and to local enhanced services being promoted by their NHS Health Boards to illustrate national and regional policy interest in this area.

> We've been doing this same thing under different names for years. It has been going on for years. It's just been called different things (PM04)

Patient safety is characterized by impermanence

The majority of participants understood patient safety as the dynamic and emergent product of many different and variable processes in health care, all in temporal relationships with each other. Many explained the impermanence of safety by referring to patient journeys within health care. They described patient journeys as unpredictable, including a wide range of health care staff with the potential to influence the 'destination', e.g. whether PSIs occurred or safe care was delivered.

> It's a whole kind of journey, and we're involved in so many aspects of it. There's safety in the physical viewing, there's safety in the medical assessment, medical administration and then the ongoing care, and I suppose secondary care. You know, you can talk about the journey into it secondary care as well. (GP07)

Patient safety is imperfect but can be improved

All but one of the participants thought PSIs were the inevitable consequence of complex clinical care provision and even if 'infinite' resources were theoretically available, they could never be completely prevented. Some therefore described the possibility of 'perfect' patient safety as a 'pipedream' or a 'wish'. Despite this, all agreed that this was not an excuse for focusing on PSI prevention or reduction and that much could still be done in this regard. They also unanimously agreed that improving patient safety was an ethical and professional responsibility for everyone working for the NHS. However, according to them, the expectations about the results of these efforts should be tempered by the acknowledgement that clinicians are 'human' and therefore imperfect and prone to err.

> *Total patient safety is [pause] will I say unachievable? I don't think it's ever going to be achievable, but I think there's a lot of things can be done to change things, but I don't think you'll ever get 100% perfect - you've got too many ingredients for that, too many ingredients (PN08)*

Factors perceived as important contributors to PSIs

Participants identified many different factors which they felt contributed to PSIs. These can be summarized in five main groups: (i) chance; (ii) inadequate time and resources to deal with increasing workloads; (iii) lack of care continuity; (iv) patient-related factors; and (v) clinician-related factors.

Chance

Most considered 'chance' or 'luck' to be the most important contributing factor to many PSIs and the resultant harm severity. Consequently, many respondents expressed feeling helpless and unable to prevent these types of PSIs in the future because, as one GP explained, *'if she were to have that same day again, probably the same thing would happen again. It's just a set of circumstances... you might be lucky, you might be unlucky'* (GP02). However, all participants acknowledged that chance was not always implicated, nor the main contributing factor for every PSIs.

Inadequate time and resources to deal with increasing workloads

All of the participants described how they, and the rest of their practice teams, were struggling to safely manage their existing workloads which continued to increase. They responded to the increasing workloads with a range of formal and informal adaptive behaviours, including changing appointment systems, working additional, unpaid hours and choosing to forego breaks and meals. Despite these behaviours, they were aware that potential safety threats still remained and in some instances had even increased. For example, participants reported the potential for inappropriate patient triage, prescriptions being signed without being reviewed and reception staff sometimes offering patients appointments with team members who were not clinically appropriate to their needs. Acceptable and feasible solutions were difficult to implement, as procuring additional time and staff directly

reduced the income and livelihood of the partners and could, in some, instances make the practice non-viable.

> *The pressure that is on practices to churn out patients and churn out facts, figures, returns - it's phenomenal (PM02)*

> *At my lunch break I'm putting information on the computer (PN03)*

Lack of care continuity

Continuity was generally perceived as an important contributing factor to safe care. Conversely, a lack of continuity was perceived to have a negative impact, particularly during care transitions between health care providers and at the interface between different organizations. Many participants were concerned that care continuity was being eroded at a practice level, which they attributed to increasing workloads, patient expectations of same-day consultations and the increasing reliance on locum staff.

> *Sometimes we've had issues over the last few years and I think really it's because people are darting in and out and don't really know what's going on (PM12)*

Patient-related factors

The majority of participants – and especially the practice managers - felt patient expectations and health care needs had increased to the point where it was difficult or impossible to meet these and this now posed a potential threat to effective and efficient care delivery. This feeling was reportedly compounded by some patients who were perceived as not taking at least some responsibility for their own health, patients with significant clinical complexity and the increasing prevalence of multimorbidity in ageing practice populations. The clinicians reported struggling, and often failing, to effectively and safely manage the *'shopping lists'* (PN08) of patients in 10 min consultations. However, while some patients were perceived as demanding, participants acknowledged that the majority of patient requests and expectations were appropriate and that clinicians and practices were responsible for meeting them.

> *I think they [patients] have some real unrealistic expectations of what doctors can and can't do (PM03)*

Clinician-related factors

Participants described a wide range of factors relating to the behavior and attitudes of clinicians that may contribute to but also help to prevent PSIs. In some cases, clinicians were making unintentional assumptions about care, although it was recognized that *'Assumptions aren't good for safety'* (GP02). In other cases, clinicians were making intentional changes that were not part of system recommendations or procedures. Reasons for assumptions and violations included workload, ongoing distractions or competing priorities for time.

The systems are there. People either don't follow the systems or don't have time so try to cut corners with the systems, and that's why things fail (PM07)

One of the more insidious factors that some participants reported contributed to PSIs was the issue of 'personalities' in their teams. Participants used the word 'personality' euphemistically to explain their observations that the specific characteristics of a few clinicians seemingly increased the risk of PSIs occurring in the practice. These characteristics included being 'afraid to ask for help'; lacking insight about their own knowledge and skill deficiencies; and interpersonal relationships and communications skills that made it challenging for others to raise concerns about potential safety threats with them.

[There is] huge variance from practice to practice and I guess it's all about the GPs that you work with (PM08)

Nobody is perfect ever, so you have to be aware of your limitations (PN09)

Existing and potential future improvement actions

Participants described many potential methods and tools that they were aware of or had used to improve patient safety. These included formal and informal interventions and their scope ranged from small changes for a single patient to changing or creating new policies and procedures for the practice. Examples of the different types of improvement actions participants described are provided in Table 2 and illustrated with selected quotes.

When asked to suggest high-priority patient safety areas for future intervention, the majority of participants identified two specific issues. The first issue was medication and medication-related processes. Participants were concerned about the very large volume of repeat prescriptions generated on a daily basis, usually by administrative team members, which were then typically signed without clinical review by GPs. They felt that more, and more thorough, medication reviews would be useful to help prevent PSIs. The second issue was ensuring housebound patients receive high-quality care, with some participants suggesting the creation of nursing roles specifically to care for this group of patients or incentivising practices to provide this service.

Despite recognizing potential areas for improvement, participants unanimously agreed that they had no time, resources or spare capacity to even consider implementing these suggestions, or *any* other new interventions. They also doubted whether any other general practice team could feasibly undertake any additional, unfunded work. Some participants also expressed concern that quality improvement interventions may increase workload and

Table 2 Examples of improvement methods and actions participants already use

Action or method	Selected verbatim quotes
'Formal' actions	
Significant event analysis (SEA)	We do significant events regularly... we will meet to discuss it (PM06)
Clinical audit	We do lots of audits around [access] and check that it's still as good as we think it is, and we occasionally have to tweak the amount of triage (PM08)
Protocols	Over the last few years with being a training practice we have tried to put a lot of protocols and systems in place to protect it (PN05)
CPD, appraisal and revalidation	Individually you are doing the best for the patient that you have and that is your responsibility, so there is a bit about professional development, CPD and maintaining your knowledge and recognising your weaknesses (GP08)
'Formal' and informal actions	
Involving patients	We're calling it 'complaints, comments and compliments' and what we're asking, we'll go out regularly and speak to the patients and say 'how do you feel about how we're doing? Is there anything we can improve on?' How do we know we're completely safe? I think this is maybe a way of us checking are we doing enough (PM02)
Informal actions	
Raising awareness of safety critical issues	People are making others aware of what has happened and that is the way forward and we will just continue to do that, and hopefully we will get better and better at it (PM06)
Sharing information / peer feedback	I think being able to discuss things with my nursing colleague - on a Wednesday I start at one, we have an hour's handover - I find that really useful (PN02)
Mitigation, esp. pharmacists and patients	I think there are lots of sources that stop us from falling short more of the time, to be honest (GP03)

paradoxically decrease patient safety by reducing their time to provide clinical care. One respondent explained that this was why *'it [patient safety initiative] can be seen as hassle for some'* because *'it takes us out from the day to day practice when I have still got other patients and normal work carries on'* (GP06).

Discussion

The study sought to understand the views of general practice staff with respect to patient safety in routine practice. All agreed that patient safety is important and understood it to be an integral part of the care they provide. Participants identified many factors that they felt were important contributors to PSIs, many of which could potentially be detected and mitigated. However, most also felt that a proportion of PSIs are an inevitable consequence of complex care delivery, and therefore not amenable to any intervention. Despite this perception, they unanimously agreed that patient safety can and should be improved. Most participants were aware of and could describe a wide range of strategies that have been used in their practices to improve standards of care. They were also able to recommend specific 'high risk' areas which they felt should be prioritized for safety improvement interventions in the future. However, everyone strongly agreed this would only be feasible if additional resources were provided.

Comparison with existing literature

The contributing factors to PSIs identified in this study are similar to those reported by clinicians in other health care settings or working in different countries. For example, a qualitative study in the USA explored the recollections of family physicians ($n = 53$) of their most memorable errors and the perceived causes through in-depth interviews. Similar to this study, many different possible contributing factors ($n = 34$) were considered, which the authors categorized as: physician stressors and characteristics; process-of-care factors; and patient-related factors [19]. Additionally, a survey of clinicians ($n = 848$) working in outpatient settings in the USA identified many cognitive and system factors considered to be related to diagnostic errors [20].

Inadequate resources, including lack of time, and increasing workloads were not only perceived as important safety threats by the study participants, but were also understood to have a negative impact on the performance and wellbeing of clinicians and staff. This finding is comparable with the international patient safety literature. In a focus-group study of primary care physicians ($n = 32$), lack of resources and time pressures were perceived as particularly important impediments to care quality, with the authors' reporting that inadequate resources *'often force physicians to compromise standards of care'* [21].

Insufficient time to provide all of the necessary care patients require is a well-recognized and important contributing factor to PSIs. A framework identifying specific types of 'time problems' in general practice was recently proposed and include the 'office tempo', which describes and quantifies the amount of time clinicians have available to provide care for patients [22]. All the participants in this study identified this 'tempo' as a particularly important risk factor for PSIs.

The two 'high-risk' areas for PSIs identified as being particularly suitable for future interventions were medication-related processes and housebound patients. These perceptions are similar to those of GPs in the Netherlands who indicated in a web-based survey that prescribing and monitoring of medication and patient age over 75 years were the most important safety risks [23]. These issues have comprehensively been described in the international patient safety literature and are widely recognized as important areas for further research [24].

The prevailing perception in this study that some PSIs are inevitable and cannot be prevented may seem overly pessimistic or even fatalistic to some, depending on their understanding of patient safety. From a 'psychological' perspective PSIs can be explained as the linear cause-and-effect results of individual human error, which in turn can be attributed to finite physiological and psychological resources [25]. Accordingly, *all* health care workers are susceptible to err, the likelihood of error increases as the number of 'demands' on human resources increase, and the frequency and type of errors are largely predictable – and therefore manageable. However, this simplistic explanation fails to acknowledge that human error is a necessary and important mechanism through which we all learn.

An alternative perspective about the contributing factors to PSIs would be that they result from technical and systems failures. These failures can be represented by linear models in which it is possible to identify simple, complex and cascading causes, contributing factors and outcomes [26]. A PSI is explained as the product of a series of events which occur in a specific and (retrospectively) recognizable manner and therefore allows knowledge about the future. The implication is that some PSIs may be prevented by detecting and eliminating potential threats proactively and by designing, incorporating and strengthening health care system defences.

Practical implications

The finding in this study that only a few participants were able to provide a formal definition of patient safety is comparable to the international literature. In a qualitative study of GPs ($n = 22$) and practice nurses ($n = 7$) in the Netherlands, none of the respondents provided a definition of patient safety, although they were able to offer a wide range of descriptions and perceptions of this concept when asked [27]. One implication of this finding is that the way in which researchers and policy makers define patient safety may not have any practical meaning for frontline care staff. In order for improvement interventions to be successfully implemented, it may therefore be necessary to first align the understanding of all stakeholders about patient safety.

The fact that all participants could provide practical examples of how they already use improvement tools and methods could be interpreted as evidence of their willingness to consider other, new interventions. On the other hand, there is a danger that any new intervention may be perceived as 'just' another tool in a toolbox that is already full. However, one of the key findings of this study is that for future interventions to be feasible, additional resources would first have to be provided.

Limitations and strengths
Approximately a third of all Scottish general practices provide GP specialty training for registrars [28], while the majority of practices in this study had training status. This was because of our sampling strategy, which was a pragmatic choice based on the resources available and access to general practices through their association with NHS Education for Scotland. The perceptions of the sample may therefore not be representative of all general practices in Scotland or other countries in the UK. On the other hand, practices were selected from two NHS Health Boards and included training and non-training, small (single practitioner) and larger practices from urban and semi-rural geographical locations.

By its nature, interview data confines analysis to what people report or their perceptions associated with the phenomenon under inquiry. However, interviews were candid, detailed and in-depth, all participants had considerable professional autonomy and the interviews were conducted by a clinical peer. It is therefore unlikely that they offered socially desirable responses. The reflexivity and rigour of the research was increased through data clinics to refine the coding framework. The perceptions and experiences of three different staff groups were explored in order to reflect the multidisciplinary reality of modern general practice. The perceptions of the vast majority of participations were highly congruent despite their different roles. While the sample size was determined beforehand, thematic saturation was achieved and more interviews would not have materially strengthened the main findings.

Conclusion
The perceptions of participants in this study are comparable with the international patient safety literature, namely that patient safety is important, integral to the delivery of care and that there are potential opportunities for improvements in general practice systems and

procedures. However, any further improvements at the level of individual general practices in the UK are contingent on investment of additional resources. The study findings also suggest a need for a more integrative approach to patient safety improvement efforts at a national level, i.e. incorporating components from human factors, systems and resilience engineering.

Acknowledgements
We would like to thank the study participants for their contributions.

Funding
Two of the authors (CdW and PB) were salaried employees of NHS Education for Scotland (NES). NES provided funding for the professional fees that were provided to participating practices and a nVivo licence.

Authors' contributions
The authors jointly designed the study, analysed the data and prepared the manuscript. CdW conducted the interviews. CdW and COD coded the data independently. All authors read and approved the final manuscript.

Authors' information
CdW worked as a general practitioner in the West of Scotland from 2007 to 2014 and was a part time PhD student with Glasgow University from 2011 to 2017. PB and COD both have extensive experience of primary care research and education and were CdW's educational supervisors. CdW's surgery was in Lanarkshire, a health board adjacent to the general practices in this study. He had met a small number of the participants in passing prior to the study while attending different educational events, but there had been no significant previous social or professional interactions.

Competing interests
The authors declare that they have no competing interests.

Author details
[1]Medical Directorate, NHS Education for Scotland, Glasgow, UK. [2]General Practice & Primary Care, Institute of Health & Wellbeing, College of Medical, Veterinary and Life Science, University of Glasgow, Glasgow, Scotland. [3]School of Medicine, Griffith University, Southport, Gold Coast, Australia.

References
1. Panesar SS, deSilva D, Carson-Stevens A, Cresswell KM, Salvilla SA, Slight SP, et al. How safe is primary care? A systematic review. BMJ Qual Saf. 2016;25(7):544–53.
2. Singh H, Schiff GD, Graber ML, Onakpoya I, Thompson MJ. The global burden of diagnostic errors in primary care. BMJ Qual Saf. 2016;26(6):1-11. http://qualitysafety.bmj.com/content/26/6/484.
3. Lorincz CY, Drazen E, Sokol PE, Neerukonda KV, Mezger J, Toepp MC, et al. Research in Ambulatory Patient Safety 2000–2010: A 10-year review. Chicago: American Medical Association (AMA). 2010. p. 1-198. https://c.ymcdn.com/sites/npsf.site-ym.com/resource/resmgr/PDF/Research-in-Amb-Pat-Saf_AMAr.pdf.

4.   Healthcare Improvement Scotland. SPSP Primary Care. Scotland: Healthcare Improvement Scotland; 2016.

5.   Cooper A, Chuter A. Patient safety research in primary care: where are we now? BJGP. 2015;65(641):622–3.

6.   Verstappen W, Gaal S, Esmail A, Wensing M. Patient safety improvement programmes for primary care. Review of a Delphi procedure and pilot studies by the LINNEAUS collaboration on patient safety in primary care. EJGP. 2015;21(sup1):50–5.

7.   Healthcare Improvement Scotland. SPSP Acute Adult - end of phase report. Scotland: Healthcare Improvement Scotland; 2016.

8.   Kirk S, Parker D, Claridge T, Esmail A, Marshall M. Patient safety culture in primary care: developing a theoretical framework for practical use. Qual Saf Health Care. 2007;16(4):313–20.

9.   de Wet C, Spence W, Mash R, Johnson P, Bowie P. The development and psychometric evaluation of a safety climate measure for primary care. Qual Saf Health Care. 2010;19(6):578–84.

10. de Wet C, O'Donnell C, Bowie P. Developing a preliminary 'never event' list for general practice using consensus-building methods. Br J Gen Pract. 2014;64(620):e159–67.

11. Bowie P, McNab D, Ferguson J, de Wet C, Smith G, MacLeod M, et al. Quality improvement and person-centredness: a participatory mixed methods study to develop the 'always event' concept for primary care. BMJ Open. 2015;5(4):e006667.

12. de Wet C, Bowie P. Screening electronic patient records to detect preventable harm: a trigger tool for primary care. Qual Prim Care. 2011;19(2):115–25.

13. de Wet C, Black C, Luty S, McKay J, O'Donnell CA, Bowie P. Implementation of the trigger review method in Scottish general practices: patient safety outcomes and potential for quality improvement. BMJ Qual Saf. 2016;26: 259-60.

14. McKay J, Bradley N, Lough M, Bowie P. A review of significant events analysed in general practice: implications for the quality and safety of patient care. BMC Fam Pract. 2009;10:61.

15. Bowie P, Ferguson J, MacLeod M, Kennedy S, de Wet C, McNab D, et al. Participatory design of a preliminary safety checklist for general practice. Br J Gen Pract. 2015;65(634):e330–43.

16. Allen D, Braithwaite J, Sandall J, Waring J. Towards a sociology of healthcare safety and quality. Sociol Health Illn. 2016;38(2):181–97.

17. Verbakel NJ, de Bont AA, Verheij TJM, Wagner C, Zwart DLM. Improving patient safety culture in general practice: an interview study. BJGP. 2015;65(641):e822.

18. Braun V, Clarke V. Using Thematic Analysis in Psychology; 2006. p. 77–101.

19. Ely JW, Levinson W, Elder NC, Mainous AG 3rd, Vinson DC. Perceived causes of family physicians' errors. J Fam Pract. 1995;40(4):337–44.

20. Sarkar U, Bonacum D, Strull W, Spitzmueller C, Jin N, Lopez A, et al. Challenges of making a diagnosis in the outpatient setting: a multi-site survey of primary care physicians. BMJ Qual Saf. 2012;21(8):641–8.

21. Manwell LB, Williams ES, Babbott S, Rabatin JS, Linzer M. Physician perspectives on quality and error in the outpatient setting. Wisc Med J. 2009;108(3):6.

22. Amalberti R, Brami JJ. 'Tempos' management in primary care: a key factor for classifying adverse events, and improving quality and safety. BMJ Qual Saf. 2011;21:729–36.

23. Gaal S, Verstappen W, Wensing M. Patient safety in primary care: a survey of general practitioners in the Netherlands. BMC Health Serv Res. 2010;10:21.

24. Elliott RA, Putman KD, Franklin M, Annemans L, Verhaeghe N, Eden M, et al. Cost effectiveness of a pharmacist-led information technology intervention for reducing rates of clinically important errors in medicines management in general practices (PINCER). PharmacoEconomics. 2014;32(6):573–90.

25. Parker D. Psychological contribution to the understanding of adverse events in health care. Qual Saf Health Care. 2003;12(6):453–7.

26. Woolf SH. A string of mistakes: the importance of Cascade analysis in describing, counting, and preventing medical errors. Ann Fam Med. 2004;2(4):317–26.

27. Gaal S, van Laarhoven E, Wolters R, Wetzels R, Verstappen W, Wensing M. Patient safety in primary care has many aspects: an interview study in primary care doctors and nurses. J Eval Clin Pract. 2010;16(3):639–43.

28. Mackay D, Watt GC. General Practice size determines participation in optional activities: cross-sectional analysis of a national primary care system. Prim Health Care Res Dev. 2010;11(3):271–9.

4

Expanding the role of clinical pharmacists on interdisciplinary primary care teams for chronic pain and opioid management

Karleen F. Giannitrapani[1*], Peter A. Glassman[2,3], Derek Vang[4], Jeremiah C. McKelvey[5], R. Thomas Day[1], Steven K. Dobscha[6,7] and Karl A. Lorenz[1,8,9]

Abstract

Background: Facilitating appropriate and safe prescribing of opioid medications for chronic pain management in primary care is a pressing public health concern. Interdisciplinary team-based models of primary care are exploring the expansion of clinical pharmacist roles to support disease management for chronic conditions, e.g. pain. Our study aims to 1) identify roles clinical pharmacists can assume in primary care team based chronic pain care processes and 2) understand the barriers to assuming these expanded roles.

Methods: *Setting*: Veterans Health Administration (VA) has implemented an interdisciplinary team-based model for primary care which includes clinical pharmacists. *Design*: We employed an inductive two part qualitative approach including focus groups and semi-structured interviews with key informants. *Participants:* 60 members of VA primary care teams in two states participated in nine preliminary interdisciplinary focus groups where a semi-structured interview guide elucidated provider experiences with screening for and managing chronic pain. To follow up on emergent themes relating to clinical pharmacist roles, an additional 14 primary care providers and clinical pharmacists were interviewed individually. We evaluated focus group and interview transcripts using the method of constant comparison and produced mutually agreed upon themes.

Results: Clinical pharmacists were identified by primary care providers as playing a central role with the ongoing management of opioid therapy including review of the state prescription drug monitoring program, managing laboratory screening, providing medication education, promoting naloxone use, and opioid tapering. Specific barriers to clinical pharmacists role expansion around pain care include: limitations of scopes of practice, insufficient institutional support (low staffing, dedicated time, insufficient training, lack of interdisciplinary leadership support), and challenges and opportunities for disseminating clinical pharmacists' expanded roles.

Conclusions: Expanding the role of the clinical pharmacist to collaborate with providers around primary care based chronic pain management is a promising strategy for improving pain management on an interdisciplinary primary care team. However, expanded roles have to be balanced with competing responsibilities relating to other conditions. Interdisciplinary leadership is needed to facilitate training, resources, adequate staffing, as well as to prepare both clinical pharmacists and the providers they support, about expanded clinical pharmacists' scopes of practice and capabilities.

Keywords: Pain, Pain management, Clinical pharmacists, Team based care, Interdisciplinary teams, Qualitative research

* Correspondence: Karleen@stanford.edu
[1]VA Palo Alto Health Care System, Center for Innovation to Implementation (Ci2i), Menlo Park, CA 94025, USA
Full list of author information is available at the end of the article

Background

Pain is a complex condition impacted by various biological, psychological, and social factors and is usually a high treatment priority for patients seeking care [1, 2]. Due to its complexity, chronic pain can be incredibly difficult to manage. Improving processes of care for chronic pain is a public health priority [3]. This is due to both the high prevalence of chronic pain diagnoses as well as the risks associated with inadequate management [4]. Since a majority of chronic pain is managed in primary care settings, primary care teams are increasingly overburdened by and not fully equipped to manage all of the complex, competing demands of patients with pain [5, 6]. With expanded patient panel sizes (the number of patients assigned to a specific provider) and limited appointment times, clinicians face prioritizing individual demands of specific medical conditions over other patient concerns.

These complex challenges can be particularly problematic in the Veteran's Health Administration (VA) where providers are working with populations that experience high rates of chronic disease, including pain and other comorbid conditions [7]. The VA is the largest integrated health care system in the United Sates. VA cares for over nine million Veterans and is comprised of 170 medical centers and 1063 outpatient clinics [8]. In 2010, the VA implemented an interdisciplinary team-based model of primary care called patient-aligned care teams (PACTs). These teams include primary care providers (PCPs), nurses, and administrative staff, and are supported by other clinicians including licensed clinical pharmacists [9–12]. Expanding roles of clinicians such as advanced practice nurses and clinical pharmacists, to include top of license tasks such as prescribing, is conceptualized as central to improving chronic disease management while minimizing the burden on individual PCPs.

One strategy being explored to support chronic disease management involves embedding clinical pharmacists in primary care to facilitate patient education, supplemental patient interaction, and population management activities [11, 13–16]. Population management comprises reviewing the entire population of patients and proactively identifying risks; risk of inappropriate opioid use for pain management is an important public health concern. Some of the expanded clinical responsibilities a clinical pharmacist can assume around pain care include: ongoing reassessment, monitoring, and management of opioid therapy in conjunction with medication renewal, review of state prescription drug monitoring programs, and medication education. Some clinical pharmacists are specializing in pain management to support teams with complex pain patients, opioid risk management, opioid education, opioid titration, opioid screening, and naloxone distribution [15]. When clinical pharmacists are involved in an interdisciplinary team, clinics have reported a decrease of burden on PCPs and improved patient satisfaction [17].

To inform future implementation efforts we queried all providers involved in primary care based pain management to better understand clinical pharmacists' current and potential roles with pain management. Further, the clinical pharmacists we interviewed included several layers of pharmacy leadership, which helped us explore system level barriers to assuming expanded roles. Existing literature suggests that expanding pharmacist's clinical roles for chronic pain care may minimize adverse effects patients experience and thus improve patient care [18]. Our study aims to 1) identify roles clinical pharmacists can assume in primary care team based chronic pain care processes and 2) understand the barriers to assuming these expanded roles.

Methods

Overview

The data for this qualitative analysis was collected as part of the Effective Screening for Pain (ESP) study, a mixed methods analysis of pain screening, assessment, and management methods [19]. All study procedures were approved by the VA central Institutional Review Board (IRB Project ID 13–08). Under ESP we had multiple waves of primary data collection. Verbal consent to participate and record all focus groups and interviews was obtained at the beginning of each session.

Setting

This study was conducted in the context of the VA. The VA relied on the patient centered medical home model (PCMH) to provide out-patient primary care. The VA's version of PCMH is called patient aligned care teams (PACT). Under PACT, interdisciplinary providers work together to provide continuous, coordinated, high quality care. PACT patients are assigned to a specific interdisciplinary care team (including a primary care provider, registered nurse, licensed practical nurse, and clerk). These small interdisciplinary teams are supported by other providers such as behavioral and mental health providers, social workers, and licensed clinical pharmacists. Clinical pharmacists are those who participate in prescribing, patient education, population management activities, and possibly academic detailing or education to other providers on evidence based prescribing practices.

Wave one data

In wave one, we conducted nine focus groups including a total of 60 providers working on interdisciplinary primary care teams in two large VA Medical Centers in

California and Oregon, as well as associated community based outpatient clinics [20–22]. Interdisciplinary team members invited to participate in the focus groups included PCPs, registered nurses, licensed practical nurses, clerks, psychologists, social workers and clinical pharmacists. Focus groups occurred between 2013 and 2014 and lasted approximately one hour.

Focus group analysis

Trained facilitators used a semi-structured interview guide to elucidate provider experiences with screening, assessment, and management of chronic pain. All focus groups were audio recorded, professionally transcribed, and transcripts were cleaned to remove identifying information. All analyses were conducted using qualitative analytic software ATLAS.ti. [23]. An initial code list was developed and iterated via the dual coding of two transcripts. The final code list was then systematically applied to every transcript. After primary coding, secondary coders reviewed each transcript for inconsistencies. Team meetings fostered consensus for code development and facilitated resolutions for coding discrepancies. ESP investigators evaluated transcribed interviews using the method of constant comparison [24] and produced mutually agreed upon themes. The method of constant comparison continued until we reached theoretical saturation on each theme. Presentation of results to PACT team primary care providers served as a member check and confirmed content validity. Expansion of clinical pharmacist roles emerged as a supportive factor to PACT pain management. As a result of this early finding we conducted further investigation through a second wave of interviews.

Wave two data

The second wave of interviews consisted of individual semi-structured interviews with 14 key participants. The participants included: PCPs (general internists and nurse practitioners) as well as multiple types of clinical pharmacists (primary care, mental health, pain management, and pharmacy leadership). These semi-structured interviews occurred at Portland and Palo Alto in 2016. The interview guild included specific probes about how clinical pharmacists are involved in chronic pain management (see Table 1). Key stakeholders were identified using a snowball sampling approach [25], and we relied heavily on referrals for recruitment. Snowball sampling represented the best method we had to access the clinical pharmacists, as we did not have a master list of people in this role. Through introductions we were able to recruit a meaningful number that we may not have have been able to access via cold calling or emails.

Wave two analysis

Informed by grounded theory [24], investigators [KG and DV] then used an open coding approach on the

Table 1 Focus Group and Interview Guide Questions

Wave One Focus group questions
Who in your opinion is the most appropriate person to screen for pain and why?
Who in your opinion is the most appropriate person to assess pain and why?
Other than the finding that the patient has pain, what information about a patient's pain is most useful to you in:
    a) preparing to assess pain
    b) actually assessing pain
    c) guiding your treatment/management plan for pain
What are the roles of different staff members [PCP, RN, LVN, Clerk, Mental health, Pharmacist etc...] in getting pain information? Assessing pain? Managing pain?

Wave Two Semi-structured interview probes relating to pharmacist role expansion
How are pharmacists involved in primary care chronic pain management currently?
How could their role expand?
What are the barriers to role expansion?
Would they need additional training or licenses?
How does the pharmacist interact with the rest of the team about pain?
For what types of conditions and concerns are they involved?
What is the role of the academic detailer relating to pain medications?
Do you have any thoughts about how we could improve pharmacist directed pain management of 'at risk' Veterans?
What do you think about pharmacists taking on responsibility for monitoring and providing medications to such Veterans?
Do you anticipate any challenges for pharmacists taking on that role?
Are there others on the team who would be better equipped to take it on? Who (Nurses, Social workers, etc.)?

wave two interview transcripts to identify emergent themes. This method was selected to help us divide the textual data into conceptual components. Specifically, through iteration and consensus the entire investigator team reviewed all quotes associated with barriers and characterized emergent themes around barriers to the clinical pharmacists' role expansion. This process continued until theoretical saturation was reached on each barrier. After the interviews were completed, one clinical pharmacist interviewee [JM] joined the investigator team during the analytic phase to provide expert guidance on contextualizing the results.

Results

Respondents included 60 focus group participants in nine focus groups and 14 semi-structured interview respondents. Below we present first the results of the focus groups which explain the roles a clinical pharmacist can - assume, second, we present results from the induvial interviews which cluster into three themes.

Focus group results

The focus groups with different providers revealed substantial support across professions for an enhanced role of clinical pharmacists. PACT providers advocated for pharmacists to assume responsibility in the team process.

"Overall if by the time I saw a patient they had been pre-screened or processed and behind the scenes somebody in pharmacy… had run the CURES reports [CURES: California's Controlled Substance Utilization Review and Evaluation System] and arranged for the interval of tox screens [urine toxicology screening] … [and] were aware of any escalations in terms of early refill-if that information was available… [Then] I didn't have to worry about it, that'd be helpful." [PCP]

Additionally, PCPs felt having the clinical pharmacists involved in refill management for patients on long term opioid therapy may offer a team strategy to minimize the risk of drug abuse.

"If the pharmacy believes that they're not due for them, they will not give it [opioid pain medication] to them. Because you have some patients that they just got the pain medication today, come back the following day…. Because it was lost or they robbed their house. Of all the valuables, it's only the Vicodin that was stolen? It's very common… Our pharmacy department, they are very smart, too. So they tell them [patient], "Okay. Then come back every week." And if they lose it again, "Then come back every day." Instead of giving them the whole supply." [PCP]

PCPs also described including clinical pharmacists on the team as particularly useful for reconciling prescriptions from providers in multiple departments. In cases where acute pain, dental pain for example, combines with chronic pain, clinical pharmacist involvement can prevent patients exhibiting drug seeking behavior from accessing inappropriate quantities of opioid medications.

"We've recently had a patient— complaining he was in pain. But the first thing he said was, "I'm not a drug addict, I have a family of four, I'm gainfully employed, I go to school," … he was placed on Tramadol… He took the Tramadol [home]… He came back a week later; he [should] still have more Tramadol, [but] claimed he hadn't used it. He said he had a [new] dental problem, went up to Dental, requested something stronger. He had an extraction; he was ordered Tylenol #3. He took that, but he had gotten the Vicodin the three days before… he came back … Requesting more Vicodin. He also went to the pharmacist, and the pharmacist said, "You can't get it. It's not due." [PCP]

PCPs also highlighted the valuable contribution clinical pharmacist run clinics make in coordinating care with pain and substance abuse specialists.

"For the chronic pain patients… they [clinical pharmacists] have the chronic or renewal clinics for pain medications and they actually do the assessments there… those clinics are pharmacist run, but they work very closely with both the actual pain clinic and the substance abuse clinics." [PCP]

"So if the substance abuser has issues, they can actually go easily right into the pain clinic and if a pain clinic patient has a problem they go right easily into the substance treatment program and then the [clinical pharmacist run] renewal clinic does a lot of monitoring-they monitor the tox screens, they monitor the CURES reports, they monitor the pain levels if something needs to be adjusted." [PCP]

Interview results

Three core themes were identified: limitations of scopes of practice, insufficient institutional support, and challenges and opportunities for disseminating clinical pharmacists' expanded roles. The quotes we present below come from the clinical pharmacist interviews and these themes were also present in the PCP interviews.

Theme 1: Limitations of scopes of practice
1.1 Including pain management in a scope of practice
Some clinical pharmacists do not have a local scope of practice for pain management.

"Currently my scope is only for the disease states I mentioned earlier [diabetes, dyslipidemia, hypertension or poly-pharmacy] and I don't have a scope for pain." [Clinical Pharmacist]

"We've tried to get some of the PACT pharmacists to help [with checking CURES report]; but, like I said, that pushback -not written within our scope- has been there." [Pharmacy Leadership]

Variation in scopes of practice relating to prescribing
Some clinical pharmacists were not scoped to prescribe controlled substances.

"We [clinical pharmacists] can't order the [controlled] medications. It just seems like something that would be kind of [helpful] in terms of time-wise and provider-wise" [Clinical Pharmacist]

In some states clinical pharmacists can prescribe controlled substances, but providers may be unaware of clinical pharmacists' scopes of practices.

I met with a new provider the other day for addiction treatment services and was explaining my role as a pharmacist, and a lot of them just aren't even sure that we have scopes of practice, that we actually see patients and prescribe. [Clinical Pharmacist]

Theme 2: Insufficient institutional support
Low staffing
Staffing levels pose a challenge for clinical pharmacists who wish to spend time doing additional training for having pain in their scope of practice.

"Another problem is... the staffing... in order to take on additional training, then I would have to be taken away from my responsibilities in order to get the hours in to get the scope [to work on pain]." [Clinical Pharmacist]

Insufficient local staffing may limit the time a clinical pharmacist has to address both chronic disease and opioid management.

"I don't think we have the manpower to...deal with the chronic diseases—diabetes, hypertension, and lipids—and also troubleshoot the [opioid] medication. So don't have much time to deal with this pain thing." [Clinical Pharmacist]

Dedicated time
Clinical pharmacists consistently reported that lack of time was a barrier to taking on additional tasks such as managing pain medication and reporting.

"For CURES [reporting] I don't think that would be the lack of training [to take on that work]. I think that's just maybe the time. They say that there's a time limitation." [Clinical Pharmacist]

Clinical pharmacists identified that given their limited time, they would benefit from guidance around where their support would be best directed.

"We know that when it comes to coag [anticoagulation] management and lipid management that they're [PACT clinical pharmacists] not needed as much as they were, so there is time freeing up...what other disease states does the health care system want them to help with, whether it's heart failure, COPD, pain. Where does pain...fall in that?" [Clinical Pharmacist]

Some clinical pharmacists report that managing an assortment of medical conditions can make it difficult to become more involved with pain care.

"Right now we are responsible for... the anticoag portion... It's not something that I could just defer [to work on pain]... now we decentralized anticoagulation, so I'll just follow all the Warfarin patients who belong to my providers... it's a little bit difficult because... I try to schedule it as best as I can, but you just can't really control when patients come in or when new patients go to the ER with a new blood clot. We do have set clinic hours for pharm care, like, when we do see diabetics but, other than that, I just have to fill in all my anticoags whenever I can." [Clinical Pharmacist]

Insufficient training
Some clinical pharmacists reported that they did not think their experiences and skills were adequate to work with pain management.

"There's not much courses or a lecture on pain management...also, I don't have that much experience [with pain] in terms of clinic to kind of learn from my experience." [Clinical Pharmacist]

Clinical Pharmacists also reported limited training opportunities in pain management.

"I [clinical pharmacist with pain specialty training] would assume it's [pain management] beyond what their [PACT clinical pharmacists] current training is and that they would need education." [Clinical Pharmacist]

Lack of interdisciplinary leadership support
Support from leadership can facilitate implementing interdisciplinary team-based approaches to pain management.

"It's been several things... Great leadership. So our associate chief of primary care, as well as our nursing leadership and myself [clinical pharmacist] and primary care behavioral health, there's four of us that get together. We put education together and we go on the road and we meet with everybody on a regular basis, and we just start piecing things together and we would identify who on the teams could help." [Clinical Pharmacist]

Theme 3: Challenges and opportunities for disseminating clinical pharmacists' expanded roles
Perceived capabilities
Clinical pharmacists believe some PCPs may have limited awareness of their capabilities.

"I had stated at a meeting that we were piloting this program and then I had sent out an email, but it still

seemed like the providers weren't familiar with what we [clinical pharmacists] could do and what our involvement could be, so I guess that dissemination of education to the providers about what we could do [would be helpful]." [Clinical Pharmacist]

Clinical pharmacists believe some PCPs do not know what clinical pharmacists can take on and have preconceived ideas as to what their roles are and can be.

"I met with a new provider the other day for addiction treatment services and was explaining my role as a pharmacist, and a lot of them just aren't even sure that we have scopes of practice, that we actually see patients and prescribe. I think a lot of providers might still be stuck in the idea that we're still behind the counter in the pharmacy, actually dispensing the medications. So yeah, maybe more clarity on the different types of pharmacists and their actual roles and how we can collaborate together." [Clinical Pharmacist]

Self-advocate

Clinical pharmacists may have to self-advocate and remind PCPs of their capabilities.

" I've met with the majority of them [PCPs] in either staff meetings or one-on-one, and I've provided them with my contact information so whether it's Instant Messaging, GUI, Outlook or calling me. Some of them attach me on a note, but I pretty much always try to say, "If you have any issues," and even because I'm not a pain specialist, that's not my area of expertise, but I try to resolve whatever barrier and seeing how can I assist? That's just me kind of putting my face out there and trying to let them know that this resource is available." [Clinical Pharmacist]

Promoting awareness of the referral process

Clinical pharmacists highlight the need to make PCPs aware of the referral process to involve clinical pharmacists for pain medication management.

"Making sure that they're [PCPs] aware of the referral process to either have the pharmacist completes an e-consult or a chart review with recommendations or they can even refer patients to physically see the pain pharmacist in clinic." [Clinical Pharmacist]

Discussion

The implementation of expanded roles for clinical pharmacists offers a central strategy to addressing the expanding need for primary care provision in the context of an impending physician workforce shortage. On the other hand, role expansions are complex undertakings. They require dedicated resources, training, and leadership support to successfully transition the roles of clinical pharmacists and surrounding PCPs with whom they share care for complex patients. The PCMH model highlights the ideal of "sharing the care" [26]. Explicitly "sharing the care" for chronic pain patients with embedded clinical pharmacists may ultimately improve patient satisfaction with care and outcomes while reducing PCP burnout associated with being alone in dealing with complex patient concerns.

In this qualitative study we set out to characterize interdisciplinary provider perspectives of how clinical pharmacists have several opportunities to fulfill enhanced roles in relation to chronic pain management in interdisciplinary primary care teams. We enumerate multiple barriers clinical pharmacists face. The strategies that may address emergent barriers included expanding primary care clinical pharmacist training so that they had a better understanding of pain as well as ensuring the team had access to a clinical pharmacist with pain expertise. Both PCPs and clinical pharmacists alike indicated the importance of having a pain trained clinical pharmacist, other providers could consult.

Given how quickly clinical pharmacy practice is evolving, it is not surprising that clinical pharmacists experience a number of barriers to expanding roles around chronic pain care. To understand pharmacist role expansion it is important to consider the historical distinctions between medicine and pharmacy practices. Our results indicate it is crucial to prepare for educating physicians about potential top of license tasks for clinical pharmacists as these may challenge current pre-conceived understandings of clinical pharmacist capabilities [27]. The barriers we identify in this study, namely low external awareness of clinical pharmacist capabilities, capacity, and prescribing authority, echo findings in other current studies [28, 29]. To overcome low awareness, interdisciplinary dialogue about clinical pharmacist roles is essential.

A central tenant of implementation science is the belief that if we understand and characterize individual barriers, we can develop targeted implementation strategies to address them [30]. In addition to training, resources, and staffing which indicate health system level strategies, the issue of how best to prioritize PCP and clinical pharmacist time for addressing chronic pain requires further consideration. Additionally, decentralization of care for some conditions (e.g. all clinical pharmacists cover a few anticoagulation patients each) versus use of clinical pharmacist dedicated clinic time for a specific condition (e.g. pain) can cause tension around clinical pharmacists' workload distribution.

What we learned from the provider focus groups is pain is a condition where having multiple diverse providers involved can add value, particularly in regard to patient safety and monitoring activities. Known mitigation strategies of opioid overuse include regular monitoring and reassessment to provide opportunities to minimize risks. Periodic reassessment allows the opportunity for tapering or discontinuing opioids [3]. Our providers indicated that clinical pharmacists can clearly play a key role in this monitoring process. In addition to having technical expertise, clinical pharmacists added value to the team by giving PCPs a way to say no about prescribing high doses to patients. Simply having someone available representing the hospital policies or guidance on safe prescribing, was supportive to primary care providers trying to navigate difficult conversations with drug seeking patients.

Additional strategies that have been called for to reduce inappropriate opioid prescribing include updated protocols and clinical guidelines [31]. In many states clinical pharmacists can prescribe controlled substances and could take on the role of prescribing per protocol. Clinical pharmacist led, academic detailing campaigns have been demonstrated to reduce high-dose opioid prescribing [32]. Clinical pharmacists scoped to deal with pain may also have the ability to support patients through tapering and medication changes.

At present, few medical schools offer sufficient training on addiction and pain management [33]. Consequently, the average PCP may be underequipped to deal with substance seeking patients with pain in primary care. This is of concern as much of the prescribing for chronic pain is occurring in primary care [5]. Having clinical pharmacists on the interdisciplinary team to help navigate complex situations and minimize risk of addiction in chronic pain patients, could represent part of a solution.

Our findings should be considered in the context of the following limitations. First our study was conducted within the VA health care system alone. The VA, however, while not generalizable to other settings does have a population with a high prevalence of pain and an extensive history of addressing chronic pain in the primary care setting [34]. This makes the VA a strong setting in which to investigate pain practice processes. Secondly, this study represents the sub analysis of a greater study meaning that all of the methods are not specifically tailored for this inquiry. For example, the initial focus group data was collected for broader purposes. We do, however, think that the benefits of hypothesis generation (i.e. exploring the role of clinical pharmacists) outweigh the limitations of being unable to identify what specific team members were included. Third, although we conducted a limited number of focus groups, sites varied by

location (rural, suburban, and urban), academic status, and size, allowing us to describe the perspectives of providers based in multiple environments. Another major limitation is that fundamentally, we do not know the exact roles of participants in the focus groups. We sought participation from all members of interdisciplinary pact teams, including clinical pharmacists, but do not know if clinical pharmacists were among those who participated. This approach was supported by the IRB. We were able to encourage broad participation of the PACT team members, allowing them to be honest and critical, because we did not collect any information on who they were.

Due to this ambiguity in the focus groups, one of the main reasons we conducted wave two of interviews was to explicitly capture the perspectives of clinical pharmacists on emergent themes. We interviewed providers as well and their comments confirm the perspectives of the clinical pharmacists. We chose to include only clinical pharmacists' quotes in the wave two results section of the paper because they were the most descriptive. Though our sample of clinical pharmacists is relatively small, it represents the majority of clinical pharmacists at a single VA region as well as additional clinical pharmacists from a second geographic region. We would also note that in this study, we do not capture the perspectives of patients; this can be an important focus of future work.

The two potential sources of bias that may impact our results are that we included an interviewee as an author and that we employed a snowball sampling approach to identify clinical pharmacists. We invited a pharmasist investigator [JM] to participate on the manuscript after data collection was completed and after initial thematic analysis was drawn on the results. We chose to do this after collecting the data when it became apparent that we needed a clinical pharmacist expert to comment on our results with full depth of understanding. Further, we appreciate that snowball sampling has some inherent limitations in that it may attract like-minded individuals. However, it is the best method we had to access the clinical pharmacists. We did not have a master list of people in this role, so we requested introductions. Through this, we were able to recruit a meaningful number that we may not have gotten via cold calling or emails.

Conclusions

These findings indicate that both providers and clinical pharmacists see an importance to expand clinical pharmacist roles in supporting management of complex pain patients. The potential benefits include reduced burdens on physicians and better guideline concordant opioid based pain care. Implementation barriers to their role expansion are not insignificant, but with appropriate targeted strategies, can be addressed. Roles and scopes of practice need to be clarified in advance. Primary care providers who work with clinical pharmacists need to then be made aware of clinical pharmacist scopes and capabilities. Interdisciplinary collaboration and communication between the medicine and pharmacy services will be essential to successful clinical pharmacist role expansion and shared team prioritization.

Acknowledgements
We would like to thank Hannah Schreibeis-Baum for her coordination of the focus groups and Matt McCaa for coordination of semi-structured interviews. We are grateful to Nancy Plath MD for reviewing findings and to the other members of the Effective Screening for Pain team including Agnes Jenson, Holly Williams, and Jesse Holliday for research support. Erin Krebs MD, Robert Kerns PhD, and Sangeeta Ahluwalia PhD should be acknowledged as other investigators on the greater team. We appreciate M. Shawn McFarland, Pharm.D., FCCP, BCACP and Terri Jorgenson, RPH, BCPS, for reviewing drafts of the manuscript. We would like to thank Natalie Lo and Raziel Gamboa for their help with manuscript preparation. Finally, we want to and thank all the primary care clinicians and staff who agreed to participates in our focus groups and interviews.

Funding
This analysis was funded through the VA CREATE program: VA HSR&D CRE 13–020.

Author's contributions
KG and KL designed the study. KG, SD, and KL designed the semi-structured interview guide and data collection process. DV and RTD served as the primary coders on the interview transcripts. KG, PG, and JM reviewed output and produced an initial draft of themes. KG and DV produced a draft of the manuscript with critical revisions from PG, SD, and KL. JM reviewed the findings and contributed expertise from the clinical pharmacist perspective including an understanding of the relevant literature. All authors read and approved the final version of the manuscript.

Competing interests
The authors declare that they have no competing interests.

Author details
[1]VA Palo Alto Health Care System, Center for Innovation to Implementation (Ci2i), Menlo Park, CA 94025, USA. [2]VA Greater Los Angeles Health Care System, Center for the Study of Healthcare Innovation, Implementation, and Policy (CSHIIP), Los Angeles, CA 90073, USA. [3]David Geffen School of Medicine, University of California, Los Angeles, 10945 Le Conte Ave, Los Angeles, CA 90024, USA. [4]VA Minneapolis Center for Chronic Disease Outcomes Research (CCDOR), 5445 Minnehaha Avenue South, Minneapolis, MN 55417, USA. [5]VA Northern California Health Care System, 10535 Hospital Way, Mather, CA 95655, USA. [6]VA Portland Health Care System, Center to Improve Veteran Involvement in Care (CIVIC), 3710 SW US Veterans Hospital Rd, Portland, OR 97239, USA. [7]Department of Psychiatry, Oregon Health and Science University, 3181 SW Sam Jackson Park RD, Portland, OR 97239, USA. [8]Stanford Medical School, Palo Alto, CA 94305, USA. [9]RAND Corporation, 1776 Main Street, Santa Monica, CA 90401, USA.

References
1. Melzack R, Wall PD. Pain mechanisms: a new theory. Science. 1965; 150(3699):971–9.
2. Goldberg DS, McGee SJ. Pain as a global public health priority. BMC Public Health. 2011;11:770.
3. Dowell D, Haegerich TM, Chou R. CDC guideline for prescribing opioids for chronic pain—United States, 2016. JAMA. 2016;315:1624.
4. Brennan F, Carr DB, Cousins M. Pain management: a fundamental human right. Anesth Analg. 2007;105(1):205–21.
5. Lasser KE, Shanahan C, Parker V, Beers D, Xuan Z, Heymann O, et al. A multicomponent intervention to improve primary care provider adherence to chronic opioid therapy guidelines and reduce opioid misuse: a cluster randomized controlled trial protocol. J Subst Abus Treat. 2016;60:101–9.
6. Upshur CC, Bacigalupe G, Luckmann R. "They don't want anything to do with you": patient views of primary care management of chronic pain. Pain Med. 2010;11(12):1791–8.
7. Richardson LM, Hill JN, Smith BM, Bauer E, Weaver FM, Gordon HS, et al. Patient prioritization of comorbid chronic conditions in the veteran population: implications for patient-centered care. SAGE Open Medicine. 2016;4:2050312116680945.
8. Veterans Health Administration. About VHA. U.S. Washington DC: Department of Veterans Affairs; 2018. https://www.va.gov/health/aboutVHA.asp. Accessed 2 Feb 2018.
9. Reiss-Brennan B, Brunisholz KD, Dredge C, Briot P, Grazier K, Wilcox A, et al. Association of integrated team-based care with health care quality, utilization, and cost. JAMA. 2016;316(8):826–34.
10. Dobscha SK, Corson K, Perrin NA, Hanson GC, Leibowitz RQ, Doak MN, et al. Collaborative care for chronic pain in primary care: a cluster randomized trial. JAMA. 2009;301(12):1242–52.
11. VHA Patient Aligned Care Team (PACT). Handbook. Washington, DC: Affairs V; 2014.
12. VHA Directive 1139: Palliative Care Consult Teams (PCCT) and VISN Leads. Washington DC: Department of Veterans Affairs; 2017.
13. DeBar LL, Kindler L, Keefe FJ, Green CA, Smith DH, Deyo RA, et al. A primary care-based interdisciplinary team approach to the treatment of chronic pain utilizing a pragmatic clinical trials framework. Translational behavioral medicine. 2012;2(4):523–30.
14. Atkinson J, de Paepe K, Sánchez Pozo A, Rekkas D, Volmer D, Hirvonen J, et al. What is a pharmacist: opinions of pharmacy department academics and community pharmacists on competences required for pharmacy practice. Pharmacy. 2016;4(1):12.
15. VHA. Handbook 1108.11: Clinical Pharmacy Services; 2017.
16. VHA. Directive 2009–053: Pain Management; 2009.
17. Rapoport A, Akbik H. Pharmacist-managed pain clinic at a veterans affairs medical center. Am J Health Syst Pharm. 2004;61(13):1341–3.
18. Jouini G, Choinière M, Martin E, Perreault S, Berbiche D, Lussier D, et al. Pharmacotherapeutic management of chronic noncancer pain in primary care: lessons for pharmacists. J Pain Res. 2014;7:163–73.
19. Effective Screening for Pain Study. Clinicaltrials.gov. 2013; Identifier: NCT01816763.
20. Giannitrapani K, Ahluwalia S, McCaa M, Pisciotta M, Dobscha S, Lorenz K. Barriers to using nonpharmacologic approaches and reducing opioid use in primary care. Pain Med. 2017. [Epub ahead of print].
21. Giannitrapani KF, Ahluwalia SC, Day RT, Pisciotta M, Dobscha S, Lorenz K. Challenges to teaming for pain in primary care. Healthcare. 2018;6:23–7.
22. Ahluwalia SC, Giannitrapani KF, Dobscha SK, Cromer R, Lorenz KA. "It Encourages Them to Complain": a qualitative study of the unintended consequences of assessing patient-reported pain. J Pain. 2018;19:562–8.
23. ATLAS.ti Scientific Software Development GmbH, Berlin, Version 7.1.0.
24. Glaser BJ, Strauss AL. The discovery of grounded theory: strategies for qualitative research. NY: Adeline Publishing Company; 1967.
25. Bernard HR. Research methods in anthropology: qualitative and quantitative methods. Walnut Creek, CA: AltaMira Press; 2002.

26. Ghorob A, Bodenheimer T. Share the care: building teams in primary care practices. J Am Board Fam Med. 2012;25(2):143–5.
27. Smith M, Bates DW, Bodenheimer T, Cleary PD. Why pharmacists belong in the medical home. Health Aff. 2010;29(5):906–13.
28. Cox N, Tak CR, Cochella SE, Leishman E, Gunning K. Impact of pharmacist previsit input to providers on chronic opioid prescribing safety. J Am Board Fam Med. 2018;31:105–12.
29. Jacobs SC, San EK, Tat C, Chiao P, Dulay M, Ludwig A. Implementing an opioid risk assessment telephone clinic: outcomes from a pharmacist-led initiative in a large veterans health administration primary care clinic, December 15, 2014-march 31, 2015. Subst Abus. 2016;37(1):15–9.
30. Bauer MS, Damschroder L, Hagedorn H, Smith J, Kilbourne AM. An introduction to implementation science for the non-specialist. BMC Psychology. 2015;3(1):32.
31. Haegerich TM, Paulozzi LJ, Manns BJ, Jones CM. What we know, and don't know, about the impact of state policy and systems-level interventions on prescription drug overdose. Drug Alcohol Depend. 2014;145:34–47.
32. Kattan JA, Tuazon E, Paone D, Dowell D, Vo L, Starrels JL, et al. Public health detailing—a successful strategy to promote judicious opioid analgesic prescribing. Am J Public Health. 2016;106(8):1430–8.
33. Volkow ND, Koob GF, McLellan AT. Neurobiologic advances from the brain disease model of addiction. N Engl J Med. 2016;374(4):363–71.
34. Mitchinson AR, Kerr EA, Krein SL. Management of chronic noncancer pain by VA primary care providers: when is pain control a priority? Am J Manag Care. 2008;14(2):77–84.

5

Optimising treatment in opioid dependency in primary care: results from a national key stakeholder and expert focus group

Marie Claire Van Hout[1,2]* ⓘ, Des Crowley[2], Aoife McBride[2] and Ide Delargy[2]

Abstract

Background: Treatment for opioid dependence in Ireland is provided predominantly by general practitioners (GP) who have undergone additional training in opioid agonist treatment (OAT) and substance misuse. The National Methadone Treatment Programme (MTP) was introduced in 1998, and was designed to treat the opioid dependent population and to regulate the prescribing regimes at the time. The past two decades have seen the increased prescribing of methadone in primary care and changes in type of opioid abused, in particular, the increased use of over the counter (OTC) and prescription medications. Despite the scaling up of OAT in Ireland, drug related deaths however have increased and waiting lists for treatment exist in some areas outside the capital, Dublin. Two previous MTP reviews have made recommendations aimed at improving and scaling up of OAT in Ireland. This study updates these recommendations and is the first time that a group of national experts have engaged in structured research to identify barriers to OAT delivery in Ireland. The aim was to explore the views of national statutory and non-statutory stakeholders and experts on current barriers within the MTP and broader OAT delivery structures in order to inform their future design and implementation.

Methods: A single focus group with a chosen group of national key stakeholders and experts with a broad range of expertise (clinical, addiction and social inclusion management, harm reduction, homelessness, specialist GPs, academics) (*n* = 11) was conducted. The group included national representation from the areas of drug treatment delivery, service design, policy and practice in Ireland.

Results: Four themes emerged from the narrative analysis, and centred on *OAT Choices and Patient Characteristics; Systemic Barriers to Optimal OAT Service Provision; GP Training and Registration in the MTP,* and *Solutions and Models of Good Practice: Using What You Have.*

Conclusion: The study identified a series of improvement strategies which could reduce barriers to access and the stigma associated with OAT, optimise therapeutic choices, enhance interagency care planning within the MTP, utilise the strengths of community pharmacy and nurse prescribers, and recruit and support methadone prescribing GPs in Ireland.

Keywords: Opioid dependence, Opioid agonist treatment (OAT), Methadone treatment Programme, General practitioner (GP), Ireland

* Correspondence: m.c.vanhout@ljmu.ac.uk; marieclaire.vanhout@icgp.ie
[1]Public Health Institute, Liverpool John Moore's University, Liverpool, UK
[2]Substance Misuse Programme, Irish College of General Practitioners, Dublin, Ireland

Background

Opioid dependence is a chronic, relapsing disorder with permanent metabolic deficiency [1], and characteristically complex in terms of patient care, pharmacological, psycho-social and relapse prevention modalities, and treatment outcomes [2, 3]. Ireland currently provides opioid agonist treatment (OAT) to those suffering from opioid dependence within a model of care which acknowledges the central role of the specialist trained general practitioner (GP) in primary care. In Ireland OAT is commenced by suitably trained specialist (GPs) in either addiction clinics or general practice settings (Level 2 GP). Once the patient is stabilised on OAT, referral to Level 1 GPs working in the community for on-going management can occur. Recent studies in 2013 and 2016 indicate a generally positive attitude of prescribing GPs toward methadone treatment. This was also underpinned by their belief that primary care prescribing of methadone is an essential service to drug users in the community, and one that supports a good relationship between the patient and GP [4, 5]. Prescribing GPs work closely with both statutory (funded and operated by the Health Services Executive, HSE) and non-statutory (part funded by the HSE through a service level agreement, SLA) organisations to optimise OAT delivery. Many of the non-statutory groups provide support and advocacy groups and a number of the larger agencies provide residential detoxification facilities. A number of the non-statutory agencies have a national brief and have been pivotal in the expansion of harm reduction and OAT in Ireland. These groups have also advocated for the decriminalisation of drug use along with the setting up of drug consumption rooms. They play a key role in drug policy and advocate for prompt and easy access to OAT.

In terms of OAT pharmacological options, substitution treatment using methadone is the most common formulation, with buprenorphine-naloxone currently available on a limited named patient basis only. Methadone has been available in Ireland since 1992, and was initially restricted in availability to the capital, Dublin. The 'Report of the Expert Group on the Establishment of a Protocol for the Prescribing of Methadone' was conducted in 1993. In 1998, the 'Misuse of Drugs (Supervision of Prescription and Supply of Methadone) Regulations' was set up and has since stipulated regulatory structures for treating opioid dependent patients using methadone. The Methadone Treatment Programme (MTP) protocol designed in 1998 guides OAT treatment delivery in primary care, in terms of protocols for methadone prescribing, guidelines and standards for patient management and care, specialist training requirements for GPs, and protocols for clinical audit [6]. Several reviews of the MTP have been conducted, both internally in 2005 by the 'Methadone Prescribing Implementation Committee' itself and externally in 2010 [7]. These reviews recommended improved prescribing and quality of practice in both community and primary care, in order to optimise treatment reach and access across the country, and with support from inter-agency referral pathways. All patients on methadone are listed on the confidential Central Treatment List (CTL) with each patient linked to one specific prescriber and a single dispensing site.

The Irish College of General Practitioners (ICGP) provides the specialist addiction training for GPs who prescribe OAT and plays a central role in the provision and auditing of the MTP. Training consists of an on-line training module in order to qualify for a Level 1 contract. A longer course consisting of workshops, on-line modules and a practice improvement project is required to obtain a Level 2 GP contract. Both Level 1 and Level 2 contracts attract additional remuneration for GPs looking after patients on OAT and ongoing audit of patient care is an essential requirement for maintenance of the contract. Since 1998, the number of prescribing GPs has risen steadily each year and there are currently (mid 2017), a total of 345 Level 1 GPs and 57 Level 2 GPs providing OAT treatment in primary care.

Since the introduction of the MTP greater prescribing of methadone in primary care is observed (Central Treatment List). As mentioned, during the early years of the MTP, heroin use and treatment were mainly confined to the capital, Dublin. In more recent times, the opioid misuse problem has spread to outside the capital, and regional OAT structures have struggled to meet the demand resulting in waiting lists in areas outside of Dublin. There have also been increasing drug related deaths and changes in the type of opioid abused (over the counter and prescription medications). Given that GPs currently provide the clear majority of OAT in Ireland across a variety of settings, the ICGP conducted a focus group study to investigate national stakeholder views around current provision of the MTP, barriers experienced and perspectives around how to improve its design and implementation in Ireland.

Methods
Aim

The aim was to explore the views of national statutory and non-statutory stakeholders and experts on current barriers within the MTP and broader OAT framework in order to inform their future design and implementation.

Approach

A qualitative study using a single focus group with a purposive sample of national key stakeholders and experts, with a broad range of expertise (clinical, addiction and social inclusion management, harm reduction, homelessness, specialist GPs, academics) was conducted. The research team selected participants to ensure national representation. Seven of the eleven experts have a national brief to their roles and oversee OAT design and implementation across the entire country. Eight of the eleven participants participate at a national level in drug related policy. The participants were also selected to ensure that non-statutory agencies were adequately represented and that these groups had a national brief (*n* = 3). The focus group was conducted in Dublin to facilitate the largest number of participants but teleconferencing facilities were made available to those unable to travel (*n* = 3). A focus group guide using four broad questions (see Additional file 1) was designed by the team, which consisted of the Director and Assistant Director of the Substance Misuse Programme (SMP) at the ICGP, the Clinical Audit Facilitator (CAF), who is also an academic, and the administrator of the SMP. The guide explored the identification of patient, system and clinical barriers and enablers to accessing and engaging with OAT, immediate and long term solutions to enhancing OAT provisions in the community, and models of good practice and lessons learnt which could be shared nationally and incorporated into the revised MTP.

Ethical and study procedure

Ethical approval was granted by the ICGP. Chosen stakeholders were sent an email with information around the focus group aims and objectives, procedures around anonymity and voluntary withdrawal assurances, and with an invitation to attend the focus group. The focus group took place at the ICGP premises in the Irish capital, Dublin. For non-attenders (*n* = 2) teleconferencing facilities were made available All participants signed a consent form permitting audio-recording. The focus group was facilitated jointly by author one and author four. Following the focus group, the audio recording was transcribed and destroyed. All data in the transcript was anonymised.

Data analysis

A content analysis of the data was undertaken by author one and two, which involved open, axial and selective coding resulting in the generation of listing of key concepts, ideas, words and phrases, formulating main and sub categories, and generating overarching themes.

Results

Both statutory (ST) and non-statutory agencies (NST) with a gender balance were represented (*n* = 11). Six males and five females participated in the focus group, with four specialist GPs, four ST (funded and operated by the HSE) and three NST stakeholders (part funded by the HSE through an SLA) represented. Four themes emerged from the analysis of narratives, and are presented here with illustrative quotes.

OAT choices and patient characteristics

Initial discussions centred on the stigma toward OAT in Ireland, and the general public and drug users' negative attitude towards it. Comments were made around the lack of choice in OAT in Ireland, with methadone available nationally for the majority of patients and buprenorphine-naloxone (trade name Suboxone) restricted to specific patient cohorts. In contrast to the stigma attached to methadone, patients appeared to have more favourable attitudes with regard to Suboxone, which is seen as a medical treatment.

'We need to have Buprenorphine available through the pharmacies nationally and not to prohibit its use.' [SpGP1]

Additional changing patterns in opioid drug abuse were observed by the group, with a shift toward increased dependence on prescription and over the counter opioid based analgesics. These changing OAT patient characteristics in terms of those with presenting with prescription and OTC opioid abuse (as opposed to heroin), and the difficulties for such patients given the stigma and location in accessing mainstream addiction clinics which generally treat heroin addiction were discussed and central to the requirement to expand choice in OAT.

'Patterns are changing, over the counter painkillers, reduction in heroin users but our models of treatment haven't changed accordingly.' [SpGP1]

Concerns were voiced around issue of OAT patient co-dependence on other substances generally alcohol, and benzodiazepines and Z-hypnotics, both prescribed and sourced on the street. Participants described difficulties in management of these poly dependencies. National assessment, referral and detoxification pathways for benzodiazepine and Z-hypnotic drug abuse and dependence were described as lacking. Efforts to manage the problem centred on some service providers refusing to prescribe these drugs to their methadone patients. Patients were described as circumventing this by accessing a GP other than their methadone prescriber.

'One of the things that puts GPs off even though it is not directly related to methadone it's a whole big mess of benzo and tablet problems.' [SpGP3]

Behavioural issues due to poly substance intoxication was also viewed as problematic for primary care and community pharmacy staff who dispense methadone, and at times requiring security measures.

'There is a problem particularly for pharmacies as well as GPs...pharmacies are a business and they can't afford to have someone coming in and causing chaos in a pharmacy'[SpGP2]

Some problems are evident with regard to all female GP practices and the supervision of drug screening for male methadone patients.

'We have no men in our practice at the moment. So supervising men is a problem for us'. [SpGP3]

Long term methadone patients along with the aging methadone patient population were viewed as creating a draw on services. Discussions centred on the adaptation of service models given the aging population of both drug users and methadone patients.

'We have to recognise it is an ageing model and in Dublin...I think we need to be very careful about setting up new models that are potentially very expensive for a profile that may not exist in 10 or 15 years time.' [SpGP1]

Participants described the complexities of treating and engaging with homeless drug users, and the difficulties around long term methadone treatment. In terms of attempting to reduce patients and taper off methadone, participants described the need for a broader de-medicalised approach to recovery. Debate occurred with regard to the Irish stipulation for opioid free urines prior to accessing a detoxification centre.

'People have to have 3 or 4 urines that are opioid-free before they can be admitted to a centre...if they are able to manage 3 or 4 urines that are opioid-free then they don't need to go into the detox centre in the first place...' [NS2]

Systemic barriers to optimal OAT service provision

National provision of OAT and dispensing of methadone was described as patchy, and largely concentrated in the capital, Dublin, and larger urban areas. Some participants voiced concern around the need for more Health Service Executive dispensing centres as a way of dealing with national demand, particularly in the context of de-stabilisation of patients and the current requirement to resume initiation of treatment in the clinics. Other logistical complexities for patients centred on lack of rural GPs and community pharmacies willing to prescribe and dispense methadone, rural residences and cost of transport, particularly outside of the capital. As outlined in the previous theme, stigma of methadone, and the lack of choice with large methadone clinics in some areas offering the only route to treatment were viewed as representing fundamental systemic barriers to OAT access. Service level barriers to access for individuals experiencing opioid dependence were described as centring on the complexities around the patients address of residence with regard to options to access stabilisation OAT in clinics or by a Level 2 GP, their general preferences to attend primary care for OAT, and lack of availability of Level 2 GPs in the community. Many participants described long waiting lists and under capacity of local

services to deal with the issue of opioid dependence, and provide the current requirement for regularity of consultations.

'There is a problem with waiting lists and I think nationally there needs to be a more robust, systematic review of waiting lists and if a patient is waiting for more than 3 months for treatment there needs to be a proper analysis'. [SpGP1]

'If there were more Methadone prescribers within the GP community then there would be no need for these people there in the country to travel to access treatment'. [NS2]

Other blocks centred on homeless patients seeking treatment with no fixed address, and the treatment influx from parts of the country outside the capital.

'Where are the homeless people going? This is not a good model of care. Having them sent to multiple pharmacies and multiple centres causes violence and antisocial behaviour, and in fact you are creating more problems and the treatment is bringing problems with it.' [SpGP1]

The MTP given its stipulation to stabilise patients in addiction clinics or by Level 2 GPs prior to referral to the community Level 1 GP was viewed as not operating efficiently. The restriction of numbers of patients managed by Level 1 GP ($n = 15$) in the community was central to this issue and was viewed as contributing to long waiting lists.

'Information we are getting is that everybody and everything has to go through the clinic...we have Level 2 GPs... I would be saying why are we not utilising the L2 GPs to the max and not be creating waiting lists.' [SpGP4]

GP training and registration in the MTP

Participants discussed the specialist Level 1 and 2 training and Health Service Executive registration complexities as systemic barriers to providing optimal OAT in Ireland. Stigma of OAT within medical practice and education was viewed as affecting training uptake. Those involved in GP training (and who prescribe methadone) described the willingness of younger doctors to engage in training when exposed to OAT, and particularly when hosted by larger GP practices involved in methadone prescribing. GP registrars not exposed to the opioid dependent patient cohort were described as not willing, and similar was described with regard to newly qualified pharmacists.

'You would like to think that GP trainers would be the frontline for educating people being open to the idea that all patients are equal...... the majority of GP trainers that we have do not do methadone and would not entertain methadone treatment. There are messages like that going out to trainees' [SpGP4]

Difficulties centred on the lack of uniform approach to mentoring younger GPs, and the current requirement for methadone contracts to be assigned to a practice address, not the prescriber. The Level 1 and Level 2 structures were viewed as complex and difficult, particularly for newly qualified GPs entering employment and securing employment in primary care practices not part of the MTP.

'It is an incredible missed opportunity, every GP trainee in the country should be obliged to do Methadone training like they are obliged to do the Women's Health. [SpGP3]

Another systemic issue in the MTP was described as centring on the significant effort, organisation and commitment in the contractual difficulties to become and register as a Level 2 prescriber which was viewed as deterring some Level 1 GPs from progressing.

'Its too difficult to get to a Level 2 scenario...if you have done the Level 1 training, to get to a Level 2 prescriber is too difficult. It's a long process.' [SpGP2]

Complexities of the GPs role in supporting the opioid dependent patient were discussed in terms of length of patient consultation, the myriad of additional health conditions and social challenges. In some areas Level 1 GPs were under resourced despite the funding allocation for OAT patients, and unable and not willing to take on more complex patients.

'Methadone is well remunerated... I don't begrudge any of our methadone users the time they take up. But new GPs won't start because it's so complicated,' [SpGP3]

Solutions and models of good practice: Using what you have

Firstly, participants discussed potential solutions and best practices for shared learning. Several key areas were identified, with first centring on the requirement for all GP registrars to be trained in methadone prescribing and the treatment of opioid dependence and related health problems. The ICGP has long held the view that all GPs should be in a position to provide methadone and other opioid agonist treatment in primary care *'to be part of routine GP primary care'*. Encouraging GPs to change attitudes, and engage in the specialist training via mentoring of more experienced GPs was discussed, and appeared to represent a way of reducing fears and concerns around engaging with the methadone patient cohort.

'I'd like to see that Level 2 would become more specialised and that Level 1 would almost become normal for GPs so that they have facilities for benzos and for other addictions.' [SpGP2]

Secondly, the group discussed how to optimise the available resources within the current MTP. Finding ways for supporting OAT patients via shared care planning with available community agencies was viewed as vital within the MTP. Addiction clinics were viewed as having a range of supports available to patients. Avenues for potential support for community practitioners centred on the available outreach, social, community and psychological support services, and engaging with case workers from local Drug Task Forces.

'There is a perception among GPs like me who are doing methadone versus the clinics is that the clinics have a lot of services that we don't get so easily, like the counselling services, ...if you were able to offer GPs some of those supports...once a month or something like that, that would be just as good as having a full blown clinic'. [SpGP3]

Informal meetings between staff were viewed as important to help share issues and support each other within the practice, particularly if GPs were working part time.

'The work is too complex to be able to manage it on your own'. [SpGP3]

'We tend to be the key worker, because we are the only person that these people are seeing.' [SpGP1]

Using family support systems where possible from treatment onset was also viewed as a potential lesson learnt. Complexities arise when patients have no family or are homeless. Shared care and key working was viewed as very important.

'Resources out there that are probably underutilized at the moment...for example, voluntary based services around the corner from the GP. It is about getting to know the person. It is about case management in all areas of their life.' [NS1]

Thirdly, given the logistical barriers for patients in rural areas, or areas with no Level 2 GP, the group discussed the potentials for utilising community pharmacy and nurse prescribing in the community. Complexities centred on this recommendation, and current service level agreements.

'I would see a lot of what's done by the doctor, could be done by the nurses...and the doctor then can be able to prescribe more ...and be able to look after more in terms of the monitoring, the supervision, the diagnosis of mental illness.' [SpGP1]

Lastly, the remit of community pharmacy could expand to support work in primary care in terms of extended dispensing, education and vaccination of drug users. Community pharmacies could expand to take on the role of patient vaccination (Hepatitis A and B) within their role in providing needle and syringe exchange.

'Another job that pharmacists might take on is Hepatitis A & B vaccination in pharmacies. It's not an immediately practical thing but something definitely to think of in the future'. [SpGP2]

'Down the country, why not augment the community pharmacies with extra staff. The 7 day pharmacies that are open.'[SpGP1]

Discussion

The study illustrates the complexities around the MTP within primary care in Ireland, along with the systemic failures in optimal service provision for opioid dependent individuals, and challenges encountered in managing opioid drug users. Primary care providers can take a proactive role in treatment of opioid dependence [8–10] and so enhance health care provision [11, 12]. Integration of OAT into primary care via different models can expand access to treatment [13]. Mainstreaming of OAT into primary care can also help to reduce stigma as a barrier to treatment uptake [14, 15]. Systemic barriers observed by these national stakeholders and experts in Ireland were similar to those reported elsewhere and centre on stigma, lack of therapeutic choice in Ireland, reluctance of GPs to prescribe OAT, and complex reimbursement systems [16–21]. Lack of MTP coverage across the country was illustrated and represents a systemic barrier to access for patients living in rural areas, homeless patients without a residential address, and those seeking treatment due to long waiting lists. Similar issues have been reported in other countries exploring the expansion of OAT into community and primary care [13, 21, 22]. The expansion of buprenorphine-naloxone availability could overcome this barrier. In many jurisdictions buprenorphine-naloxone availability in primary care has allowed for the rapid expansion of OAT. Buprenorphine's use as a combined product with naloxone has allowed for a safe reduction in supervision requirements and increased utility in patients living in isolated areas with poor access to medical and pharmacy services. The use of tele-medicine linking less experienced rural GPs with their more specialist colleagues could further increase OAT coverage nationally.

Participants described the complexities of the current Irish opioid dependent population in terms of long term and aging patients, co-dependencies on other drugs such as benzodiazepines and Z-hypnotics, abuse of prescription and OTC opioid analgesics, and homelessness. These complexities of opioid dependent patients in terms of psychiatric co-morbidity, and co- dependencies are well evidenced in the literature [10]. Similar to other countries, primary care practice based pressures centre on patient behavioural issues and resources required to support longer consultation times due to the health and social care challenges of these patients. Studies have reported on GP reluctance to prescribe methadone due to their fears around patient behavioural issues, the complexities of opioid dependent patients, concerns around workload and the time required to manage such patients, and staff safety [4, 6, 16, 17, 23–29]. Van Hout

and Bingham [4] have underscored the multiplicity of roles (patient advocate, medical supervisor and detoxification gate keeper) that GPs have when involved in prescribing methadone.

Strategies to address systemic barriers centre on the expansion of training, increased use of community pharmacists, development of the nurse prescribing role and promoting the easy access to GPs via key working [13]. Shared care with available community based services was viewed as vital in terms of family support, key working, outreach and psycho-social support. The lack of therapeutic choice in Ireland needs to be addressed. Buprenorphine is underutilised in Ireland due its restricted availability, but has been reported as safe and effective in OAT in primary care [21]. Providing this OAT option could lessen the draw on resources and support OAT patients across the country. Other potential solutions using the available resources in the MTP centred on expanding the remit of the community pharmacy in terms of patient education and vaccination, and the role of the nurse prescriber. Nurse prescribers can overcome systemic barriers and failures and improve access to OAT [21]. Technology using E-consultation and e-prescribing to support patients who have to travel long distances for treatment could also be considered and would facilitate access to Level 2 GP services.

Similar to research in the United States [10] and building on the primary care model now widely accepted in Europe, mainstreaming of OAT has many advantages, and success will depend on service delivery models and the improved and expanding training of doctors in Ireland. GPs are ideally placed to diagnose patients with substance related problems and require a specific skill set to provide clinical care. The focus group highlighted the need to ensure newly qualified GPs are trained in OAT and to support those interested in securing Level 1 and Level 2 contracts. Participants echoed views reported by the ICGP in 2016, where a need for continued support of prescribing GPs (Level 1 and 2), training of new GPs and encouragement of further specialisation to Level 2 were identified [5]. Issues around encouraging newly qualified GPs to engage in provision of the MTP service were described, and support research reporting on newly qualified GPs having a more positive attitude toward opioid dependent patients and self-awareness of competencies to treat this condition [30, 31]. Training at undergraduate and registrar levels is warranted [10]. No Irish medical school has any elective or integrated training in addictions, and with no documented drug and alcohol teaching sessions [32, 33]. Particularly in undergraduate training, addiction as a disease should be integrated into pre-clinical course material, and careful emphasis on development of positive attitudes to working with addicted patients is warranted [34–36]. Hussein

Rassool [37] has indicated that substance misuse training can contribute to an increase in confidence in participants in working with substance misusing patients. Research elsewhere has underscored the need to integrate addiction medicine into medical and primary care registrar education, given the public health cost of medical, behavioural and social problems associated with substance use, and also given the frequent lack of recognition of substance abuse and failure to provide appropriate treatment on the part of general practitioners [38–43].

The use of the focus group methodology in this study allowed for the efficient collection of the views of a very diverse group of Irish addiction experts in relation to the blocks and facilitators to OAT in Ireland. The inclusion of both statutory and non-statutory experts allowed for robust and insightful discussion and the focus group methodology is recognised as a good research method to capture the richness of these discussions. The inclusion of experts in the area of policy development and implementation along with experts in treatment design and delivery allowed for an in-depth exploration of the issues.

There are a number of limitations to this study. The findings are limited to the data collected from only one focus group which contained only 11 experts. While the research team endeavoured to ensure national representation it is reasonable to assume that this group is not fully representative of all regions and there are deficits in recognising all the barriers and enablers to OAT in Ireland. The focus group did not include patients or patient representatives. A further limitation is that the focus group was conducted by, or included, those who have responsibility for the SMP. The researchers recognised this and attempted to limit this conflict of interest by picking researcher 1 as the group facilitator. This researcher would have had the least prior involvement with the focus group participants. Lastly, the involvement of the members of the SMP in the focus group may have impacted on participants' willingness to share their views fully for fear of antagonising or upsetting these SMP members.

Conclusion
The study is a first step in a process to identify barriers to optimal OAT provision by GPs in Ireland. It has successfully identified a number of previously unrecognised issues that will be progressed through a number of national drug treatment and policy groups. Key national stakeholders and experts identified a series of improvement strategies which can reduce OAT stigma and barriers to access, optimise therapeutic choice, enhance interagency care planning within the MTP, utilise the strengths of community pharmacy and nurse prescribers,

and recruit and support methadone prescribing GPs. The ICGP will advance the implementation of these recommendations through a number of national drug treatment and policy groups and will plan and undertake a series of independently run expert focus groups across the country to gain further insight into this topic and add to these recommendations.

Abbreviations
CAF: Clinical Audit Facilitator; CTL: Central Treatment List; GP: General Practitioner; HSE: Health Service Executive; ICGP: Irish College of General Practitioners; MTP: Methadone Treatment Programme; NST: Non Statutory Stakeholder; OAT: Opiate Agonist Treatment; SLA: Service Level Agreement; SMP: Substance Misuse Programme; ST: Statutory Stakeholder

Funding
The study was funded by the Irish College of General Practitioners.

Authors' contributions
All authors (MCVH, DC, AM, ID) were involved in the study design, had full access to the survey data and analyses, and interpreted the data, critically reviewed the manuscript and had full control, including final responsibility for the decision to submit the paper for publication. All authors read and approved the final manuscript.

Authors' information
MCVH is Professor of Public Health Policy and Practice at the Public Health Institute of Liverpool John Moores University, United Kingdom. She also holds the Clinical Audit Facilitator role at the Irish College of General Practitioners, Ireland.
DC is Assistant Director of the Substance Misuse Programme at the Irish College of General Practitioners, Ireland.
AM is the Administrator of the Substance Misuse Programme at the Irish College of General Practitioners, Ireland.
ID is Director of the Substance Misuse Programme at the Irish College of General Practitioners, Ireland.

Competing interests
The authors declare that they have no competing interests.

References
1. Dole VP, Nywsander M. A medical treatment for diacetylmorphine (heroin) addiction. A clinical trial with methadone hydrochloride. JAMA. 1965;23: 646–50.
2. Amato L, Minozzi S, Davoli M, Vecchi S. Psychosocial combined with agonist maintenance treatments versus agonist maintenance treatments alone for treatment of opioid dependence. Cochrane Database Syst Rev 2011;DOI:10.1002/14651858. CD004147.pub4
3. Bonhomme J, Shim R, Gooden R, Tyus D, Rust G. Opioid Addiction and Abuse in Primary Care Practice: A Comparison of Methadone and Buprenorphine as Treatment Options. J Natl Med Assoc. 2012;104:342–50.
4. Van Hout MC, Bingham T. A qualitative study of prescribing doctor experiences of methadone maintenance treatment. Int J Ment Health Addict. 2013;12:227–42.
5. Delargy I, O'Shea M, Van Hout MC, Collins C. General Practitioners perspectives on and attitudes toward the Methadone Treatment Protocol in Ireland. Heroin Addict and Relat Clin Probl. 2016;18:43–50.
6. Butler S. The making of the methadone protocol: The Irish system?'. Drugs: Educ Prev Polic. 2002;9:311–24.

7. Farrell M, Barry J. The introduction of the Opioid Treatment Protocol. Dublin: Health Service Executive; 2010. www.drugsandalcohol.ie/14458. Accessed 14 Dec 2011

8. Weaver MF, Jarvis MA, Schnoll SH. Role of the primary care physician in problems of substance abuse. Arch Intern Med. 1999;159:913–24.

9. McLellan AT, Lewis DC, O'Brien CP, Kleber HD. Drug dependence, a chronic medical illness: implications for treatment, insurance, and outcomes evaluation. JAMA. 2000;284:1689–95.

10. Krantz MJ, Mehler PS. Treating opioid dependence. Growing implications for primary care. Arch Intern Med. 2004;164:277–88.

11. O'Connor PG, Selwyn PA, Schottenfeld RS. Medical care for injection-drug users with human immunodeficiency virus infection. N Engl J Med. 1994;33:1450–9.

12. Stein MD, Urdaneta ME, Clarke J, Maksad J, Sobota M, Hanna L, Markson LE. Use of antiretroviral therapies by HIV-infected persons receiving methadone maintenance. J Addict Dis. 2000;19:1985–94.

13. Korthuis T, McCarty D, Weimer M, Bougatsos C, Blazina I, Zakher B, Grusing S, Devine B, Chou R. Primary Care–Based Models for the Treatment of Opioid Use Disorder: A Scoping Review. Ann Intern Med. 2017;166:268–78.

14. McCaffrey BR. Methadone treatment: our vision for the future. J Addict Dis. 2001;20:93–101.

15. Merrill JO, Jackson R. Treatment of heroin dependence. Ann Intern Med. 2001;134:165–6.

16. Langton D, Hickey A, Bury G, Smith M, O'Kelly F, Barry J, Sweeney B, Bourke M. Methadone maintenance in general practice: impact on staff attitudes'. Irish J Med Sci. 2000;169:133–6.

17. Abouvanni G, Stevens LJ, Harris MF, Wickes W, Ramakrishna SS, Ta E. Knowlden, S.M. GP attitudes to managing drug- and alcohol-dependent patients: a reluctant role. Drug Alcohol Rev. 2000;19:165–70.

18. Watson F. Models of primary care for substance misusers: the Lothian experience. Drugs: Educ, Prev, Polic. 2000;7:223–34.

19. Keen J. Primary care treatment for drug users: the Sheffield experience. J Primary Care Mental Health. 2001;5:4–7.

20. McKeown A, Matheson C, Bond C. A qualitative study of GPs' attitudes to drug misusers and drug misuse services in primary care. Fam Pract. 2003;20:120–5.

21. Jenkinson J, Ravert P. Underutilization of Primary Care Providers in Treating Opiate Addiction. J Nurse Pract. 2013;9:516–22.

22. Chou R, Korthuis PT, Weimer M, Bougatsos C, Blazina I, Zakher B, Grusing BS, Devine B, McCarty D. Medication-Assisted Treatment Models of Care for Opioid Use Disorder in Primary Care Settings. 2016. Rockville: Agency for Healthcare Research and Quality (US); 2016 Dec. (Technical Briefs, No. 28.) Available from: https://www.ncbi.nlm.nih.gov/books/NBK402352/

23. Gruer L, Wilson P, Scott R, Elliott L, Macleod J, Harden K, Forrester E, Hinshelwood S, McNulty H, Strang J. General practitioner centred scheme for treatment of opiate dependent drug injectors In Glasgow. BMJ. 1997;314:1730–5.

24. McGillion J. GPs' attitudes towards the treatment of drug misusers. Br J Gen Pract. 2000;50:385–6.

25. Gabbay M, Shiels C, van den Bos A. Turningthe tide': influencing future GP attitudes to opiate misusers. Educ Gen Pract. 2001;12:144–52.

26. Matheson C, Pitcairn J, Bond CM, van Teijlingen E, Ryan M. (2003). General practice management ofillicit drug users in Scotland: a national survey. Addiction 2003;98:119–126.

27. Gjersing L, Waal H, Caplehorn JRM, Gossop M, Clausen T. Staff attitudes and the associations with treatment organisation, clinical practices and outcomes in opioid maintenance treatment. BMC Health Serv Res. 2010;10:194.

28. Lloyd C. Sinning and Sinned Against: The Stigmatisation of Problem Drug Users. York: Universityof York; 2010.

29. Shapiro B, Coffa D, McCance-Katz E. A Primary Care Approach to Substance Misuse. Am Fam Physician 2013;88:113–21.

30. Carnwath T, Peacock J, Huxley P, Davies A, Bowers L. Are all districts equally ready for "shared care" of drug misusers? Addict Res. 1999;6:307–18.

31. Glanz A, Taylor C. Findings of a national survey of the role of general practitioners in the treatment of opiate misuse: Extent of contact with opiate misusers. BMJ 1986;293:427–30.

32. Klimas J, Rieb L, Bury G, Muench J, O'Toole J, Rieckman T, Cullen W. Integrating addiction medicine training into medical school and residency curricula. Addict Sci Clin Pract. 2015;10:A28.

33. Wilson M, Cullen W, Klimas J. Off the record: substance related disorders in the undergraduate medical curricula in Ireland. J Substance Use. 2016;21:598–600.

34. Gorman D. A theory-driven approach to the evaluation of professional training in alcohol abuse. Addict. 1993;88:229–36.

35. Haber P, Murnion B. Training in Addiction Medicine in Australia. Subs Abuse. 2011;32(2):115–9.

36. Barron R, Frank E, Gitlow S. Evaluation of an Experiential Curriculum for Addiction Education Among Medical Students. J Addict Medicine. 2012;6:131–6.

37. Hussein Rassool G. Curriculum Model, Course Development, and Evaluation of Substance Misuse Education for Health Care Professionals. J Addict Nursing. 2004;15:85–90.

38. Klamen D. Integration in Education for Addiction Medicine. J Psychoactive Drugs. 1997;29:263–8.

39. Miller N, Sheppard L, Colenda C, Magen J. Why Physicians Are Unprepared to Treat Patients Who Have Alcohol- and Drug-related Disorders. Acad. Med. 2001;7:410–8.

40. O'Connor P, Nyquist J, McLellan T. Integrating Addiction Medicine Into Graduate Medical Education in Primary Care: The Time Has Come. Ann Intern Med. 2011;154:56–9.

41. De Jong C, Luycks L, Delicat JW. The Master in Addiction Medicine Program in The Netherlands. Subst Abus. 2011;32:108–14.

42. Carroll J, Goodair C, Chaytor A, Notley C, Ghodse H, Kopelman P. () Substance Misuse teaching in undergraduate medical education. BMC Med Educat. 2014;14:34.

43. Kothari D, Gourevitch M, Lee J, Grossman E, Truncali A, Tavinder K, Kalet A. Undergraduate Medical Education in Substance Abuse: A Review of the Quality of the Literature. Acad Med. 2011;86:98–112.

6

The effect of a new lifetime-cardiovascular-risk display on patients' motivation to participate in shared decision-making

Nikita Roman A. Jegan[1]*[ID], Sarah Anna Kürwitz[1], Lena Kathrin Kramer[1], Monika Heinzel-Gutenbrunner[2], Charles Christian Adarkwah[1,3], Uwe Popert[1,4] and Norbert Donner-Banzhoff[1]

Abstract

Background: This study investigated the effects of three different risk displays used in a cardiovascular risk calculator on patients' motivation for shared decision-making (SDM). We compared a newly developed time-to-event (TTE) display with two established absolute risk displays (i.e. emoticons and bar charts). The accessibility, that is, how understandable, helpful, and trustworthy patients found each display, was also investigated.

Methods: We analysed a sample of 353 patients recruited in general practices. After giving consent, patients were introduced to one of three fictional vignettes with low, medium or high cardiovascular risk. All three risk displays were shown in a randomized order. Patients were asked to rate each display with regard to motivation for SDM and accessibility. Two-factorial repeated measures analyses of variance were conducted to compare the displays and investigate possible interactions with age.

Results: Regarding motivation for SDM, the TTE elicited the highest motivation, followed by the emoticons and bar chart ($p < .001$). The displays had no differential influence on the age groups ($p = .445$). While the TTE was generally rated more accessible than the emoticons and bar chart ($p < .001$), the emoticons were only superior to the bar chart in the younger subsample. However, this was only to a small effect (interaction between display and age, $p < .01$, $\eta^2 = 0.018$).

Conclusions: Using fictional case vignettes, the novel TTE display was superior regarding motivation for SDM and accessibility when compared to established displays using emoticons and a bar chart. If future research can replicate these results in real-life consultations, the TTE display will be a valuable addition to current risk calculators and decision aids by improving patients' participation.

Keywords: Shared decision-making, Risk, Risk assessment, Decision aid, Comprehension

Background

Risk calculators for cardiovascular events (CE), such as myocardial infarction or stroke have been recommended by German [1], American [2] and British [3] guidelines to aid patients in understanding their quantitative risk and the possible benefits of various interventions. They make an individual calculation of risk and the recommendation of treatments, such as lipid-lowering medication possible. When used as part of a decision aid, such as the arriba™ protocol, risk calculators can improve patients' knowledge, increase participation in the decision-making process (shared decision-making, SDM [4, 5]) and lead to decisions that are more congruent to their values [6].

Multivariate risk functions provide the absolute 5- or 10-year risk for suffering a CE. Apart from the numerical result, cardiovascular risk calculators may also present the risk in different graphical formats [3]. Icon arrays depict risk as a natural frequency (X of 100). In this type of display, emoticons are often used to communicate the number of people with the outcome of interest. Other frequently used forms are vertical bar charts comparing the individual risk to the mean or median risk, or distribution graphs of the risk across all age groups. These

---

* Correspondence: jegan@staff.uni-marburg.de
[1]Department of General Practice and Family Medicine, Philipps-University Marburg, Karl-von-Frisch-Str. 4, 35032 Marburg, Germany
Full list of author information is available at the end of the article

formats vary in complexity. Therefore, they should be chosen according to the level of graphical literacy and preference of each patient [3, 7].

Decision-making based on the absolute risk for a defined timespan, such as ten years, has been criticized [8–10]. Younger individuals with high-risk behaviour, such as smoking or unhealthy diet, have relatively small absolute risks for CEs, although their lifetime risk is high [8–12]. This stems from the fact that absolute risk calculations are largely influenced by age [10]. When absolute risks are calculated, the benefits of early interventions most relevant to this age group such as diet and regular physical activity do not become evident. Therefore, risk calculators based only on absolute risk do not provide adequate information for this age group to help them make well-informed decisions. To address this problem, research recommends using lifetime-risk calculations [3, 8, 9] or, more specifically, the number of years free from a CE and the number of years gained by an intervention, i.e., time-to-event (TTE) [10].

A well-established and evaluated risk calculator and decision aid in Germany is arriba™ [13–17]. It uses a modified Framingham formula to calculate the absolute 10 year risk for a CE [18, 19]. So far, arriba™ has provided three graphical displays with increasing complexity to inform patients about their risk: 1) a 10 by 10 field of icon arrays portrayed as emoticons; 2) a vertical bar chart showing the individual risk and the median risk of the same age and gender group; 3) a distribution graph of the risk across all age groups. Arriba™ is predicated on the philosophy of SDM with an explicit script to be used during consultation. Following this protocol results in higher satisfaction, higher participation and lower decisional regret with primary care patients [14].

We have developed a TTE display to be incorporated into arriba™. It shows in how many years and at what age a CE is likely to occur in an individual patient. A horizontal bar depicts the total lifespan. The point in time with the highest risk for an event is marked by a different colour. The possible gain by interventions is shown in a second horizontal bar. In order to present individualized TTE predictions, we developed a Markov-based microsimulation model based on cardiovascular risk factors.

This new display has already been compared qualitatively with the established arriba™ displays in a preliminary study (Kürwitz et al.: Playing on fears - Family physician's comparative evaluation of a new risk format presenting cardiovascular risk, in preparation; Kürwitz et al.: Such a display can be hard enough!- Patients evaluation of a new risk format: cardiovascular risk presented as time-to-event, submitted). In this study, different displays based on

fictional case vignettes were shown to patients and general practitioners (GPs). Respondents were asked to comment on comprehensibility, risk perception, motivation to participate in SDM, and ethical defensibility. The new TTE display received the most favourable feedback, with emoticons and a bar chart following and the distribution graphs lagging behind.

In this article, we first present the quantitative evaluation of these three displays regarding their ability to elicit motivation for SDM in patients. Second, we test the hypothesis that the TTE display leads to a higher motivation for SDM than the other two displays in younger patients when compared to older patients. This hypothesis is based on the assumption, that an increased lifetime risk of young patients should become more apparent in the TTE display, creating a higher subjective feeling of risk. In other words, we evaluate a possible interaction with the age of responding patients. Finally, we asked patients which of the three displays was the most understandable, helpful and trustworthy ('accessible').

Methods
Design
We contacted 100 GPs in the northern region of Hesse, Germany for participation. A total of 30 agreed to participate while 19 declined. The remaining 51 did not reply. Those who agreed were asked to consecutively recruit 20 patients among those presenting for a health check. In case the recruitment goal could not be reached by a single GP, patients visiting as part of the diabetes type 2 Disease Management Program were also allowed to be included. Recruited patients had to be between 35 and 70 years old, with 35 being the earliest eligible age for an adult health check provided by public healthcare in Germany. After giving their written consent, patients completed a questionnaire, which covered sociodemographic characteristics and their reactions to different risk presentation formats. They were introduced to one of three fictional case scenarios, namely low, medium or high cardiovascular risk). The low risk vignette portrayed a 47-year-old healthy, non-smoking female with normal weight, consulting her GP after reading a news article about cholesterol. The medium risk vignette portrayed a 50 year old smoking male (12 cigarettes per day), physically inactive, and with a high fat and high sugar diet being sent to his GP by his worried wife. Finally, the high-risk vignette described a 50-year-old heavy-smoking male with a high workload and imbalanced diet, reporting to his GP after hospitalisation due to a heart attack. The vignette was then followed by the three displays (emoticons, bar chart and TTE, Fig. 1) showing the cardiovascular risk and the achievable change by lipid lowering (statin) treatment. Each display was presented along with a verbal description of the displayed risk. The patients were

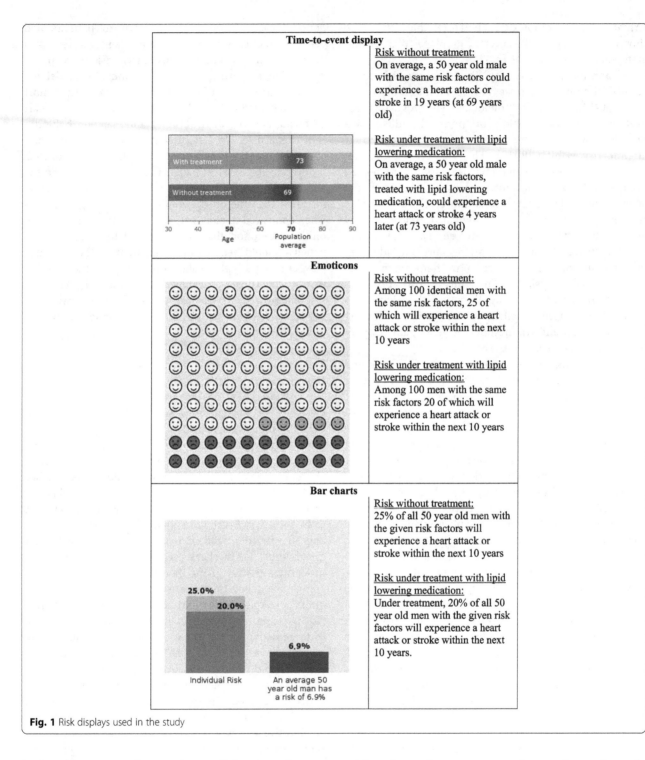

Fig. 1 Risk displays used in the study

instructed to answer the questions as if they were the person described in the fictional case.

The sequence of displays was varied randomly to avoid systematic sequence effects. Moreover, low, medium, and high-risk scenarios were evenly distributed in each practice. Finally, the order of fictional cases and permutations of displays was varied systematically from practice to practice.

After six weeks, we contacted a random subsample again to evaluate the test-retest reliability of the scale measuring motivation for SDM.

Measures

Sample description

We assessed sociodemographic patient data by asking about age, gender, education, and migrant status [20].

GPs were asked to specify known cardiovascular risk factors for each patient and state if the patient has been exposed to counselling with arriba™ before.

Motivation for SDM

Due to the lack of scales measuring the motivation to participate in SDM [21, 22], we created eight items asking about the motivation to perform behaviours that are crucial for the participation in making a well-informed decision. Patients were asked to rate their agreement with each statement on a five-point Likert scale. Then, we calculated the means across all items for each display. Internal consistency and retest-reliability-coefficients (six week interval) were initially moderate (Cronbach's α = .589–.684, r_{tt} = .485–.834). Eliminating two items improved the results (Cronbach's α: .867–.877, r_{tt} = .562–.890) and led to the six- item solution we used for further analysis (Table 1).

Accessibility

To measure the subjective accessibility of the information, we used the accessibility scale developed by Gaissmaier and colleagues. The scale includes five items asking for subjective judgements regarding comprehensibility, usefulness, seriousness, and intuitive accessibility on a five-point Likert scale [23].

Sample size calculation and statistical analysis

We calculated the required sample size a priori with G*Power (Ver.3.1.5) [24]. Our main hypothesis was tested with a repeated measures analysis of variance with three measurements (displays) and two groups (young vs. old patients, median split) for the main outcome "motivation for SDM". Assuming a small effect-size of Cohen's f = 0.10 [25] for the interaction term, we calculated a required sample size of n = 324 to achieve an α-error of 5% and a power (1-β) of 0.8. Taking into account a 90%participation rate and a 10% data loss due to missing values, we would need to approach 405 patients.

All calculations were conducted with IBM SPSS (Version 21) [26]. We calculated means, standard deviations and frequencies for variables of interest. After splitting the sample at the median age, we compared the two age groups regarding demographic variables and risk factors with χ^2-, Fisher's exact and t-tests. The internal consistency of the motivation-for-SDM scale was determined by calculating Cronbach's α coefficients [27] and the test-retest-reliability was quantified by Pearson correlations. The comparison of the displays in terms of motivation for SDM and possible differential influences on the age groups was tested with a two-factorial repeated measures analysis of variance. We used the same procedure to analyse the secondary outcome "accessibility". In case of significant main or interaction effects, we calculated pairwise comparisons with post-hoc Scheffé tests to account for multiple testing.

Results
Sample characteristics

In total, 409 patients were asked for participation, of which 22 patients declined. The remaining 387 patients completed the questionnaire immediately after consultation. However, 34 of them were older than 70 years and were subsequently excluded from the analysis (Fig. 2). The baseline characteristics of the analysed sample (n = 353) along with the subsamples after splitting at the median age (52 years) can be seen in Table 2. Young and old patients differed in educational background (a higher proportion of basic education and lower proportion of higher education in the older patients), as well as in the number of cardiovascular risk factors (both p-values < .001). When calculating the statistical tests, we had to exclude a small number of cases due to missing values in the outcomes (motivation for SDM: 20 cases; accessibility: 46 cases). For each outcome, we compared the patients with complete data sets to those with incomplete data sets. No statistical differences could be found except for migrants who had more frequently missing values than Germans (motivation for SDM: 16.7% vs.

Table 1 Motivation for shared decision-making scale; final six-item version (translated from German for the purpose of this article)

If I was the patient being shown the information…	Not at all (1)	Not Likely (2)	Partially (3)	Likely(4)	Very much (4)
1. …I would be motivated to think further about my risk.					
2. …I would be motivated to request further information from my family doctor.					
3. …I would be motivated to use other sources to learn more about my risk.					
4. …I would feel sufficiently informed by the display to make a decision for or against an intervention.					
5. …I would be motivated to talk with my doctor about the decision for or against therapy.					
6. …I would be sufficiently informed to decide together with my doctor whether I should receive treatment.					

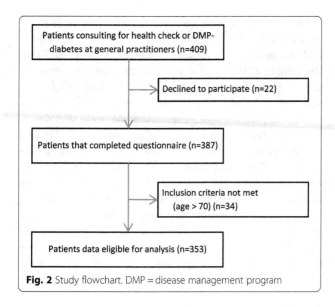

Fig. 2 Study flowchart. DMP = disease management program

4.7% ($p = .021$); accessibility: 26.7% vs. 11.4% ($p = .038$); $n = 346$ due to seven missing values in immigration data, see Additional file 1). Furthermore, we compared patients receiving the small, medium, and high-risk case vignettes to control for possible group imbalance and found no differences in any of the demographic variables (see Additional file 2).

Primary and secondary outcomes
Examining the primary outcome "Motivation for SDM", all three display types differed from each other (medium to large effect size; all results shown in Table 3 and Fig. 3). The TTE display received significantly higher ratings than emoticons and bar charts. In addition, the emoticons were rated higher than the bar chart. This applied irrespective of age (interaction effect age * display not significant). In general, older patients felt a higher motivation for SDM than younger patients, irrespective of the display type (small to moderate effect size).

The analysis for the secondary outcome "accessibility" showed significant results for age and display (Table 3

Table 2 Baseline characteristics of patient sample and subsamples after splitting at the median age (52 years)

Variable	Total sample (n = 353)	Young patients (n = 178)	Old patients (n = 175)	Young vs. old p-value
Female, n (%)	197 (55.8%)	112 (62.9%)	85 (48.6%)	.007[a]
Mean age in years*, M (SD)	53.5 (9.0)	45.9 (4.7)	61.2 (4.8)	<.001[b]
Migrant status, n (%)				
No (German)	316 (89.5%)	157 (88.2%)	159 (90.9%)	.495[a]
Yes	30 (8.5%)	16 (9.0%)	14 (8.1%)	
Insufficient data	7 (2.0%)	5 (2.8%)	2 (1.1%)	
Education*, n (%)				
Basic education (up to 9 years)	114 (32.4%)	36 (20.3%)	78 (44.6%)	< .001[a]
Medium education (10–11 years)	138 (39.2%)	81 (45.8%)	57 (32.6%)	
Higher education (12 years and more)	100 (28.4%)	60 (33.9%)	40 (22.9%)	
Reason for Consultation, n (%)				
Health check	337 (95.5%)	175 (98.3%)	162 (92.6%)	.009[a]
Disease management for diabetes	16 (4.5%)	3 (1.7%)	13 (7.4%)	
Number of risk factors besides age*, M (SD)	0.56 (0.8)	0.28 (0.6)	0.83 (0.94)	<.001[b]
Existing risk factors				
Existing coronary heart disease	12 (3.4%)	3 (1.7%)	9 (5.1%)	.085[c]
Prior myocardial infarction	8 (2.3%)	2 (1.1%)	6 (3.4%)	.172[c]
Prior stroke	14 (4.0%)	2 (1.1%)	12 (6.9%)	.006[c]
Peripheral artery disease	7 (2.0%)	1 (0.6%9	6 (3.4%)	.066[c]
Diabetes	40 (11.3%)	7 (3.9%)	33 (18.9%)	<.001[a]
Hypertension	115 (32.6%)	35 (19.7%)	80 (45.7%)	<.001[a]
Contact with arriba™ prior to examination, n (%)	54 (15.3%)	23 (12.9%)	31 (17.7%)	.211[a]

SD standard deviation, *CVD* cardiovascular disease;
* = difference between old and young patients is significant by $p < .001$;
[a] = χ^2-test; [b] = t-test; [c] = Fisher's exact test

Table 3 Comparison of young and old patients' ratings of the three displays

Variable / Sample	Bar chart M (SD)	Emoti-cons M (SD)	Time-to-event M (SD)	Total M (SD)	Display p-value ($\eta^{2\,a}$)	Age p-value ($\eta^{2\,a}$)	A*D[b] p-value ($\eta^{2\,a}$)	Post-hoc tests[c]
Motivation for SDM[d]								
Young (n = 169)	3.40 (0.89)	3.47 (0.86)	3.59 (0.83)	3.49 (0.79)	<.001 (0.035)	< .001 (0.084)	.445 (0.002)	T > E, E > B, T > B
Old (n = 164)	3.88 (0.81)	3.92 (0.77)	4.00 (0.74)	3.94 (0.70)				
Total (n = 333)	3.64 (0.89)	3.69 (0.85)	3.79 (0.81)					
Accessibility[d]								
Young (n = 155)	3.35 (0.88)	3.69 (0.79)	3.81 (0.73)	3.62 (0.65)	< .001 (0.102)	< .001 (0.045)	.005 (0.018)	T > E, E > B, T > B
Old (n = 152)	3.79 (0.76)	3.88 (0.76)	4.02 (0.68)	3.90 (0.64)				T > E, T > B
Total (n = 307)	3.57 (0.85)	3.79 (0.78)	3.92 (0.71)					

SDM shared decision-making, M mean, SD standard deviation, E emoticons, B bar chart, T time-to-event display

[a]η^2 = effect size; 0.01 = small effect; 0.06 = medium effect; 0.14 = large effect

[b]Interaction between age group and display. Significance means that the displays' ratings relate differently to each other in each group

[c]Post-hoc Scheffé pairwise comparisons of display types in case of significant main effect or interaction: > means significantly higher rating

[d]Range 1–5; higher numbers reflect higher perceived ability to motivate patients to participate in SDM, or a higher perceived accessibility, respectively

and Fig. 3). Again, older patients rated all displays higher than younger patients, but this time with a smaller effect. In addition, there was an interaction effect between age and display: both of the two patients groups (young and old) rated the TTE display higher than emoticons and the bar chart. The latter, however, was rated lower than the emoticons by the younger patients. The effect size for this interaction was small.

Discussion

Our results suggest that the displays differently influence the patients' motivation to participate in the SDM process. The novel TTE display showed the highest potential, followed by emoticons and the bar chart. The differences between displays, however, were small. Older patients generally reported a higher motivation for SDM, but there was no difference in how

the displays affected motivation for SDM among older and younger patients. It is notable that the order the displays are ranked (TTE first, followed by emoticons and the bar chart) is the same for "motivation for SDM" and "accessibility" (see Fig. 3).

To date, literature on the effect of TTE predictions on patient decision-making is scarce. In fact, while looking for explanations for the different effects of the displays on the motivation to participate in SDM, we were unable to find any previous work exploring this issue. However, existing literature shows that TTE formats are superior to other formats in terms of a subjective perception of understandability of the presented risk information [28–30].

In a Danish study, participants were asked how difficult it was for them to understand a presented information about a fictional drug treatment postponing heart

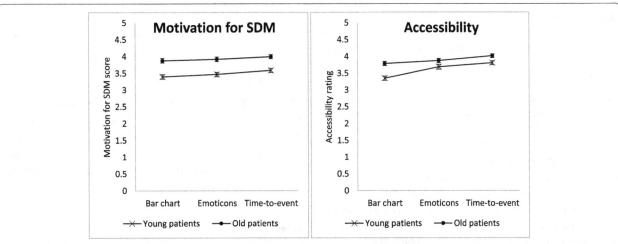

Fig. 3 Motivation for SDM and accessibility ratings of young and old patients for each display. Patient sample was split at the median age (52 years); SDM = shared decision-making

attacks. The information was presented in a verbal TTE format. There was no comparison with another risk format, but overall level of understandability was high with 81% of all participants judging the information as "not difficult to understand" [28].

Another study compared the effects of a hypothetical osteoporosis intervention either presented in numbers-needed-to-treat, or a verbal TTE format, presenting the duration a hip fracture could be postponed. The TTE information was associated with lower subjective uncertainty about the meaning of the presented information [29].

A web-based study presented the benefit of a fictional antibiotic in one of several formats to healthy individuals [30]. Among them was a TTE display that showed the duration of symptoms with and without treatment. It was judged the easiest format to understand.

In summary, these results show that patients prefer risk information presented in a TTE format. Moreover, it was perceived as easier to understand than traditional absolute risk information. It can be assumed that an improved feeling of understanding translates into higher enablement to form a decision and, therefore, a higher motivation to participate in the decision-making process. This might be the case for our results as well.

As demonstrated in Fig. 2, the pattern showing the displays ranking is identical to that for "motivation for SDM" and "accessibility". In this way, the TTE display might elicit the highest motivation to participate in SDM because the feeling of understanding is also highest in the display that is judged as easier to understand. This hypothesis, however, cannot be proven with our results. A future study could include a measurement of enablement or certainty and examine how this is related to the displays and the motivation to participate in SDM.

The fact that older patients rated the displays more accessible and felt more motivated by them in our study can be explained by differences in experience dealing with risk. Since the older patients had significantly more risk factors and, therefore, a longer history of consultations, they might have more background knowledge and thus be more involved and motivated to participate in the decision regarding their health [31].

The lack of interaction between the displays and age might have methodical reasons. Patients were either presented a low, medium, or high-risk scenario, all depicting cases of the same age group (49–50 years old). They were instructed to imagine themselves in the place of the fictional person and answer the questions as if they were that person. Therefore, even if the groups differed in the actual age of the participants, they did not differ in the age of the case vignettes with which participating

patients were expected to identify with. As a result, there might have actually been no difference in subjective risk between the groups and, therefore, no interaction effect. In order to avoid this effect, future investigations based on vignettes should use vignettes featuring different age groups and be compared irrespective of the actual age of the participants. On the positive side, this indicates that patients were able to understand and follow the instructions as we intended.

This study has several limitations. First, even though patients were able to identify with the fictional cases, their involvement might be different when confronted with their own risk and related decisions. Second, for technical reasons we presented the risk information in a paper-based form with a static picture for each display. In reality, the information is presented on a computer screen and can be changed interactively to show differences in risk due to interventions. This could actually lead to a higher participation since the patients can engage more in the process. Third, since there is a lack of scales measuring motivation to participate in SDM, we developed a new scale for this study. Although we achieved good reliability, the actual validity of the scale remains to be shown since we did not use other scales to measure divergent and convergent validity. Ideally the scale would be validated in real-life consultations together with ratings of the actual behaviour and involvement in the decision-making [32]. In our point of view, despite these limitations, the following conclusions can be drawn from our findings.

Conclusions

In a survey of primary care patients, a TTE display increased motivation to participate in decisions regarding cardiovascular risk modification. In this, TTE displays were superior to absolute risk displays such as emoticons and bar charts. Since we asked patients to assess fictional cases, future studies should compare risk displays with patients being informed about their own risk and having to make real life decisions. Since patients also judged the TTE display as easier to understand, more useful and more serious (i.e. more accessible) than emoticons and bar charts, the new TTE display is be a valuable addition to current risk calculators and decision aids.

Abbreviations
CE: General Practitioners; SDM: Shared Decision-Making; TTE: Time-to-event

Acknowledgements

The study was made possible by the participating GPs who generously recruited patients during their everyday tasks. We also thank our research associates Dr. Elisabeth Szabo, Muazzez Ilhan, and Marion Herz-Schuchart for their excellent contribution to recruitment and data collection. We also would like to thank Juliette Rautenberg and Jasmin Buller for providing English-language editing, improving the precision and fluency of the manuscript.

Funding

The German Federal Ministry of Education and Research (Grant #01GX1045) funded the study.

Authors' contributions

Authorship has only been granted to individuals who have contributed substantially to the research and manuscript. All authors have read and approved the final version of the manuscript. NRAJ and MHG have done the statistical work for the project. NRAJ, along with SAK, LKK and CCA, have developed, carried out and coordinated the study design, recruitment, data collection, interpretation, and discussion of the results. UP and NDB were involved in the initial design of the project and the application for funding. Additionally, NDB oversaw the study as head of the department. Besides the authors, two study nurses assisted us in our work by sending out invitation letters, conducting initiation and conclusion visits, and transferring the completed questionnaires into a digital database. All authors read and approved the final manuscript.

Competing interests

NRAJ, SAK, I KK, CCA and MHG were paid by the government grant provided for carrying out the study. UP has nothing to disclose. NDB is on the editorial board of this journal. He is Co-CEO of the Gesellschaft für Patienten-zentrierte Kommunikation (Organization for Patient-centred Communication). This is a registered non-profit entity contracting with health insurers and providers aiming at the dissemination of arriba™ decision support software. He obtains no financial revenue from this organisation apart from travel expenses.

Author details

[1]Department of General Practice and Family Medicine, Philipps-University Marburg, Karl-von-Frisch-Str. 4, 35032 Marburg, Germany. [2]MH Statistical Consulting, Marburg, Germany. [3]Department of Health Services Research, Maastricht University, Maastricht, the Netherlands. [4]Department of General Practice, Georg-August-University, Göttingen, Germany.

References

1. Ludt S, Angelow A, Baum E, Chenot J-F, Donner-Banzhoff N, Egidi G, et al. Hausärztliche Risikoberatung zur kardiovaskulären Prävention: S3-Leitlinie. Berlin; 2017.
2. Goff DC, Lloyd-Jones DM, Bennett G, Coady S, D'Agostino RB, Gibbons R, et al. 2013 ACC/AHA Guideline on the Assessment of Cardiovascular Risk. J Am Coll Cardiol. 2014;63:2935–59. https://doi.org/10.1016/j.jacc.2013.11.005.
3. JBS3 Board. Joint British Societies' consensus recommendations for the prevention of cardiovascular disease (JBS3). Heart. 2014;100(Suppl 2):ii1–ii67. https://doi.org/10.1136/heartjnl-2014-305693.
4. Charles C, Gafni A, Whelan T. Shared decision-making in the medical encounter: what does it mean? (or it takes at least two to tango). Soc Sci Med. 1997;44:681–92. https://doi.org/10.1016/S0277-9536(96)00221-3.
5. Makoul G, Clayman ML. An integrative model of shared decision making in medical encounters. Patient Educ Couns. 2006;60:301–12. https://doi.org/10.1016/j.pec.2005.06.010.
6. Stacey D, Légaré F, Col NF, Bennett CL, Barry MJ, Eden KB, et al. Decision aids for people facing health treatment or screening decisions. In: Stacey D, editor. Cochrane database of systematic reviews. Chichester: John Wiley & Sons, Ltd; 2014. https://doi.org/10.1002/14651858.CD001431.pub4.
7. Garcia-Retamero R, Galesic M. Who profits from visual aids: overcoming challenges in people's understanding of risks corrected. Soc Sci Med. 2010; 70:1019–25. https://doi.org/10.1016/j.socscimed.2009.11.031.
8. Elward KS, Simpson RJ, Mendys P. Improving cardiovascular risk reduction for primary prevention–utility of lifetime risk assessment. Postgrad Med. 2010;122:192–9. https://doi.org/10.3810/pgm.2010.07.2186.
9. Sniderman AD, Toth PP, Thanassoulis G, Pencina MJ, Furberg CD. Taking a longer term view of cardiovascular risk: the causal exposure paradigm. BMJ. 2014;348:g3047. https://doi.org/10.1136/bmj.g3047.
10. Ulrich S. What is the optimal age for starting lipid lowering treatment? A mathematical model. BMJ. 2000;320:1134–40. https://doi.org/10.1136/bmj.320.7242.1134.
11. Marma AK, Berry JD, Ning H, Persell SD, Lloyd-Jones DM. Distribution of 10-year and lifetime predicted risks for cardiovascular disease in US adults: findings from the National Health and nutrition examination survey 2003 to 2006. Circ Cardiovasc Qual Outcomes. 2010;3:8–14. https://doi.org/10.1161/CIRCOUTCOMES.109.869727.
12. Di Castelnuovo A, Costanzo S, Persichillo M, Olivieri M, de Curtis A, Zito F, et al. Distribution of short and lifetime risks for cardiovascular disease in Italians. Eur J Prev Cardiol. 2012;19:723–30. https://doi.org/10.1177/1741826711410820.
13. Krones T, Keller H, Sönnichsen AC, Sadowski EM, Baum E, Donner-Banzhoff N. Partizipative Entscheidungsfindung in der kardiovaskulären Risikoprävention: Ergebnisse der Pilotstudie von ARRIBA-Herz, einer konsultationsbezogenen Entscheidungshilfe für die allgemeinmedizinische Praxis. Z Med Psychol. 2006;15:61–70.
14. Krones T, Keller H, Sonnichsen A, Sadowski E-M, Baum E, Wegscheider K, et al. Absolute cardiovascular disease risk and shared decision making in primary care: a randomized controlled trial. Ann Fam Med. 2008;6:218–27. https://doi.org/10.1370/afm.854.
15. Krones T, Keller H, Becker A, Sönnichsen A, Baum E, Donner-Banzhoff N. The theory of planned behaviour in a randomized trial of a decision aid on cardiovascular risk prevention. Patient Educ Couns. 2010;78:169–76. https://doi.org/10.1016/j.pec.2009.06.010.
16. Sadowski EM, Eimer C, Keller H, Krones T, Sönnichsen AC, Baum E, Donner-Banzhoff N. Evaluation komplexer Interventionen: Implementierung von ARRIBA-Herz , einer Beratungsstrategie für die Herz-Kreislaufprävention. Z Allg Med. 2005;81:429–34. https://doi.org/10.1055/s-2005-872475.
17. Hirner B, Rehwald U, Geserick R. Newsletter Thema Allgemeinmedizin: Gesundheitsforschung. Berlin: Forschung für den Menschen; 2007.
18. D'Agostino RB, Vasan RS, Pencina MJ, Wolf PA, Cobain M, Massaro JM, Kannel WB. General cardiovascular risk profile for use in primary care: the Framingham heart study. Circulation. 2008;117:743–53. https://doi.org/10.1161/CIRCULATIONAHA.107.699579.
19. Donner-Banzhoff N, Popert U. Hausärztliche Beratung zur kardiovaskulären Prävention (Version 4.2). 2007. http://arriba-hausarzt.de/downloads/arriba_broschuere.pdf. Accessed 24 May 2018.
20. Schenk L, Bau A-M, Borde T, Butler J, Lampert T, Neuhauser H, et al. Mindestindikatorensatz zur Erfassung des Migrationsstatus. Bundesgesundheitsblatt-Gesundheitsforschung. 2006;49:853–60. https://doi.org/10.1007/s00103-006-0018-4.
21. Scholl I, MK-v L, Sepucha K, Elwyn G, Légaré F, Härter M, Dirmaier J. Measurement of shared decision making – a review of instruments. Zeitschrift für Evidenz, Fortbildung und Qualität im Gesundheitswesen. 2011;105:313–24. https://doi.org/10.1016/j.zefq.2011.04.012.
22. Simon D, Loh A, Härter M. Measuring (shared) decision-making – a review of psychometric instruments. Z Arztl Fortbild Qualitätssich. 2007;101:259–67. https://doi.org/10.1016/j.zgesun.2007.02.029.
23. Gaissmaier W, Wegwarth O, Skopec D, Müller A-S, Broschinski S, Politi MC. Numbers can be worth a thousand pictures: individual differences in understanding graphical and numerical representations of health-related information. Health Psychol. 2012;31:286–96. https://doi.org/10.1037/a0024850.

24. Faul F, Erdfelder E, Buchner A, Lang A-G. Statistical power analyses using G*power 3.1: tests for correlation and regression analyses. Behav Res Methods. 2009;41:1149–60. https://doi.org/10.3758/BRM.41.4.1149.

25. Cohen J. Statistical power analysis. Curr Dir Psychol Sci. 1992;1:98–101. https://doi.org/10.1111/1467-8721.ep10768783.

26. IBM Corp. IBM SPSS Statistics for Windows. Armonk: IBM Corp.; 2012.

27. Cronbach LJ. Coefficient alpha and the internal structure of tests. Psychometrika. 1951;16:297–334. https://doi.org/10.1007/BF02310555.

28. Dahl R, Gyrd-Hansen D, Kristiansen IS, Nexøe J, Bo Nielsen J. Can postponement of an adverse outcome be used to present risk reductions to a lay audience? A population survey. BMC Med Inform Decis Mak. 2007;7: 8. https://doi.org/10.1186/1472-6947-7-8.

29. Christensen P. A randomized trial of laypersons' perception of the benefit of osteoporosis therapy: number needed to treat versus postponement of hip fracture. Clin Ther. 2003;25:2575–85. https://doi.org/10.1016/S0149-2918(03)80318-1.

30. Carling CLL, Kristoffersen DT, Flottorp S, Fretheim A, Oxman AD, Schünemann HJ, et al. The effect of alternative graphical displays used to present the benefits of antibiotics for sore throat on decisions about whether to seek treatment: a randomized trial. PLoS Med. 2009;6:e1000140. https://doi.org/10.1371/journal.pmed.1000140.

31. Say R, Murtagh M, Thomson R. Patients' preference for involvement in medical decision making: a narrative review. Patient Educ Couns. 2006;60: 102–14. https://doi.org/10.1016/j.pec.2005.02.003.

32. Kasper J, Hoffmann F, Heesen C, Köpke S, Geiger F, Reindl M. MAPPIN'SDM – the multifocal approach to sharing in shared decision making. PLoS One. 2012;7:e34849. https://doi.org/10.1371/journal.pone.0034849.

7

Patients' experiences of motivation, change, and challenges in group treatment for insomnia in primary care

Christina Sandlund[1,2*], Kimberly Kane[1,2,3], Mirjam Ekstedt[4,5] and Jeanette Westman[1,2]

Abstract

Background: The majority of patients who seek help for insomnia do so in primary health care. Nurse-led group treatment in primary care based on cognitive behavioral therapy for insomnia (CBT-I) can lead to improvements in both day- and nighttime symptoms. This study aimed to explore patients' experiences of nurse-led group treatment for insomnia in primary health care.

Methods: Seventeen patients who had participated in the group treatment program were interviewed in five focus groups. Interview transcriptions were analyzed with qualitative content analysis.

Results: Four themes emerged that described patients' experiences of the group treatment program. *Involvement and trust open the door for change*: Motivation to engage in treatment arose from patients' own desire for change, from being together with others who shared or understood their struggles, and from feeling emotionally affirmed and trustful. *Competence arising from deeper understanding*: Patients obtained knowledge and made it their own, which enabled them to develop functional sleep habits and let go of sleep performance and worry. The ability to impact their insomnia increased patients' trust in their own efficacy and helped them persist in behavioral change. *Struggling with vulnerability and failure*: Treatment was tough, and patients could feel challenged by external circumstances. Moreover, they could distrust their own efficacy. *Tailoring treatment to individual needs*: Patients experienced different life circumstances and adapted the techniques to their needs and abilities by focusing on what felt right for them.

Conclusions: Patients went through a process of motivation, change, and challenges. They experienced certain aspects of treatment as essential to changing behavior and achieving improvements. Examples included being in a group with others who shared similar experiences, gaining knowledge about sleep, keeping a sleep diary, and practicing the sleep restriction technique. The study provides insights into patients' struggles during treatment, both those related to external circumstances and those related to feelings of vulnerability and failure. It also highlights the importance of adapting treatment to patients' differing needs, underscoring the value of person-centered care.

Keywords: Behavioral change, General practice, Group therapy, Health behavior, Motivation, Nursing, Patient education, Self-efficacy, Sleep initiation and maintenance disorders

* Correspondence: christina.sandlund@ki.se
[1]Department of Neurobiology, Care Sciences and Society, Karolinska Institutet, Stockholm, Sweden
[2]Academic Primary Health Care Centre, Stockholm County Council, Solnavägen 1 E, Box 45436, 104 31 Stockholm, Sweden
Full list of author information is available at the end of the article

Background

Sleep plays a vital role in good health and well-being and living with insomnia affects overall health. Its impact on health is reflected in physical and mental illnesses, cognitive decline, and reduced quality of life [1–3]. Nine to 15% of people worldwide have insomnia [4, 5], which is experiential in nature and diagnosed on the basis of a person's own perceptions of sleeping difficulties and the daytime impairments they associate with these difficulties [6, 7]. Qualitative studies show that people who live with insomnia can experience impaired cognitive, emotional, and physical functioning on a daily basis, as well as limitations in work performance, social participation, and life aspirations [8]. It is these experiences that cause people to seek treatment, typically in primary care [9]. Patients who seek primary health care for insomnia commonly receive hypnotic drugs even though the recommended treatment is cognitive behavioral therapy for insomnia (CBT-I) [10, 11].

Because of the experiential nature of insomnia, qualitative evaluations can provide insight into treatments that quantitative evaluations cannot, illuminating patients' experiences of the treatment, symptom change or stability, and processes through which improvements did or did not occur. Such explanations for how and why psychological and behavioral treatments work are important, as a better understanding of key mechanisms can facilitate the design of more effective and efficient therapies [12, 13].

Few studies have explored patients' experiences of insomnia treatment. Most qualitative studies on insomnia focus on people's experiences of living with the disorder, professionals' experiences of treating patients with insomnia, and patients' experiences of health care professionals' attitudes toward the disorder and its treatment [14]. However, one study has explored patients' experiences of long-term treatment with hypnotic drugs [15]; another, patients' experiences of mindfulness-based group treatment for insomnia [16]; and a third, patients' experiences of sleep restriction therapy, one technique included in CBT-I [17]. On the other hand, there have been numerous explorations of patients' experiences of individual psychotherapy for problems other than insomnia [18]. Some have focused on experiences of treatment-related change [19, 20] and others on helpful [21, 22] or unhelpful aspects of treatment [23, 24].

Although CBT-I is the recommended treatment for insomnia, primary care patients' access to it is limited. We therefore conducted a randomized control trial in Swedish primary health care to investigate whether a nurse-led, CBT-I based group treatment program for insomnia could be effective in treating patients with insomnia who seek primary care [25]. The 2011-2104 trial included 165 patients with insomnia aged 20 to 90 years (mean age

54 years), mostly women (72.7%). Analyses showed that the group treatment significantly improved insomnia symptoms (insomnia severity, sleep, and daytime symptoms), and decreased hypnotic drug use [25, 26]. However, some patients improved more than others, and some may not have improved at all. Because qualitative approaches can illuminate the lived experiences behind quantitative results [27], we reasoned that a qualitative study could potentially reveal patients' experiences of key mechanisms that underlay the quantitative findings, helping us improve the efficiency of the intervention.

In the present study, we thus aimed to explore patients' experiences of the nurse-led group treatment program for insomnia in primary health care.

Methods

Study design

We performed focus group interviews with patients who had participated in the nurse-led group treatment program for insomnia in primary health care. The interviews took place in Stockholm County, Sweden, from 2013 to 2015. Focus groups promote the expression of differing views, which can lead to further discussion and exploration of experiences [28]. Qualitative content analysis as described by Graneheim and Lundman was used to analyze the interviews [29, 30]. This method is appropriate for illuminating lived experience and has a well-defined analytical process and clear concepts for discussing trustworthiness [30].

Participants

Seventeen patients who had taken part in the group treatment program participated in this study. To participate in group treatment, patients had to be 18 years or older and meet the criteria for insomnia disorder [31]. Inclusion and exclusion criteria are described in detail elsewhere [25]. Patients who participated in the focus group interviews had been in the control group in the randomized controlled trial [25] and received treatment as usual (mainly hypnotic drugs) while waiting three to 4 months for group treatment.

All focus-group participants had attended treatment together and thus knew one another. We expected patients' shared experiences of treatment and familiarity with each other to facilitate group discussions [28]. All patients who participated in treatment between 2013 and 2015 were asked to take part in the focus groups (n = 23).

Five focus groups were conducted. Each group included three or four patients, and all were women. Their median age was 57.9 years (25 to 75 years). Nine were employed and eight were retired. Their mean Insomnia Severity Index score before treatment was 18.9 (range

14-25; possible scores 0-28) [32]. Scores above 11 indicate clinical insomnia [33].

Five patients (four women and one man) who had participated in the group treatment did not take part in the interviews. Three were sick on the day of the interview, one was traveling, and one was taking care of a sick relative.

Group treatment program for insomnia

Patients met at their primary health care center for seven 2-h group treatment sessions over the course of 10 weeks. The first six sessions were weekly and were followed by a final session 4 weeks later. The group treatment program was based on the theoretical framework and techniques of CBT-I [32, 34–36]. CBT-I targets mental and physical hyperarousal, maladaptive cognitions (e.g., rumination), and maladaptive behaviors (e.g., irregular sleep habits) [37]. It includes educational components and behavioral and cognitive techniques that aim to change these cognitions and behaviors, improve sleep, and increase ability to cope with insomnia [38].

Educational components of the program included information about sleep and sleep regulation and theoretical frameworks for understanding insomnia. Patients kept a sleep diary throughout the program and used their entries as the basis of reflections during group sessions. At each session, the nurse who led the group introduced one or more techniques that patients applied as homework between the sessions (relaxation, worry time, paradoxical intention, sleep restriction, stimulus control, reduction of hypnotic drugs, sleep hygiene, identifying and arguing against unhelpful thoughts, stress reducing techniques, and techniques to cope with daytime symptoms). At the last session, each patient identified treatment gains and created an individual program to prevent relapse and maintain benefits. A comprehensive description of the treatment program is found elsewhere [25].

The nurses who led the groups were district nurses, registered nurses with a 1-year master's degree in primary health care nursing. Together with physicians, district nurses make up the largest group of professionals in Swedish primary care. In partnership with patients and in close collaboration with other health care professionals, they work to meet patients' basic needs (e.g., sleep and rest), promoting health, preventing illness, and alleviating suffering [39]. The nurses who led the treatment program had taken part in a 16-h training course that covered the causes and diagnosis of insomnia and how to deliver the treatment. None had previous experience of CBT-I, but all were experienced in nursing (median 29 years).

Focus group interviews

Each interview took place at the end of the last treatment session (session seven). In two of the focus groups (groups 2 and 5), the moderator was also the nurse who had led the treatment sessions (CS). In the other groups, the nurse who led the group left prior to the start of the interview. Each interview took approximately 70 min and was audio recorded and transcribed verbatim.

The moderator (CS) used a semi-structured interview guide with open-ended questions. The guide was developed for the study. The interview started with opening questions, such as "Can you tell me about how it was before you started the group treatment?" and "Can you tell me about a night, how it was, how it felt, how it affected you during the day, and what you did so you could sleep?" The moderator then used the following questions to guide the interviews: 1) "How do you experience your sleep after the treatment?" 2) "Is there anything special that helped you?" 3) "What changes have you made?" 4) "What was it that got you to make these changes?" 5) "Was there something that didn't work so well?" 6) "Was there something about the treatment that you thought was hard? That didn't fit you? Why do you think that was?" and 7) "What do you think could be done to improve this program?" Probing questions and statements were used to clarify or deepen the discussion, including, "What did you do then?" "What could have helped you to act or feel otherwise?" "What do you think that was due to?" and "Tell me more about that."

Data analysis

The transcriptions were analyzed using qualitative content analysis [30]. Patients' experiences were explored at a manifest and descriptive level close to the text and a latent, more abstract and interpretative level [29, 30].

We took an inductive approach [40], generating our ideas on the basis of the interview texts. In the beginning of the process, we read the texts several times to get a sense of the whole. After reading, we divided the text into meaning units that were relevant to the aim. Next, we shortened the meaning units to condensed meaning units, taking care to preserve the core meaning and context. These condensed meaning units were labeled with codes that expressed the content of the meaning unit. The codes were then sorted on the basis of similarities and differences and abstracted into conceptual categories. Twelve subthemes emerged from the categories and were abstracted to four themes that captured the essence of patients' experiences of the group treatment for insomnia. Throughout the entire analytical process, we moved back and forth among all levels of analysis, from the original text to the themes.

The researchers took several steps to achieve trustworthiness. CS and KK each conducted their own initial coding and analysis of the transcribed interviews before coming together to compare their findings. All researchers engaged in ongoing discussion and reflection throughout the process of analysis until consensus was reached. Prior understanding of insomnia, nursing, and the intervention were important topics of the ongoing discussions throughout the entire analytical process.

Results

Four themes emerged that described patients' experiences of the group treatment: involvement and trust open the door for change, competence arising from deeper understanding, struggling with vulnerability and failure, and tailoring treatment to individual needs. The themes and the subthemes that lay behind them are presented in Table 1.

Involvement and trust open the door for change
Desiring positive change

Patients experienced a desire for positive change grounded partly in health concerns, such as the belief that high blood pressure could be a result of insomnia. The non-pharmacological nature of the treatment could also lie behind patients' engagement. They said that it felt appealing that the group treatment addressed their overall problem and that they saw the opportunity to escape the need to take hypnotic drugs for their entire life. Moreover, patients described having come to the end of their rope. They felt they had tried everything, and it had not solved the problem.

I think it was that I gave up, that I'm so tired of it, and that it's gone on so awfully many years, and that I felt that I had tried everything except the strongest

Table 1 Overview of subthemes and themes

Subthemes	Themes
Desiring positive change	Involvement and trust open the door for change
Being together with others pushes you forward	
Feeling emotionally affirmed and trustful	
Obtaining knowledge and making it your own	Competence arising from deeper understanding
Developing functional sleep habits	
Letting go of sleep performance and worry	
Trusting in own efficacy	
Finding treatment tough	Struggling with vulnerability and failure
Challenged by external circumstances	
Distrusting own efficacy	
Experiencing different life circumstances	Tailoring treatment to individual needs
Focusing on what feels right	

sleeping pills. That yeah, now it's the last chance, like: let's do this. (Patient [P] 3, Group [G] 5)

Moreover, patients felt a commitment to themselves. Once they chose to do something about their problem, they felt obligated to follow through.

Being together with others pushes you forward

Patients described how meeting in person and having someone who led them was supportive. It pushed them forward, helping them initiate and persist in behavioral change. They also felt a commitment to the group which pushed them toward behavioral change.

And once you've started in this kind of a group, you can't let it down. Instead, you have to do your bit. If you had done it by yourself, you might have thought that no, this was too tough. But if you start it, you have to complete it, so to speak. (P1, G2)

Feeling emotionally affirmed and trustful

Patients found that living with insomnia in a world of good sleepers could be lonely; meeting others who had the same problem or who understood it made them feel less "weird." In the group treatment context, where they were surrounded by people who knew what it was like to live with insomnia, the patients felt understood and less lonely: "We, like, experienced each other's wakeful nights and everyone just, 'God, I know, I know, it's terrible, it's terrible!' And then when someone had slept more, it was like everyone just, 'Oh, it's unbelievable, oh!'" (P3, G3). Patients also experienced engagement, both from other group members and the group leader, and thus felt taken care of and seen. The small size of the groups helped patients feel heard. Feeling involved and feeling that others were involved helped them go on with treatment.

Trust in authorities (society, primary health care, and primary health care professionals) helped motivate patients to take part in the treatment. As the primary health care center was offering this program, they thought it must be good. Moreover, patients found it convenient and motivating to meet at their own health care center because they felt at home there. If their doctor had suggested the treatment, patients wanted to follow their doctor's advice. Their trust in the group leader let them dare to "go for it" and try new behaviors.

Competence arising from deeper understanding
Obtaining knowledge and making it your own

Patients experienced knowledge as a key ingredient in treatment. They gained this knowledge via the educational components of the treatment and particularly highlighted the importance of learning about sleep and how it works. Patients said they were familiar with some of the information presented but came to understand it at a deeper level during the course of treatment.

The introduction of techniques one at a time kept patients from feeling overwhelmed, and by practicing the techniques, patients learned what worked for them. This kind of learning by doing allowed them to try new paths and break old patterns. Their intellectual learning was strengthened by the bodily experience that came as a result of practicing the techniques, which confirmed what they had learned about the sleep process. One patient expressed it this way: "You got your body to cooperate purely physically, it wasn't just up here, instead the physical, too, that got you to understand, your body to understand" (P2, G2).

Patients described how repeating and discussing information and practicing techniques over the 10-week treatment period helped them process the information and achieve deeper understanding. By sharing experiences with each other, the patients gained new perspectives: "It's a little like brain washing. You repeat things, and we sit here, and you tell us, and we talk about it here, and then we repeat things the whole time. And finally, it sinks in somehow" (P1, G3).

Moreover, patients said they gained perspective and achieved insight by reflecting on their own thinking and behavior. For instance, one described the realization that it was her mind rather than her body that caused her sleep problems. The techniques of worry time and identifying and arguing against unhelpful thoughts helped patients in this process. Additionally, keeping a sleep diary helped the patients reach a deeper level of understanding by giving them an overview of their behavior. "It's the sleep diary, I feel, that makes it sink in. Because you document it. And you see some kind overarching picture of your behavior. Otherwise you just muddle around" (P3, G3).

Developing functional sleep habits

Patients described achieving more functional sleep habits during treatment. Practicing techniques (e.g., sleep restriction) enabled them to break old patterns of unhelpful sleep habits, and by trying out what worked for them, they began to adopt new sleep habits in their daily lives. One of these was a more regular sleep schedule. Another was spending less time in bed. They felt that these new habits consolidated their sleep, and that the more efficient sleep meant they were not as tired during the day.

> Sleep quality has become totally different. I'm up at over 80% [sleep efficiency] now. I'm really very satisfied about this, and I go to bed, somehow, I've found that I got to bed between 12:00 and 1:00 and

usually wake up around 6:00. And it works, and I'm not tired during the day. (P4, G3)

They found that spending less time awake in bed left less room for worry and rumination and talked about how going to bed later felt liberating and gave them more spare time. Patients also cut down on the time they spent sleeping during the afternoon. Instead they took short daytime naps. These naps could have a positive impact on nighttime sleep and could make them feel more alert. Moreover, taking short naps facilitated a more regular nighttime sleep schedule and reduced worry.

> Yeah, that power nap is probably pretty good for me. It feels like a little reward there in the middle of the day before 3:00, that, "Now I'm actually a little tired. I do this now, and I'll feel better. When I pick up the grandkids, then I'm a little more alert." (P3, G2)

Letting go of sleep performance and worry

Patients talked about how they became able to dedramatize sleep and insomnia by accepting the situation and letting go of the idea that they had to force themselves to sleep. By gaining perspective on their sleep problems, the pressure they put on themselves to achieve perfect sleep diminished. For instance, one said, "'Screw it, I don't have the energy to be angry anymore.' And then it just let go, there was something that let go then" (P2, G2). Patients also grew more relaxed in their attitudes toward feelings of tiredness and sleepiness. They talked about how before group treatment, tiredness and sleepiness felt entirely negative. Now these feelings were less like enemies and more like allies that could help them sleep well. Moreover, they were able to let go of sleep-related worries because their perspectives on sleep had become more relaxed.

> It was a really big relief for me, this insight that it's not dangerous to lie awake, and it's not dangerous if I only got five hours. It's given me a much more relaxed way to handle it all. So it made a really big difference. Because before I could stress myself: "God, now I'm going to get a migraine. Oh God, oh!" I lay there and my thoughts ran around in circles and got more and more irritated and stressed that I couldn't sleep, and then of course you can't sleep. I often lay awake like that. But I think that that this part has been a huge ah-ha help for me. (P4, G4)

Knowing that they had strategies reduced worry. For instance, one patient said that just knowing she could choose to get up for a while if she could not sleep made her less worried about sleeplessness. Moreover, the relaxation exercise helped patients achieve mental and bodily relaxation, and worry time helped them gain perspective on worry. Patients said they developed routines, and in doing so, experienced how the routines let the body meet its needs, which in turn made it easier to handle worry and relax. Developing routines resulted in a more regular amount of sleep every night, which gave patients a feeling of flow and energy. They could experience relief by focusing on practical matters rather than feelings and relying on routines instead of trying so hard emotionally.

P3: But now I have a good flow, I sleep. I have these routines. Then maybe I don't sleep so much, it's just five hours, but even so, it's given me some kind of overall energy that's good. . . . So that's what I feel, that during the actual night I've been able to handle my worry a little more, thanks to the fact that my body got its needs met with routines and all. It's been a nice insight—that like the body needs its harmony.

P2: The body really likes its routines. That's become really clear.

P3: Exactly. The body likes it, and it also becomes, it's nice that you don't need to influence everything, to strain your brain the whole time.

P2: Exactly. That's what I think, too.

P3: There's so much of that the whole time. That you can also affect things. I like sleep restriction. It's a good thing. (G5)

Trusting in own efficacy

Patients described an increased trust in their own efficacy. They experienced the power to act and positive feelings that were related to doing what they could: "Every time you manage to change something, you feel more like life is in your own hands" (P3, G3). Patients achieved trust in their own ability to sleep, including their body's ability to take care of its sleep needs. They found that their bodies could actually produce better sleep than drugs could, which increased their trust in their own efficacy. Patients experienced trust in the techniques; they said they felt confident in having strategies that worked. They found it helpful that the sleep restriction technique was introduced early in the treatment. It quickly had a positive effect on sleep, and the patients felt that this put them on the right track. Once they were on the right track, experiencing that "it

worked" motivated them to keep going. One put it like this: "It's obvious. When you notice it's going this way, you keep going" (P3, G4).

Struggling with vulnerability and failure
Finding treatment tough

Patients described how fear of sleeplessness and frustration about sleeplessness could interfere with the ability to stop trying to force sleep to come, to relax, and to take action and use the techniques they had learned. Physical tiredness and mental exhaustion could make it more difficult to handle problems: "It's hard to deal with things like this when you're already tired and exhausted, so then you're also more sensitive" (P2, G5).

Some difficulties were related to the sleep restriction technique, which limited patients' hours in bed and initially caused sleep deprivation, making it difficult to adhere to the technique. One patient explained: "I was going to go to bed at 1:00 at night and get up at 6:00. But I tried to keep to that as well as I could, but it hasn't gone very well for me. I was really tired sometimes, and I've gone to bed a little earlier" (P3, G1).

Challenged by external circumstances

Patients described how circumstances outside their control could make it difficult to put the techniques into practice. For instance, one patient had problems with pain. Another explained that her partner was unstable on his feet. She had trouble relaxing, as he got up several times a night and she was worried that he might fall. The environment could also make it challenging to use techniques. If it was hectic and noisy at work, for example, it could be difficult use the relaxation exercise.

The strict routines that came with sleep restriction could make it difficult to live a life that included spontaneous social events, such as staying up late with friends and/or sleeping over at someone else's house. One patient said that the late bedtime made her start eating during the evening, which she experienced as a problem.

Distrusting own efficacy

Patients could express feelings of uncertainty. They described how techniques that usually worked sometimes might not, for instance in extra stressful situations. "Like last week, work was like a disaster with tons of conflicts and pressure, and then I can lie down and breathe as much as I want, but it [relaxation] won't come" (P2, G5). Even though patients found techniques for coping with worry helpful, it might tend to come back. Moreover, they could feel that improvements were fragile and the future uncertain: "It feels fragile. What if it comes back, that it starts to be hard to sleep?" (P1, G5).

Patients could also express feelings of helplessness and failure, for example if they felt they had not improved as much as others or had not reached their own treatment goals. They could find that even though they did everything right, their situation did not improve. For instance, one said that even though she had no specific worries and had adopted functional sleep habits, her sleep did not get better. She attributed this failure to improve to herself: "So I don't have any reasonable explanation except that there's something that's wrong in my brain" (P1, G2).

Tailoring treatment to individual needs
Experiencing different life circumstances
Depending on their life circumstances, patients could view techniques as more or less important. For example, those who worked sometimes wanted more discussion about how to cope with stress, whereas those who were retired might not recognize themselves in the discussion about stress. Moreover, patients could find it stressful to repeatedly leave work early to get to the treatment sessions on time. On the other hand, some could find the multiple short sessions comfortable.

Focusing on what feels right
Patients felt they had the freedom to choose from a smorgasbord of techniques that included something for everyone: "But we've been helped by so many different things, too. So it's probably that everyone, yeah, everyone can, like, find something" (P3, G3). They focused on what felt right for them, trying things out, choosing what suited them, and using techniques in the way that worked for them. They adapted and adjusted the techniques to fit their own needs, life situations, abilities, and inclinations. Patients also described how the group leader adapted the techniques to fit the needs and circumstances of each individual. For example, patients felt that adjustments to the sleep restriction schedule made it easier to adhere to sleep restriction.

Discussion
This qualitative analysis revealed four themes that illuminate patients' experiences of a nurse-led group treatment for insomnia in primary health care [25]: involvement and trust open the door for change, competence arising from deeper understanding, struggling with vulnerability and failure, and tailoring treatment to individual needs. To the best of our knowledge, this is the first study to investigate patients' experiences of multi-component CBT-I-based group treatment for insomnia.

Discussion of findings in relation to previous research
Readiness for change can be an important step toward change [41]. In this study, patients started treatment with a desire for change, and this desire may have influenced their engagement in the treatment and their ability to achieve improvements [42, 43]. Patients described how they felt "strange," "weird," and "lonely" in a world of "good sleepers." Such feelings of isolation and alienation have been described previously by people living with insomnia [8]. In the current study, important motivators for engaging in behavioral change were feeling that you were not alone in your problems and that you had the support of other group members who shared the experience of living with insomnia. These findings echo those of previous studies of patients' experiences of mindfulness-based group treatment for insomnia [16] and of group treatment for health problems other than insomnia (obesity and diabetes) [44, 45]. Moreover, in our study, patients found that the engagement and understanding of the group leader motivated them to try new behaviors. The importance of a trustful relationship with care providers for behavioral change and health outcomes is well known, both from qualitative [16, 18] and quantitative studies [46, 47].

Our finding that the group format was important to behavioral change is in line with the findings of previous studies [48, 49]. A set of therapeutic or curative factors common to group therapy seem to be the main mechanisms behind such change [50], and many of these factors are recognizable in our findings. They include being in a safe and secure environment in which people can both listen and be heard; feelings of involvement, trust, and validation; recognizing that one's own experiences are similar to those of others; becoming more optimistic about one's own chances of success after witnessing the success of others; learning by observing the journeys of other group members; gaining knowledge from the group members and leader; gaining insight through the feedback of others; and gaining insight into what lies behind one's own feelings and behaviors [50].

Educational theory posits that lived experience is crucial to learning [51] and that learners move from gaining fact-based knowledge through experience and reflection to deeper understanding and the ability to broadly apply what they have learned [52]. Consistent with educational theory, patients in our study experienced knowledge as essential to behavioral change. They described how repeated information and discussion, shared experiences, keeping a sleep diary, and bodily experience that came from practicing techniques facilitated a deeper understanding of sleep and their own behaviors. Previous studies of group treatment [45] and of individual treatment [18] have also found that such deeper understanding facilitates behavioral change. Like our findings and in keeping with educational theory, the findings of a previous study of sleep restriction underscore the role that bodily experience plays in deeper understanding [17].

Similar to the patients in our study, patients in that study found that sleep restriction led to bodily experiences congruent with what they had learned about sleep and noticed the quality of their sleep was better.

In the present study, patients' deeper understanding of sleep and of their own behaviors made them feel competent. Feelings of competence helped patients relax and let go of sleep performance and worry, develop more regular sleep habits, and reduce the time they spent in bed. These findings are clinically important because worry—especially worry about sleep—perpetuates insomnia by inducing maladaptive sleep behaviors aimed at achieving sleep and avoiding sleeplessness, such as spending extra time in bed [34].

Our findings that feelings of involvement, trust, and competence were important to motivation and to patients' success in changing their behaviors are consistent with behavioral theory [53, 54]. These feelings are similar to those of autonomy, relatedness, and competence described in self-determination theory as crucial to the intrinsic motivation that allows people to take action and persist in behavioral change [54]. Moreover, according to the theory of self-efficacy, feelings of competence are important to motivation, and self-efficacy is crucial to how people choose to act and how they cope with challenges [53].

In addition to feeling involved, trustful, and competent, patients could also struggle with feelings of vulnerability and failure. Some vulnerabilities may have been related to insomnia. When they choose to seek help for insomnia in primary care, people have typically passed a certain threshold of symptomatology. Specifically, problems with fatigue and psychological distress are often the experiences that prompt people to seek help [9]. Some patients in the present study felt distressed because they thought they might get too little sleep. Obtaining a good night's sleep is often a major concern for people with insomnia, and this concern helps maintain the disorder [55].

People's confidence in their coping abilities affects their emotional reactions to difficult situations [53]. In the current study, some patients lacked confidence that the techniques would work for them or that they would be able to use what they learned; these patients expressed feelings of helplessness and failure. Patients with poor confidence in their coping ability might also feel less motivated to try to change their behaviors and to persist in behavioral change [54].

Sleep restriction is one of the most potent techniques in CBT-I [56]. In the present study, patients were mostly positive toward sleep restriction, but it could pose challenges. For instance, the limited sleep that came with the technique caused mental and physical tiredness, side effects that have been described previously [17, 57]. Like

our study, an earlier study found that challenges to practicing sleep restriction also included experiences of negative impact on functioning, difficulties managing sleepiness prior to bedtime, boredom during extra hours awake, and changes in appetite/hunger [17]. In addition to these challenges, we found that sleep restriction could affect patients' social life because of its inflexibility.

Patients used the techniques that felt right for them and adapted these techniques as needed. Like the findings of the current study, the findings of a qualitative meta-analysis of patients' experiences of psychotherapy highlighted how important it was for patients to feel free to adjust techniques to their individual needs [18]. In our study, group leaders' adaptation of sleep restriction to patients' needs helped patients overcome barriers posed by this challenging technique. Patients who perceive fewer barriers to sleep restriction are more likely to continue practicing it [58].

Finally, the importance of adjusting techniques to the individual underscores the value of person-centered care. In person-centered care, one of the core competencies in nursing, the patient is viewed as an expert on her or his own experiences and everyday life [59]. Person-centered care can empower patients [60] by helping them feel able to make autonomous decisions about their self-management [61].

Clinical implications

This study suggests ways in which the group treatment program for insomnia might be refined to better suit primary health care patients. Our findings indicate that certain aspects of the treatment program helped patients feel motivated and helped them achieve improvements. These included a group of people that shared the experience of insomnia, an involved and engaged leader, meeting at a convenient and trusted location, educational components, the sleep diary, regular meetings, and stepwise introduction and practice of techniques. Certain techniques seemed to be particularly helpful; for instance, sleep restriction, the relaxation exercise, power naps, reduction of hypnotic drugs, and techniques related to worry (worry time and identifying and arguing against negative thoughts).

Our findings also indicate that participation might be facilitated by fewer weekly treatment sessions. However, patients' worries about future relapse suggest that follow-up sessions might be a helpful addition to the program.

Finally, the study provides insight into challenges related to treatment. Many of the challenges experienced by patients may be inevitable because they are related to insomnia itself (e.g., worry about sleep, tiredness, and a lack of confidence in the ability to sleep), and confronting them is a part of treatment. Other challenges are inherent in the techniques but can be minimized by adjusting the techniques to the individual. Still other challenges may arise from the group format. For instance, group leaders should keep in mind that comparing oneself to others is not always helpful. Whereas some people in the group may feel encouraged by such comparison, others can feel they have failed and even blame themselves for their perceived failure.

Methodological discussion

A number of aspects of the study affected its trustworthiness. The atmosphere in the focus groups was relaxed, and it was clear that the patients felt familiar with each other. The participation of three to four patients in each focus group enabled each person to contribute to the discussion. However, larger focus groups might have offered more opportunities for active group interaction [62].

In qualitative analysis, data saturation is reached when new data no longer add novel information, but there is no consensus on how to determine when saturation has been achieved [63, 64]. In the current study, repeated interviews [65] were not carried out; we interviewed all the groups that were ongoing at the time of the study. However, the study had a relatively narrow aim, and sample specificity was high: all participants had experiences of the explored phenomenon. Moreover, we judge the dialogues to have been strong and data to have been rich within and across groups. Patients expressed a variety of experiences, characterized by both similarities and differences. We thus judge the study to have an adequate sample size in relation to information power [64]. Study findings were not presented to the study participants for validation [66].

In two of the five groups, the researcher who conducted the interview was also the group leader and had guided the participants through group treatment. This may be a limitation if patients felt they had to be particularly polite or focus on positive experiences. On the other hand, it may have helped patients feel secure because they knew the interviewer had followed their treatment process.

The prior understanding of two of the researchers was high, as they had previously led insomnia groups. Such prior understanding may have limited the analyses by affecting the interpretation of the data [67]. However, it may also have strengthened the study by conferring a deeper understanding of the explored context. To reduce the analytical limitations caused by prior understanding, all four authors participated actively in the analytical process, which involved ongoing discussion and reflection until consensus was reached. One of the authors of this study (KK) is bilingual; English is her native language. The others, like the patients, are native speakers

of Swedish. KK and CS continuously discussed the coding with each other and collaborated to translate the condensed meaning units, quotations, codes, categories, subthemes, and themes. This increased the trustworthiness of the findings.

All interview participants were women, in part because of the distribution of insomnia in the general population [5] and in part because the majority of patients in the trial from which participants came were women (73%) [25]. It is possible that men would have experienced the group treatment differently or expressed their experiences in a different way.

The patients who were interviewed had participated voluntarily in and completed the group treatment. Many had waited for this treatment for more than 3 months, and none who had waited dropped out once they started. They were thus a selected and highly motivated group. Readers should take this into account when judging the transferability of the results. However, previous studies of treatments that encourage behavioral change have found experiences that are reflected in our findings. Thus, the findings of the current study may be relevant to other, similar treatment contexts.

Conclusions

This study illuminated patients' experiences of a nurse-led group treatment program for insomnia in primary health care. Patients described a process of motivation, change, and challenges. They experienced certain components as particularly important to motivation for behavioral change and for achieving improvements. Examples include meeting at a trusted and convenient location (the patients' own primary health care center), being part of a group of people who shared similar experiences, gaining knowledge about sleep and insomnia, keeping a sleep diary, and practicing the sleep restriction technique. Moreover, this study highlights the importance of adapting treatment to differing needs and abilities and underscores the value of person-centered care. Finally, accessibility to treatment may be facilitated by fewer treatment sessions. These findings should be taken into account in future versions of the program.

Abbreviations
CBT-I: Cognitive behavioral therapy for insomnia; G: Group; P: Patient

Acknowledgements
The authors thank the patients who participated in the interviews, as well as the participating primary health care centers. We also thank Rebecca Popenoe, PhD, for useful input during the early stage of the analysis.

Funding
JW thanks the Stockholm County Council for funding the project (Public Health Grant, PPG, and Pickup). The funding body played no role in the design of the study; in the collection, analysis, and interpretation of data; or in writing the manuscript.

Authors' contributions

CS, ME, and JW planned the study. CS conducted the interviews. All authors contributed to the analysis and interpretation of the data. CS and KK performed the initial coding and data analysis and drafted the manuscript. All authors revised the manuscript critically for important intellectual content and approved the final version for publication.

Authors' information

CS, JW, and ME are registered nurses. CS and JW are also district nurses; JW and ME have formal training in cognitive behavioral therapy. KK is trained in qualitative methods and is a scientific writer. CS and ME have experience leading insomnia groups. JW and KK have no such experience.

Ethics approval and consent to participate

Ethical approval for the focus group interviews was obtained from the Regional Ethics Review Board in Stockholm (Dnr: 2013/484-32). This approval was obtained as a supplement to the approval for the randomized controlled trial of nurse-led group treatment for insomnia in primary health care (Dnr. 2011/194-31/1). The trial and focus group interviews were performed in accordance with the Declaration of Helsinki [68].
Patients provided written informed consent to participate in the trial, and 4 weeks prior to the last group treatment session and the interviews, a letter with information about the purpose of the focus group study was sent to each patient. The letter explained that if any of the invited patients declined to take part in the interview, the last session would proceed without the interview. It also stated that the interview, recording, and transcription would be treated confidentially and that patients could discontinue participation in the interview at any time without providing a reason and without any consequences for their care. The first author phoned the patients to confirm that they had received the study information and give them the opportunity to ask questions. Verbal informed consent was recorded at the beginning of the interview.

Competing interests

The authors declare that they have no competing interests.

Author details

[1]Department of Neurobiology, Care Sciences and Society, Karolinska Institutet, Stockholm, Sweden. [2]Academic Primary Health Care Centre, Stockholm County Council, Solnavägen 1 E, Box 45436, 104 31 Stockholm, Sweden. [3]Aging Research Center, Karolinska Institutet and Stockholm University, Stockholm, Sweden. [4]Department of Health and Caring Sciences, Linnaeus University, Stagneliusgatan 14, SE-392 34 Kalmar, Sweden. [5]Department of Learning, Informatics, Management and Ethics, Karolinska Institutet, Stockholm, Sweden.

References

1. Benbir G, Demir AU, Aksu M, Ardic S, Firat H, Itil O, Ozgen F, Yılmaz H, et al. Prevalence of insomnia and its clinical correlates in a general population in Turkey. Psychiatry Clin Neurosci. 2015;69(9):543–52.
2. Fernandez-Mendoza J, Shea S, Vgontzas AN, Calhoun SL, Liao D, Bixler EO, et al. Insomnia and incident depression: role of objective sleep duration and natural history. J Sleep Res. 2015;24(4):390–8.
3. Léger D, Morin CM, Uchiyama M, Hakimi Z, Cure S, Walsh JK. Chronic insomnia, quality-of-life, and utility scores: comparison with good sleepers in a cross-sectional international survey. Sleep Med. 2012;13(1):43–51.
4. Ohayon MM. Epidemiology of insomnia: what we know and what we still need to learn. Sleep Med Rev. 2002;6(2):97–111.
5. Mallon L, Broman JE, Akerstedt T, Hetta J. Insomnia in Sweden: a population-based survey. Sleep Disord. 2014;843126(10):12.
6. American Psychiatric Association. Diagnostic and statistical manual of mental disorders. 5th ed. Arlington: American Psychiatric Publishing; 2013.
7. American Academy of Sleep Medicine. International classification of Sleep disorders. 3rd ed. Darien: American Academy of Sleep Medicine; 2014.
8. Kyle SD, Espie CA, Morgan K. "...Not just a minor thing, it is something major, which stops you from functioning daily". Quality of life and daytime functioning in insomnia. Behav Sleep Med. 2010;8(3):123–40.
9. Morin CM, LeBlanc M, Daley M, Gregoire JP, Mérette C. Epidemiology of insomnia: prevalence, self-help treatments, consultations, and determinants of help-seeking behaviors. Sleep Med. 2006;7(2):123–30.
10. Riemann D, Baglioni C, Bassetti C, Bjorvatn B, Dolenc Groselj L, Ellis JG, et al. European guideline for the diagnosis and treatment of insomnia. J Sleep Res. 2017;26(6):675–700.
11. Sateia MJ, Buysse DJ, Krystal AD, Neubauer DN, Heald JL. Clinical practice guideline for the pharmacologic treatment of chronic insomnia in adults: an American Academy of sleep medicine clinical practice guideline. J Clin Sleep Med. 2017;13(2):307–49.
12. Kazdin AE. Understanding how and why psychotherapy leads to change. Psychother Res. 2009;19(4-5):418–28.
13. Gardner B, Broström A, Nilsen P, Hrubos Ström H, Ulander M, Fridlund B, et al. From 'does it work?' to 'what makes it work?': the importance of making assumptions explicit when designing and evaluating behavioural interventions. Eur J Cardiovasc Nurs. 2014;13(4):292–4.
14. Araújo T, Jarrin DC, Leanza Y, Vallières A, Morin CM. Qualitative studies of insomnia: current state of knowledge in the field. Sleep Med Rev. 2017;31: 58–69.
15. Barter G, Cormack M. The long-term use of benzodiazepines: patients' views, accounts and experiences. Fam Pract. 1996;13(6):491–7.
16. Hubbling A, Reilly-Spong M, Kreitzer MJ, Gross CR. How mindfulness changed my sleep: focus groups with chronic insomnia patients. BMC Complement Altern Med. 2014; https://doi.org/10.1186/1472-6882-14-50.
17. Kyle SD, Morgan K, Spiegelhalder K, Espie CA. No pain, no gain: an exploratory within-subjects mixed-methods evaluation of the patient experience of sleep restriction therapy (SRT) for insomnia. Sleep Med. 2011; 12(8):735–47.
18. Levitt HM, Pomerville A, Surace FI. A qualitative meta-analysis examining Clients' experiences of psychotherapy: a new agenda. Psychol Bull. 2016; 142(8):801–30.
19. Nilsson T, Svensson M, Sandell R, Clinton D. Patients' experiences of change in cognitive–behavioral therapy and psychodynamic therapy: a qualitative comparative study. Psychother Res. 2007;17(5):553–66.
20. Olivera J, Braun M, Gómez Penedo JM, Roussos A. A qualitative investigation of former Clients' perception of change, reasons for consultation, therapeutic relationship, and termination. Psychotherapy. 2013;50(4):505–16.
21. Smith AH, Norton PJ, McLean CP. Client perceptions of therapy component helpfulness in group cognitive-behavioral therapy for anxiety disorders. J Clin Psychol. 2013;69(3):229–39.
22. Straarup NS, Poulsen S. Helpful aspects of metacognitive therapy and cognitive behaviour therapy for depression: a qualitative study. Cogn Behav Ther. 2015;8:e22. https://doi.org/10.1017/S1754470X15000574.
23. Bowie C, McLeod J. 'It was almost like the opposite of what I needed': a qualitative exploration of client experiences of unhelpful therapy. Couns Psychother Res. 2016;16(2):79–87.
24. Werbart A, von Below C, Brun J, Gunnarsdottir H. "Spinning one's wheels": nonimproved patients view their psychotherapy. Psychother Res. 2015;25(5): 546–64.
25. Sandlund C, Hetta J, Nilsson GH, Ekstedt M, Westman J. Improving insomnia in primary care patients: a randomized controlled trial of nurse-led group treatment. Int J Nurs Stud. 2017;72:30–41.
26. Sandlund C, Hetta J, Nilsson GH, Ekstedt M, Westman J. Impact of group treatment for insomnia on daytime symptomatology: analyses from a randomized controlled trial in primary care. Int J Nurs Stud. 2018;85:126–35.
27. Palinkas LA. Qualitative and mixed methods in mental health services and implementation research. J Clin Child Adolesc Psychol. 2014;43(6):851–61.
28. Kitzinger J. Qualitative research. Introducing focus groups. BMJ. 1995; 311(7000):299.
29. Graneheim UH, Lindgren BM, Lundman B. Methodological challenges in qualitative content analysis: a discussion paper. Nurse Educ Today. 2017;56: 29_34.
30. Graneheim UH, Lundman B. Qualitative content analysis in nursing research: concepts, procedures and measures to achieve trustworthiness. Nurse Educ Today. 2004;24(2):105–12.

31. American Psychiatric Association. Diagnostic and statistical manual of mental disorders: DSM-IV-TR. Washington, DC: American Psychiatric Association; 2000.
32. Morin CM. Insomnia: psychological assessment and management. New York: Guilford Press; 1993.
33. Morin CM, Belleville G, Bélanger L, Ivers H. The insomnia severity index: psychometric indicators to detect insomnia cases and evaluate treatment response. Sleep. 2011;34(5):601–8.
34. Harvey AG. A cognitive model of insomnia. Behav Res Ther. 2002;40(8):869–93.
35. Jansson M, Linton SJ. Cognitive-behavioral group therapy as an early intervention for insomnia: a randomized controlled trial. J Occup Rehabil. 2005;15(2):177–90.
36. Jernelöv S, Lekander M, Blom K, Rydh S, Ljótsson B, Axelsson J, et al. Efficacy of a behavioral self-help treatment with or without therapist guidance for co-morbid and primary insomnia -a randomized controlled trial. BMC Psychiatry. 2012;12(5):12–5.
37. Riemann D, Spiegelhalder K, Feige B, Voderholzer U, Berger M, Perlis M, et al. The hyperarousal model of insomnia: a review of the concept and its evidence. Sleep Med Rev. 2010;14(1):19–31.
38. Morin CM. Cognitive-behavioral approaches to the treatment of insomnia. J Clin Psychiatry. 2004;16:33–40.
39. International Council of Nurses. The ICN code of ethics for nurses. Geneva: International Council of Nurses; 2012.
40. Hsieh HF, Shannon SE. Three approaches to qualitative content analysis. Qual Health Res. 2005;15(9):1277–88.
41. Prochaska JO, Velicer WF. The transtheoretical model of health behavior change. Am J Health Promot. 1997;12(1):38–48.
42. Matthews EE, Arnedt JT, McCarthy MS, Cuddihy LJ, Aloia MS. Adherence to cognitive behavioral therapy for insomnia: a systematic review. Sleep Med Rev. 2013;17(6):453–64.
43. Matthews EE, Schmiege SJ, Cook PF, Berger AM, Aloia MS. Adherence to cognitive behavioral therapy for insomnia (CBTI) among women following primary breast cancer treatment: a pilot study. Behav Sleep Med. 2012;10(3):217–29.
44. Tarrant M, Khan SS, Farrow CV, Shah P, Daly M, Kos K. Patient experiences of a bariatric group programme for managing obesity: a qualitative interview study. Br J Health Psychol. 2017;22(1):77–93.
45. Rise MB, Pellerud A, Rygg LØ, Steinsbekk A. Making and maintaining lifestyle changes after participating in group based type 2 diabetes self-management educations: a qualitative study. PLoS One. 2013; https://doi.org/10.1371/journal.pone.0064009.
46. Falkenstrom F, Ekeblad A, Holmqvist R. Improvement of the working alliance in one treatment session predicts improvement of depressive symptoms by the next session. J Consult Clin Psychol. 2016;84(8):738–51.
47. Fuertes JN, Toporovsky A, Reyes M, Osborne JB. The physician-patient working alliance: theory, research, and future possibilities. Patient Educ Couns. 2017;100(4):610–5.
48. Behenck A, Wesner AC, Finkler D, Heldt E. Contribution of group therapeutic factors to the outcome of cognitive-behavioral therapy for patients with panic disorder. Arch Psychiatr Nurs. 2017;31(2):142–6.
49. Behenck AS, Gomes JB, Heldt E. Patient rating of therapeutic factors and response to cognitive-behavioral group therapy in patients with obsessive-compulsive disorder. Issues Ment Health Nurs. 2016;37(6):392–9.
50. Yalom ID. The theory and practice of group psychotherapy. 5th ed. New York: Basic Books; 2005.
51. Kolb DA. Experiential learning: experience as the source of learning and development. USA: FT press; 2014.
52. Biggs J, Tang C. Teaching for quality learning at university. McGraw-hill education (UK); 2011.
53. Bandura A. Health promotion by social cognitive means. Health Educ Behav. 2004;31(2):143–64.
54. Ryan RM, Deci EL. Self-determination theory and the facilitation of intrinsic motivation, social development, and well-being. Am Psychol. 2000;55(1):68–78.
55. Espie CA, Broomfield NM, MacMahon KM, Macphee LM, Taylor LM. The attention-intention-effort pathway in the development of psychophysiologic insomnia: a theoretical review. Sleep Med Rev. 2006;10(4):215–45.
56. Miller CB, Espie CA, Epstein DR, Friedman L, Morin CM, Pigeon WR, et al. The evidence base of sleep restriction therapy for treating insomnia disorder. Sleep Med Rev. 2014;18(5):415–24.
57. Miller CB, Kyle SD, Marshall NS, Espie CA. Ecological momentary assessment of daytime symptoms during sleep restriction therapy for insomnia. J Sleep Res. 2013;22(3):266–72.
58. Vincent N, Lewycky S, Finnegan H. Barriers to engagement in sleep restriction and stimulus control in chronic insomnia. J Consult Clin Psychol. 2008;76(5):820–8.
59. Swedish Society of Nursing. Strategy for improving the quality of nursing. Stockholm: Swedish Society of Nursing; 2017.
60. Pulvirenti M, McMillan J, Lawn S. Empowerment, patient centred care and self-management. Health Expect. 2014;17(3):303–10.
61. Anderson RM, Funnell MM. Patient empowerment: myths and misconceptions. Patient Educ Couns. 2010;79(3):277–82.
62. Kitzinger J. Focus group research: using group dynamics. Qual Res Health Care. 2005;56:70.
63. Fusch PI, Ness LR. Are we there yet? Data saturation in qualitative research. Qual Rep. 2015;20(9):1408.
64. Malterud K, Siersma VD, Guassora AD. Sample size in qualitative interview studies: guided by information power. Qual Health Res. 2015; Epub ahead of print
65. Tong A, Sainsbury P, Craig J. Consolidated criteria for reporting qualitative research (COREQ): a 32-item checklist for interviews and focus groups. Int J Qual Health Care. 2007;19(6):349–57.
66. Birt L, Scott S, Cavers D, Campbell C, Walter F. Member checking: a tool to enhance trustworthiness or merely a nod to validation? Qual Health Res. 2016; Epub ahead of print
67. Malterud K. Qualitative research: standards, challenges, and guidelines. Lancet. 2001;358(9280):483–8.
68. World Medical Association Declaration of Helsinki. Ethical principles for medical research involving human subjects. JAMA. 2013;310(20):2191–4.

8

Multimorbidity patterns with K-means nonhierarchical cluster analysis

Concepción Violán[1,2]* iD, Albert Roso-Llorach[1,2], Quintí Foguet-Boreu[1,2,3], Marina Guisado-Clavero[1,2], Mariona Pons-Vigués[1,2,4], Enriqueta Pujol-Ribera[1,2,4] and Jose M. Valderas[5]

Abstract

Background: The purpose of this study was to ascertain multimorbidity patterns using a non-hierarchical cluster analysis in adult primary patients with multimorbidity attended in primary care centers in Catalonia.

Methods: Cross-sectional study using electronic health records from 523,656 patients, aged 45–64 years in 274 primary health care teams in 2010 in Catalonia, Spain. Data were provided by the Information System for the Development of Research in Primary Care (SIDIAP), a population database. Diagnoses were extracted using 241 blocks of diseases (International Classification of Diseases, version 10). Multimorbidity patterns were identified using two steps: 1) multiple correspondence analysis and 2) k-means clustering. Analysis was stratified by sex.

Results: The 408,994 patients who met multimorbidity criteria were included in the analysis (mean age, 54.2 years [Standard deviation, SD: 5.8], 53.3% women). Six multimorbidity patterns were obtained for each sex; the three most prevalent included 68% of the women and 66% of the men, respectively. The top cluster included coincident diseases in both men and women: Metabolic disorders, Hypertensive diseases, Mental and behavioural disorders due to psychoactive substance use, Other dorsopathies, and Other soft tissue disorders.

Conclusion: Non-hierarchical cluster analysis identified multimorbidity patterns consistent with clinical practice, identifying phenotypic subgroups of patients.

Keywords: Multimorbidity, Cluster analysis, Multiple correspondence analysis, K-means clustering, Primary health care, Electronic health records, Diseases

Background

In the first decade of the twenty-first century, tremendous effort was concentrated on surfacing data about multimorbidity patterns in order to increase the knowledge of how the diseases were clustered [1–3]. In everyday primary care settings, multimorbidity is more the norm than an exception, with a prevalence ranging from 13 to 95% in the global population, depending on the age group included and methodology used [2]. Therefore, establishing these clustered associations could inform Clinical Practice Guidelines (CPG) and guide decision-making in the clinical practice [4].

No consensus has been established about a standard model to determine multimorbidity patterns. Differences between studies have been observed, such as the unit of

analysis selected (patients versus diseases), the statistical method for grouping diseases (factor analysis vs. cluster analysis), diseases included (chronic or all), and number of diseases included in the models [1, 5].

To identify the multimorbidity patterns, methods that identify and separate certain population groups from others and study non-random associations between diseases in those sub-groups are needed [3, 6]. There are basically two statistical methods for grouping diseases: factor analysis and cluster analysis. Exploratory factor analysis is based on correlations between diagnoses to identify the patterns; it is used to test hypothesised relationships between observed measures and latent constructs and allows the inclusion of a diagnosis in multiple factors. In contrast, cluster analysis obtains the patterns of multimorbidity based on dissimilarities between diseases; clusters tend to contain diagnoses that are similar to each other (in terms of Euclidean

* Correspondence: cviolan@idiapjgol.org; http://www.idiapjgol.org
[1]Institut Universitari d'Investigació en Atenció Primària Jordi Gol (IDIAP Jordi Gol), Gran Via Corts Catalanes, 587 àtic, 08007 Barcelona, Spain
[2]Universitat Autònoma de Barcelona, Bellaterra, Cerdanyola del Vallès, Spain
Full list of author information is available at the end of the article

distances) and a diagnosis cannot be included in more than one cluster. Usually, factor analysis is used to study diseases and cluster analysis to study patients [7]. A recent comparison of the two methods concluded that cluster analysis is more useful than factor analysis for in-depth study of multimorbidity patterns [8].

Among cluster analysis methods, there are two main types of techniques: hierarchical (HCA) and non-hierarchical cluster analysis (NHCA) [9]. The first, often considered when choosing a clustering technique in biomedicine, attempts to identify relatively homogeneous groups of cases based on selected characteristics, using an algorithm that either agglomerates or divides entities to form clusters. HCA is organized so that one cluster can be entirely contained within another cluster, but no other kind of overlap between clusters is allowed. However, the technique is not particularly good when it comes to robust identification of patterns in data. The main limitations are that the hierarchical clusters are susceptible to outliers in the data, the final solution depends on the chosen distance measure, and the algorithms are not efficient to analyse large data sets, as they require a large distance matrix. Nevertheless, almost all studies to date have used HCA to analyse multimorbidity patterns [2, 3].

Among the NHCA methods, K-means is the most frequently used. In contrast to HCA, this approach does not involve the construction of groups via iterative division or clustering; instead, patients are assigned to clusters once the number of clusters is specified. The results are less susceptible to outliers in the data, to the influence of choosing a distance measure, or to the inclusion of inappropriate or irrelevant variables. Algorithms that do not require a distance matrix, such as k-means, can analyse extremely large data sets [9–11].

The study of biological heterogeneity requires the identification of subgroups of populations with specific combinations of coexisting diseases. This "multimorbidity patient" approach identifies phenotypes of the subgroups, describes the patterns of diseases within each one, and facilitates the development of more targeted patient management [12].

The purpose of this study was to obtain the multimorbidity patterns in adult patients with multimorbidity attended in primary care in Catalonia (Spain), stratified by sex, using a k-means cluster analysis.

Methods
Design, setting and study population
A cross-sectional study was conducted in Catalonia (Spain), a Mediterranean region with 7,434,632 inhabitants, 81% of which live in urban municipalities (2010 census). The Spanish National Health Service (NHS) provides universal coverage, financed mainly by tax revenue. The Catalan Health Institute (CHI) manages primary health care teams (PHCTs) that serve 5,501,784 patients (274 PHCT), or 74%

of the population; the remaining PHCTs are managed by other providers.

The CHI's Information System for the Development of Primary Care Research (SIDIAP) contains the coded clinical information recorded in electronic health records (EHR) by its 274 PHCTs since 2006. A subset of SIDIAP records meeting the highest quality criteria for clinical data, the SIDIAP-Q, includes 1,833,125 patients attended by the 1365 general practitioners (GPs). SIDIAP Q represents 40% of the SIDIAP population whose data recording scores contain information on the majority of the population of Catalonia, and is highly representative of the whole region in terms of geography, age, sex, and diseases. This study was limited to SIDIAP-Q, as the sample was representative of the population [13].

Prevalence of individual conditions, multimorbidity, and disease patterns varies by age. To obtain a more homogenous sample of multimorbidity, we identified 408,944 patients with multimoribidity aged 45 to 64 years [14] on 31 December 2010 (Additional file 1).

Coding and selection of diseases
Diseases are coded in SIDIAP using International Classification of Diseases version 10 (ICD-10) [15]. For this study, we selected all active diagnoses recorded in EHR as of December 31, 2010, except for R codes (symptoms, signs, and abnormal clinical and laboratory findings, not elsewhere classified) and Z codes (factors influencing health status and contact with health services). Of the 263 blocks of diagnosis in the ICD-10, excluding the R codes and Z codes yielded 241 blocks. Non-active diagnoses, based on the presence of an end date in the EHR, were excluded. These diagnoses covered a broad list of acute diseases for which the system automatically assigns an end date (e.g., 60 days after the initial diagnosis).

To facilitate information management, the diagnoses were extracted using the 263 blocks (disease categories) in the ICD-10 structure. These are homogeneous categories of very closely related specific diagnoses. For example, *Hypertensive diseases* include Essential (primary) hypertension, Hypertensive heart disease, Hypertensive renal disease, Hypertensive heart and renal disease, and Secondary hypertension. To obtain consistent and clinically interpretable patterns of association, and to avoid spurious relationships that could bias the results, we considered only diagnoses with greater than 1% prevalence in each sex. All patients with multimorbidity were included.

Multimorbidity definition
Multimorbidity was defined by the presence of two or more ICD-10 diagnoses in the EHR from the 241 blocks selected.

Variables

The unit of measurement was the diagnoses included in the 241 blocks (disease categories) of the ICD-10 structure (values: 1 if present, 0 if absent). Other variables recorded were number of diseases, age (in years), and sex (women, men).

No missing values were handled, as sex and age were recorded for all patients. Wrong sex-specific diagnosis codes and diagnoses with inconsistent dates were excluded during data cleaning. Any record with no disease diagnoses was considered as a disease-free individual.

Statistical analysis

Analyses were stratified by sex. Descriptive statistics were used to summarize overall information. Categorical variables were expressed as frequencies (percentage) and continuous variables as mean (Standard deviation, SD) or median (interquartile range, IQR). Two sample tests of proportions were used to assess sex-based differences between groups Mann Whitney was used to test the non-normally distributed variable of number of blocks of diagnoses by sex.

We identified disease patterns using two steps:

1) Multiple Correspondence Analysis (MCA): A data analysis technique for nominal categorical data, was used to detect and represent underlying structures in the data set. The method allows representation in a multidimensional space of relationships between a set of dichotomous or categorical variables (in our case, diagnoses) that would otherwise be difficult to observe in contingency tables and show groups of patients with the same characteristics [16]. MCA also allows direct representation of patients as points (coordinates) in geometric space, transforming the original binary data to continuous data (Additional file 2). The MCA analysis was based on the indicator matrix. Optimal number of dimensions extracted and percentages of inertia were determined by the means of scree plot.

2) K-means clustering: From the geometric space created in MCA, patients were classified into clusters according to proximity criteria by means of the k-means algorithm. The algorithm is composed of the following steps: 1) Place K points into the space represented by the patients that are being clustered. These points represent initial group centroids. 2) Assign each patient to the group that has the closest centroid. 3) When all patients have been assigned, recalculate the positions of the K centroids. Repeat Steps 2 and 3 until the centroids no longer move. This produces a separation of the patients into homogenous groups while maximizing heterogeneity across groups [9]. The optimal number

of clusters is the solution with the highest Calinski-Harabasz index value. To assess internal cluster quality, cluster stability of the optimal solution was computed using Jaccard bootstrap values with 100 runs [17]. Highly stable clusters should yield average Jaccard similarities of 0.85 and above [9].

Statistics of multimorbidity patterns

To describe the multimorbidity patterns in patients, frequencies and percentages of diseases in each cluster were calculated. Observed/expected ratios ("O/E-ratios") were calculated by dividing disease prevalence in the cluster by disease prevalence in the sex group. A disease was considered to be associated with the multimorbidity pattern when O/E-ratio was ≥2 [18]. Exclusivity, defined as the fraction of patients with the disease included in the cluster over the total strata patients with the disease, was also calculated. To describe the relative position of the clusters, centrality defined as the distance of the cluster centroid to the origin was calculated. Descriptive statistics of age and the median number of diagnoses for each cluster were also obtained. Clinical criteria were used to evaluate the consistency and utility of the final cluster solution. To reduce the size of the tables, only groups of diseases with a prevalence higher than 10% in the cluster were shown.

The analyses were carried out using SPSS for Windows, version 18 (SPSS Inc., Chicago, IL, USA) and R version 3.3.1 (R Foundation for Statistical Computing, Vienna, Austria).

Results

Out of 523,656 patients aged 45 to 64 years, 408,994 (78.1%) met the multimorbidity criteria. Women had a higher multimorbidity prevalence than men (82.2% vs. 73.9%, $p < 0.001$). The mean age was 54.2 years (Standard deviation [SD]: 5.8), 53.3% were women, and the mean number of diagnoses per patient was 5.7 (SD: 3.3). The analysis included 217,823 women and 191,171 men with 79 and 73 different diagnoses, respectively (Table 1 and Additional file 3).

Data were transformed using MCA (Additional file 2). K-means clustering using Calinski criterion to obtain six clusters was considered the optimal solution for both women and men. Average Jaccard bootstrap values for women and men were 0.98 and 0.90, respectively, showing highly stable solutions. A spatial representation of clusters is shown with a cluster plot for women (Fig. 1a) and men (Fig. 1b).

Six multimorbidity patterns were obtained for each sex. The three most prevalent multimorbidity patterns included 68.4% of women patients (Table 2) and 65.6% of men patients (Table 3). The number of diseases included in each pattern varied by sex; women had a

Table 1 Number of diseases for patients 45–64 years old, stratified by sex, Catalonia, 2010*

	Women n (%) 217,823 (82.2)	Men n (%) 191,171 (73.9)
Number of diagnoses†		
2	26,106 (12.0)	33,850 (17.7)
3	28,243 (13.0)	33,515 (17.5)
4	28,274 (13.0)	30,356 (15.9)
≥ 5	135,200 (62.1)	93,450 (48.9)
Median number of diagnoses (IQR)‡	5 (4–8)	4 (3–7)
Number of diagnoses included	79	73

Abbreviations: *IQR* inter-quartile range
*Included in the analysis *N* = 523,656, people with ≥2 diagnoses; 408,994 (78.1%)
†Two sample test of proportions; all *p*-values< 0.001
‡Mann-Whitney test; *P* < 0.001

higher number of diseases than men, although there was a high coincidence (matching) between them in the type of diseases grouped.

The clusters were sorted in descending order by number of individuals included. The first cluster included about 40% of the population (40.7% of women and 38.7% of men) and no O/E ratio higher than 2 was observed in these first clusters. In these first clusters, the highest exclusivity value was 46.1% for *Mental and behavioural disorders due to psychoactive substance use* (tobacco) in women and 35.3% for *Metabolic disorders* in men.

The most prevalent cluster included coincident diseases in both men and women: *Metabolic disorders, Hypertensive diseases, Mental and behavioural disorders due to psychoactive substance use, Other dorsopathies* and *Other soft tissue disorders* (Tables 2 and 3).

Four other patterns were almost coincident between the sexes: 1) Cluster 4 (women) and cluster 3 (men), composed mostly of diseases of the digestive and musculoskeletal system; 2) Cluster 2 (women) and Cluster 4 (men), connective tissue diseases; 3) Cluster 5 was composed of a cardiometabolic pattern (obesity, hypertension and diabetes) in both groups; and 4) Cluster 6, infectious and injurious diseases (see Tables 2 and 3). O/E ratios varied for each cluster, peaking at 8.99 for *Other viral diseases* and 8.24 for *Other acute lower respiratory infections* in cluster 6 (women) (Tables 2 and 3).

In both sexes, the most prevalent multimorbidity pattern in the oldest patients (Tables 2 and 3) were musculoskeletal system and connective tissue diseases in women (mean age: 57.4) and cardiometabolic pattern (obesity, hypertension, and diabetes) in men (mean age: 57.1).

Multimorbidity patterns considering only blocks of diagnoses with O/E ratio ≥ 2, ordered by exclusivity in women and men, showed that the highest exclusivity in women was observed in Cluster 6: 83.9% of the people who had a diagnosis of *Other viral diseases* are included in this cluster. They were followed by Cluster 5, which 77.0% of people with *Diabetes mellitus* belonged to. In men, 83.7% of people with *Disorders of choroid and retina* belongs to Cluster 5, and 77.6%, which includes *Viral hepatitis*, in Cluster 2 (Additional file 4).

Discussion

Non-hierarchical cluster analysis yielded an informative categorization of patients, generating reasonable multimorbity patterns from a clinical, practical perspective, and identified phenotypes for sub-groups of patients. Metabolic-circulatory-tobacco use-musculoskeletal pattern is the most common multimorbidity pattern

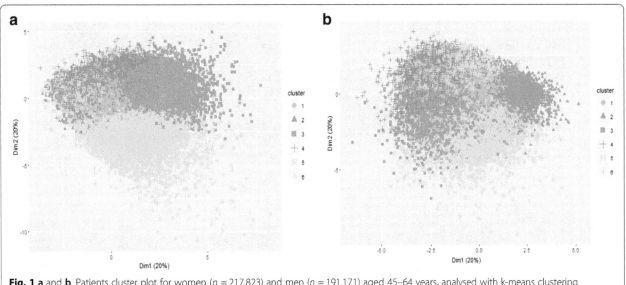

Fig. 1 a and **b**. Patients cluster plot for women (*n* = 217,823) and men (*n* = 191,171) aged 45–64 years, analysed with k-means clustering

Table 2 Three most prevalent multimorbidity patterns in women (n = 217,823) aged 45–65 years, Catalonia, 2010

Cluster n (%)[a]	Blocks of diagnoses	Prevalence in cluster (%)[b]	Prevalence in women (%)[c]	O/E ratio[d]	Exclusivity (%)	Centrality	Mean Age	Median number of diagnoses
1	E70-E90:Metabolic disorders	25.9	35.4	0.73	29.8	0.8	53.0	3
88,657 (40.7)	M50-M54:Other dorsopathies	23.6	35.8	0.66	26.9			
	F10-F19:Mental and behavioural disorders due to psychoactive substance use	21.1	18.6	1.13	46.1			
	F40-F48:Neurotic. stress-related and somatoform disorders	20.0	27.3	0.73	29.9			
	N80-N98:Noninflammatory disorders of female genital tract	17.6	24.2	0.73	29.6			
	I10-I15:Hypertensive diseases	15.6	25.6	0.61	24.9			
	M70-M79:Other soft tissue disorders	13.9	27.0	0.52	21.0			
	E00-E07:Disorders of thyroid gland	11.8	14.9	0.79	32.3			
	D10-D36:Benign neoplasms	10.4	16.2	0.65	26.3			
2	M50-M54:Other dorsopathies	55.4	35.8	1.55	23.0	1.6	57.4	7
32,249 (14.8)	E70-E90:Metabolic disorders	53.6	35.4	1.52	22.4			
	M15-M19:Arthrosis	**48.2**	**15.7**	**3.08**	**45.6**			
	M70-M79:Other soft tissue disorders	47.5	27.0	1.76	26.1			
	M80-M85:Disorders of bone density and structure	**38.7**	**11.3**	**3.41**	**50.5**			
	M20-M25:Other joint disorders	33.0	18.6	1.78	26.3			
	F40-F48:Neurotic. stress-related and somatoform disorders	30.1	27.3	1.10	16.3			
	I10-I15:Hypertensive diseases	29.3	25.6	1.14	16.9			
	I80-I89:Diseases of veins. Lymphatic vessels and lymph nodes. Not elsewhere classified	29.2	18.3	1.60	23.7			
	F30-F39:Mood [affective] disorders	20.8	14.6	1.43	21.1			
	N80-N98:Noninflammatory disorders of female genital tract	20.5	24.2	0.85	12.5			
	E65-E68:Obesity and other hyperalimentation	20.5	19.0	1.08	16.0			
	G50-G59:Nerve. nerve root and plexus disorders	**20.0**	**8.5**	**2.34**	**34.7**			
	M45-M49:Spondylopathies	**19.7**	**4.3**	**4.56**	**67.4**			
	E00-E07:Disorders of thyroid gland	17.8	14.9	1.20	17.7			
	M40-M43:Deforming dorsopathies	**15.1**	**3.8**	**3.96**	**58.6**			
	D10-D36:Benign neoplasms	12.4	16.2	0.77	11.4			
	K20-K31:Diseases of oesophagus. Stomach and duodenum	12.0	11.4	1.05	15.6			
	J30-J39:Other diseases of upper respiratory tract	11.2	9.4	1.19	17.6			
	G40-G47:Episodic and paroxysmal disorders	11.2	10.5	1.06	15.7			

Table 2 Three most prevalent multimorbidity patterns in women ($n = 217,823$) aged 45–65 years, Catalonia, 2010 *(Continued)*

Cluster n (%)[a]	Blocks of diagnoses	Prevalence in cluster (%)[b]	Prevalence in women (%)[c]	O/E ratio[d]	Exclusivity (%)	Centrality	Mean Age	Median number of diagnoses
	J00-J06:Acute upper respiratory infections	11.1	12.6	0.88	13.0			
	H90-H95:Other disorders of ear	10.2	6.3	1.60	23.7			
3	N80-N98:Noninflammatory disorders of female genital tract	48.1	24.2	1.99	25.6	1.7	53.0	8
28,024 (12.9)	M50-M54:Other dorsopathies	46.9	35.8	1.31	16.9			
	M70-M79:Other soft tissue disorders	38.8	27.0	1.44	18.5			
	M20-M25:Other joint disorders	33.6	18.6	1.81	23.3			
	D10-D36:Benign neoplasms	**32.8**	**16.2**	**2.03**	**26.1**			
	I80-I89:Diseases of veins. Lymphatic vessels and lymph nodes. Not elsewhere classified	29.3	18.3	1.60	20.6			
	L20-L30:Dermatitis and eczema	**28.4**	**9.3**	**3.05**	**39.2**			
	E70-E90:Metabolic disorders	27.7	35.4	0.78	10.1			
	F40-F48:Neurotic. stress-related and somatoform disorders	26.3	27.3	0.96	12.4			
	K00-K14:Diseases of oral cavity. Salivary glands and jaws	23.3	12.1	1.93	24.9			
	B35-B49:Mycoses	**19.8**	**5.7**	**3.46**	**44.5**			
	D50-D53:Nutritional anaemias	**19.7**	**8.3**	**2.38**	**30.6**			
	N60-N64:Disorders of breast	**19.2**	**7.5**	**2.56**	**32.9**			
	J00-J06:Acute upper respiratory infections	16.9	12.6	1.34	17.2			
	H53-H54:Visual disturbances and blindness	**16.8**	**4.4**	**3.84**	**49.4**			
	E00-E07:Disorders of thyroid gland	16.7	14.9	1.13	14.5			
	L60-L75:Disorders of skin appendages	**16.7**	**4.8**	**3.51**	**45.2**			
	I10-I15:Hypertensive diseases	15.9	25.6	0.62	8.0			
	E65-E68:Obesity and other hyperalimentation	15.4	19.0	0.81	10.4			
	J30-J39:Other diseases of upper respiratory tract	15.2	9.4	1.61	20.8			
	G40-G47:Episodic and paroxysmal disorders	14.0	10.5	1.33	17.1			
	B00-B09:Viral infections characterized by skin and mucous membrane lesions	**13.9**	**4.3**	**3.21**	**41.2**			
	H90-H95:Other disorders of ear	**12.9**	**6.3**	**2.03**	**26.2**			
	H49-H52:Disorders of ocular muscles. Binocular movement. Accommodation and refraction	**12.9**	**3.5**	**3.64**	**46.8**			
	L80-L99:Other disorders of the skin and subcutaneous tissue	**12.8**	**3.3**	**3.83**	**49.3**			
	H10-H13:Disorders of conjunctiva	**12.2**	**3.8**	**3.21**	**41.3**			
	F30-F39:Mood [affective] disorders	11.7	14.6	0.80	10.3			

Table 2 Three most prevalent multimorbidity patterns in women ($n = 217,823$) aged 45–65 years, Catalonia, 2010 *(Continued)*

Cluster n (%)[a]	Blocks of diagnoses	Prevalence in cluster (%)[b]	Prevalence in women (%)[c]	O/E ratio[d]	Exclusivity (%)	Centrality	Mean Age	Median number of diagnoses
	K55-K63:Other diseases of intestines	11.3	8.6	1.32	17.0			
	M15-M19:Arthrosis	11.1	15.7	0.71	9.2			
	K20-K31:Diseases of oesophagus. Stomach and duodenum	10.3	11.4	0.91	11.7			

[a]Individuals (% of total women) / [b]Individuals as % of cluster / [c]Individuals as % of total women)
[d]Observed / Expected Ratio. Values ≥2 in bold

identified by NHCA in both sexes. This pattern would be classified as nonspecific because it had the lowest centrality value (0.8 for both sexes). It is the most common in the population with multimorbidity aged 45–65 years. This pattern seems to be consistent with other studies which obtained similar associations of diseases with other methods of analysis [2, 3].

Other data of interest are the higher exclusivity values obtained in some clusters. For example, 77% of women who suffered diabetes mellitus have other associated diseases, such as forms of heart disease, obesity, and hypertension. These results are similar to the report from Hughes et al. that 71% of people with diabetes had multimorbidity [19]. Other coexisting diseases in the 84% of men who had disorders of choroid and retina (ischemic heart diseases, diseases of arteries, arterioles and capillaries, diabetes, other forms of heart disease, obesity, and hypertension) reflect a broad affectation of the vascular tree. Another remarkable observation in some patterns was the clustering of diseases of the same system or the presence of diseases, reflecting a complication. For example, one multimorbidity pattern consisted of seven diseases, of which five were diseases of the musculoskeletal system and connective tissue (Cluster 2, women). Another well-known example is the complications of diabetes mellitus such as disorders of choroid and retina (diabetic retinopathy) and renal failure (Cluster 5, men).

These results can be translated into clinical practice. When a disease is first diagnosed, we can suspect other associated diseases. Clinical practice guidelines could orient their recommendations toward these sub-groups (for example: arthritis, anxiety and depression). On the other hand, some results could be difficult to interpret in the context of current knowledge. Some patterns obtained included many diseases with no apparent connection between them.

In general, it is difficult to compare our results with the findings of other studies because of variations in methods, data sources and structures, populations, and diseases studied. However, there are some similarities between the current study and others. The first pattern is similar to the cardio-metabolic pattern reported by Prados et al. in adults aged 45 to 64 years (hypertension, diabetes, obesity, and lipid metabolism disorders) with an exploratory factor analysis [6]. In participants older than 50 years, another study found a cardiorespiratory factor (angina, asthma, and chronic lung disease) quite similar to our Cluster 5 in men and a mental-arthritis factor (arthritis, anxiety and depression) similar to our Cluster 2 in women [20].

The major strength of this study is the large, high-quality population database of primary care records that have been shown to be representative of a much larger population [13]. The analysis was stratified by sex and a patient-level perspective was used with NHCA. Admittedly, this analysis of almost all potential diagnoses may have added a complexity that will hinder interpretation of findings and comparison with other studies. Another major strength of this study was the operational definition of multimorbidity as the co-occurrence of multiple chronic or acute diseases [21] which allows the inclusion of the full range of diseases observed in any one patient. This is especially relevant because the boundaries between chronic and acute disease are not always clear [22, 23]. The strengths of using K-means cluster analysis is that the results are less susceptible to outliers in the data, the influence of chosen distance measure, or the inclusion of inappropriate or irrelevant variables [10]. The method can also analyse extremely large data sets as in our study, as no distance matrix is required. Some disadvantages of the method are that different solutions for each set of seed points can occur and there is no guarantee of optimal clustering [12]. To minimize this shortcoming, we tested the internal validity of our solution using bootstrap methods, and the results were highly stable (Jaccard> 0.85) [17]. In addition, the method is not efficient when a large number of potential cluster solutions are to be considered [10]; to address this limitation, we computed the optimal number using analytical indexes like Calinski Harabasz [24].

A number of limitations need to be taken into account as well. The use of MCA can produce low percentages of variation on principal axes and make it difficult to choose the number of dimensions to retain. We assumed a 5-dimension solution using the elbow rule in the scree

Table 3 Three most prevalent multimorbidity patterns in men (n = 191,171) aged 45–65 years, Catalonia, 2010

Cluster n (%)[a]	Blocks of diagnoses	Prevalence in cluster (%)[b]	Prevalence in men (%)[c]	O/E ratio[d]	Exclusivity (%)	Centrality	Mean Age	Median number of diagnoses
1	E70-E90:Metabolic disorders	38.4	42.2	0.91	35.3	0.8	53.3	3
73,979 (38.7)	I10-I15:Hypertensive diseases	28.1	32.5	0.86	33.4			
	F10-F19:Mental and behavioural disorders due to psychoactive substance use	25.4	33.6	0.76	29.2			
	M50-M54:Other dorsopathies	20.8	27.8	0.75	28.9			
	M70-M79:Other soft tissue disorders	10.7	16.9	0.63	24.6			
	E65-E68:Obesity and other hyperalimentation	10.6	14.6	0.73	28.2			
2	**F10-F19:Mental and behavioural disorders due to psychoactive substance use**	**77.3**	**33.6**	**2.30**	**34.9**	1.5	52.6	4
28,951 (15.1)	E70-E90:Metabolic disorders	26.4	42.2	0.63	9.5			
	F40-F48:Neurotic. stress-related and somatoform disorders	25.1	13.5	1.86	28.1			
	M50-M54:Other dorsopathies	23.7	27.8	0.85	12.9			
	K00-K14:Diseases of oral cavity. Salivary glands and jaws	23.2	12.0	1.93	29.2			
	J40-J47:Chronic lower respiratory diseases	**19.4**	**9.3**	**2.09**	**31.6**			
	F30-F39:Mood [affective] disorders	**17.0**	**6.3**	**2.72**	**41.2**			
	B15-B19:Viral hepatitis	**16.6**	**3.2**	**5.13**	**77.6**			
	I10-I15:Hypertensive diseases	14.2	32.5	0.44	6.6			
	K70-K77:Diseases of liver	**12.5**	**5.2**	**2.38**	**36.1**			
	K20-K31:Diseases of oesophagus. Stomach and duodenum	12.3	11.5	1.06	16.1			
	M70-M79:Other soft tissue disorders	10.4	16.9	0.62	9.4			
3	E70-E90:Metabolic disorders	43.4	42.2	1.03	12.1	1.9	55.2	6
22,458 (11.8)	**K20-K31:Diseases of oesophagus. Stomach and duodenum**	**40.0**	**11.5**	**3.47**	**40.7**			
	K40-K46:Hernia	**31.3**	**8.8**	**3.57**	**41.9**			
	N40-N51:Diseases of male genital organs	**30.9**	**12.1**	**2.54**	**29.9**			
	I10-I15:Hypertensive diseases	30.3	32.5	0.93	10.9			
	M50-M54:Other dorsopathies	29.6	27.8	1.06	12.5			
	I80-I89:Diseases of veins. Lymphatic vessels and lymph nodes. Not elsewhere classified	**29.6**	**10.0**	**2.95**	**34.7**			
	K55-K63:Other diseases of intestines	**28.2**	**6.4**	**4.39**	**51.6**			
	D10-D36:Benign neoplasms	**21.1**	**8.6**	**2.46**	**28.9**			
	F10-F19:Mental and behavioural disorders due to psychoactive substance use	20.8	33.6	0.62	7.3			

Table 3 Three most prevalent multimorbidity patterns in men ($n = 191,171$) aged 45–65 years, Catalonia, 2010 *(Continued)*

Cluster n (%)[a]	Blocks of diagnoses	Prevalence in cluster (%)[b]	Prevalence in men (%)[c]	O/E ratio[d]	Exclusivity (%)	Centrality	Mean Age	Median number of diagnoses
	F40-F48:Neurotic. stress-related and somatoform disorders	19.7	13.5	1.46	17.2			
	J30-J39:Other diseases of upper respiratory tract	**16.1**	**8.0**	**2.01**	**23.6**			
	M70-M79:Other soft tissue disorders	15.6	16.9	0.92	10.9			
	G40-G47:Episodic and paroxysmal disorders	13.1	7.4	1.77	20.8			
	N20-N23:Urolithiasis	**13.0**	**4.3**	**3.00**	**35.3**			
	J40-J47:Chronic lower respiratory diseases	12.0	9.3	1.29	15.1			
	H90-H95:Other disorders of ear	10.8	7.7	1.40	16.5			

[a]Individuals (% of total men) / [b]Individuals as % of the cluster /[c]Individuals as % of total men
[d]Observed / Expected Ratio. Values ≥2 in bold

plot to achieve the most accurate solution possible without including too many dimensions in the analysis [16]. In some clusters, an accumulative diagnosis belonging to the same chapter could be coded in multiple ways; however, use of the structure of ICD10 3-character codes that group diseases as the unit of analysis, rather than the more specific individual diagnosis, makes this improbable.

Few studies have focused on the MM patterns in patients rather than on diseases [25–27]. This methodology produced results that can be transferred to clinical practice, as they suggested that diseases are not equally associated with all phenotypes and there may be a genetic basis for patterns of multimorbidity.

Multimorbidity can present a problem for health services delivery, affecting patients, health professionals, and managers who are attempting to improve service delivery [28]. Our study offers a new methodological approach to understanding the relationships between specific diseases in individual patients, which is an essential step in improving the care of patients and health systems in organizations. Analysing patient profiles permitted the identification of subgroups of patients with different associated diseases.

This study illustrates the need to pay careful attention to the methods used to support policies and decision-making. The study results have implications for three fundamental areas of action: a) the need to change the orientation of clinical guidelines that focus on a single disease; b) the need to change health policy that is based on a disease rather than on the whole person; and c) the need to change current incentive policies that focus the health professional's attention on a disease rather than on multimorbidity, which includes not only diseases but also drug interactions, polypharmacy and the process of patient-health professional interactions.

Future studies on the current topic are therefore recommended, with a special focus on three major issues. First, the genetic typing of these multimorbidity patterns will identify genetic confluence in these patterns. Second, the delimitation of environment factors (alimentation, physical exercise, toxicity, etc.) associated with these patterns. Third, longitudinal studies should be done to establish the order of disease onset. Finally, the influence of polypharmacy, or the use of multiple drugs, could decrease treatment efficacy and cause unexpected adverse events or even the development of other diseases [29, 30].

These findings suggest that multimorbidity patterns obtained using non-hierarchical cluster analysis identified clusters more consistent with clinical practice, identifying phenotypes of certain sub-groups of patients.

Conclusion

Non-hierarchical cluster analysis identified multimorbidity patterns consistent with clinical practice, identifying phenotypic subgroups of patients.

Abbreviations
CHI: Catalan Health Institute; CPG: Clinical Practice Guidelines; EHR: Electronic Health Records; HCA: Hierarchical Clustering Analysis; ICD-10: International Classification of Diseases version 10; IQR: Interquartile Range; MCA: Multiple Correspondence Analysis; NHCA: Non-hierarchical cluster analysis; NHS: National Health Service; O/E-ratios: Observed/expected ratios; PHCTs: Primary Health Care Teams; SD: Standard Deviation; SIDIAP: Information System for the Development of Research in Primary Care

Acknowledgements
We thank the Catalan Health Institute and especially the SIDIAP Unit, which provided the database for the study. The authors also appreciate the English language review by Elaine Lilly, PhD, and are grateful to Carmen Ibáñez for administrative work.

Funding
The project has been funded by the Instituto de Salud Carlos III of the Ministry of Economy and Competitiveness (Spain) through the Network for Prevention and Health Promotion in Primary Health Care (redIAPP, RD12/0005), by a grant for research projects on health from ISCiii (PI12/00427) and co-financed with European Union ERDF funds). Jose M. Valderas was supported by the National Institute for Health Research Clinician Scientist Award NIHR/CS/010/024. The funders had no role in the study design, collection, analysis and interpretation of data, writing of the manuscript or decision to submit for publication. The views expressed in this publication are those of the author(s) and not necessarily those of the National Health Service, the National Institute for Health Research, or the National Department of Health.

Authors' contributions
All authors contributed to the design of the study, revised the article, and approved the final version. CV and QFB obtained the funding. ARL, CV, QFB and MGC contributed to the analysis and interpretation of data. CV, ARL, QFB wrote the first draft, and the rest of authors (MGC, MPV, EPR, and JMV) contributed ideas, interpreted the findings and reviewed rough drafts of the manuscript. All authors read and approved the final manuscript.

Competing interests
The authors declare that they have no competing interests.

Author details
[1]Institut Universitari d'Investigació en Atenció Primària Jordi Gol (IDIAP Jordi Gol), Gran Via Corts Catalanes, 587 àtic, 08007 Barcelona, Spain. [2]Universitat Autònoma de Barcelona, Bellaterra, Cerdanyola del Vallès, Spain. [3]Department of Psychiatry, Vic University Hospital, Francesc Pla el Vigatà, 1, 08500 Vic, Barcelona, Spain. [4]Faculty of Nursing, University of Girona, Emili Grahit, 77, 17071 Girona, Spain. [5]Health Services & Policy Research Group, Academic Collaboration for Primary Care, University of Exeter Medical School, Exeter EX1 2LU, UK.

References
1. Marengoni A, Angleman S, Melis R, Mangialasche F, Karp A, Garmen A, et al. Aging with multimorbidity: a systematic review of the literature. Ageing Res Rev. 2011;10(4):430–9.
2. Violan C, Foguet-Boreu Q, Flores-Mateo G, Salisbury C, Blom J, Freitag M, et al. Prevalence, determinants and patterns of multimorbidity in primary care: a systematic review of observational studies. PLoS One. 2014;9:e102149.
3. Prados-Torres A, Calderon-Larranaga A, Hancco-Saavedra J, Poblador-Plou B, van den Akker M. Multimorbidity patterns: a systematic review. J Clin Epidemiol. 2014;67:254–66.
4. Weiss CO, Varadhan R, Puhan MA, Vickers A, Bandeen-Roche K, Boyd CM, et al. Multimorbidity and evidence generation. J Gen Intern Med. 2014;29(4): 653–60.
5. Holzer BM, Siebenhuener K, Bopp M, Minder CE. Evidence-based design recommendations for prevalence studies on multimorbidity: improving comparability of estimates. Popul Health Metr. 2017;15(1):9.
6. Prados-Torres A, Poblador-Plou B, Calderón-Larrañaga A, Gimeno-Feliu LA, González-Rubio F, Poncel-Falcó A, et al. Multimorbidity patterns in primary care: interactions among chronic diseases using factor analysis. PLoS One. 2012;7(2):e32190.
7. Haregu T, Oldenburg B, Setswe G, Elliott J. Perspectives, constructs and methods in the measurement of multimorbidity and comorbidity: a critical review. Internet J Epidemiol. 2012;10(2):1–9.
8. Roso-Llorach A, Violán C, Foguet-Boreu Q, Rodriguez-Blanco T, Pons-Vigués M, Pujol-Ribera E, et al. Comparative analysis of methods for identifying multimorbidity patterns: a study of "real-world" data. BMJ Open. 2018;8(3): e018986.
9. Everitt BS, Landau S, Leese M, Stahl D. Cluster analysis. 5th ed. Chichester: John Wiley & Sons,Ltd; 2011.
10. Liao M, Li Y, Kianifard F, Obi E, Arcona S. Cluster analysis and its application to healthcare claims data: a study of end-stage renal disease patients who initiated hemodialysis. BMC Nephrol. 2016;17:25.
11. Ilmarinen P, Tuomisto LE, Niemelä O, Tommola M, Haanpää J, Kankaanranta H. Cluster Analysis on Longitudinal Data of Patients With Adult-Onset Asthma. J Allergy Clin Immunol Pract. 2017;S2213–2198(17):30048-X.
12. Fabbri E, Zoli M, Gonzalez-Freire M, Salive ME, Studenski SA, Ferrucci L. Aging and multimorbidity: new tasks, priorities, and Frontiers for integrated Gerontological and clinical research. J Am Med Dir Assoc. 2015;16(8): 640–7.
13. García-Gil MM, Hermosilla E, Prieto-Alhambra D, Fina F, Rosell M, Ramos R, et al. Construction and validation of a scoring system for the selection of high-quality data in a Spanish population primary care database (SIDIAP). Inform Prim Care. 2011;19(3):135–45.
14. Violán C, Foguet-Boreu Q, Roso-Llorach A, Rodriguez-Blanco T, Pons-Vigués M, Pujol-Ribera E, et al. Burden of multimorbidity, socioeconomic status and use of health services across stages of life in urban areas: a cross-sectional study. BMC Public Health. 2014;14:1–13.
15. World Health Organization: ICD-10 International Statistical Classification of Diseases and Related Health Problems 10th Revision Version for 2010. http://apps.who.int/classifications/apps/icd/icd10online/ . Accessed 20 Feb 2016.
16. Sourial N, Wolfson C, Zhu B, Quail J, Fletcher J, Karunananthan S, et al. Correspondence analysis is a useful tool to uncover the relationships among categorical variables. J Clin Epidemiol. 2010;63(6):638–46.
17. Hennig C. Cluster-wise assessment of cluster stability. Computational Statistics & Data Analysis. 2007;52:258–71.
18. Schäfer I, Kaduszkiewicz H, Wagner HO, Schön G, Scherer M, van den Bussche H. Reducing complexity: a visualisation of multimorbidity by combining disease clusters and triads. BMC Public Health. 2014;14:1285.
19. Hughes LD, McMurdo ME, Guthrie B. Guidelines for people not for diseases: the challenges of applying UK clinical guidelines to people with multimorbidity. Age Ageing. 2013;42(1):62–9.
20. Garin N, Olaya B, Perales J, Moneta MV, Miret M, Ayuso-Mateos JL, et al. Multimorbidity patterns in a national representative sample of the Spanish adult population. PLoS One. 2014;9(1):e84794.
21. Van den Akker M, Buntinx F, Knottnerus JA. Comorbidity or multi- morbidity: what's in a name? A review of literature. Eur J Gen Pract. 1996;2:65–70.
22. O'Halloran J, Miller GC, Britt H. Defining chronic conditions for primary care with ICPC-2. Fam Pract. 2004;21(4):381–6.
23. Soler JK, Okkes I, Oskam S, Van Boven K, Zivotic P, Jevtic M, et al. Revisiting the concept of 'chronic disease' from the perspective of the episode of care model. Does the ratio of incidence to prevalence rate help us to define a problem as chronic? Inform Prim Care. 2012;20(1):13–23.
24. Calinski RB, Harabasz JA. Dendrite method for cluster analysis. Comm Stat. 1974;3:1–27.
25. Guisado-Clavero M, Roso-Llorach A, López-Jimenez T, Pons-Vigués M, Foguet-Boreu Q, Muñoz MA, Violán C. Multimorbidity patterns in the elderly: a prospective cohort study with cluster analysis. BMC Geriatr. 2018;18(1):16.
26. Newcomer SR, Steiner JF, Bayliss EA. Identifying subgroups of complex patients with cluster analysis. Am J Manag Care. 2011;17:e324e32.
27. Goldstein G, Luther JF, Jacoby AM, Haas GL, Gordon AJ. A taxonomy of medical comorbidity for veterans who are homeless. J Health Care Poor Underserved. 2008;19:991e1005.
28. McPhail SM. Multimorbidity in chronic disease: impact on health care resources and costs. Risk Manag Healthc Policy. 2016;9:143–56.
29. Marengoni A, Onder G. Guidelines, polypharmacy, and drug-drug interactions in patients with multimorbidity. Br Med J. 2015;350:h1059.
30. Maher RL, Hanlon J, Hajjar ER. Clinical consequences of polypharmacy in elderly. Expert Opin Drug Saf. 2014;13(1):57–65.

9

Effectiveness of standardized nursing care plans to achieve A1C, blood pressure, and LDL-C goals among people with poorly controlled type 2 diabetes mellitus at baseline

J. Cárdenas-Valladolid[1,2,3,4*], A. López-de Andrés[4,5], R. Jiménez-García[4,5], M. J. de Dios-Duarte[6], P. Gómez-Campelo[3,4,7,8], C. de Burgos-Lunar[3,4,5,9,10], F. J. San Andrés-Rebollo[4,11], J. C. Abánades-Herranz[3,4,12] and M. A. Salinero-Fort[3,4,9,13]

Abstract

Background: No studies that have measured the role of nursing care plans in patients with poorly controlled type 2 diabetes mellitus. Our objectives were firstly, to evaluate the effectiveness of implementing Standardized languages in Nursing Care Plans (SNCP) for improving A1C, blood pressure and low density lipoprotein cholesterol (ABC goals) in patients with poorly controlled type 2 diabetes mellitus at baseline (A1C ≥7%, blood pressure ≥ 130/80 mmHg, and low-density lipoprotein cholesterol≥100 mg/dl) compared with Usual Nursing Care (UNC). Secondly, to evaluate the factors associated with these goals.

Methods: A four-year prospective follow-up study among outpatients with type 2 diabetes mellitus: We analyzed outpatients of 31 primary health centers (Madrid, Spain), with at least two A1C values (at baseline and at the end of the study) who did not meet their ABC goals at baseline. A total of 1916 had A1C ≥7% (881 UNC versus 1035 SNCP). Two thousand four hundred seventy-one had systolic blood pressure ≥ 130 mmHg (1204 UNC versus 1267 SNCP). One thousand one hundred seventy had diastolic blood pressure ≥ 80 mmHg (618 UNC versus 552 SNCP); and 2473 had low-density lipoprotein cholesterol ≥100 mg/dl (1257 UNC versus 1216 SNCP). Data were collected from computerized clinical records; SNCP were identified using NANDA and NIC taxonomies.

Results: More patients cared for using SNCP achieved in blood pressure goals compared with patients who received UNC (systolic blood pressure: 29.4% versus 28.7%, p = 0.699; diastolic blood pressure: 58.3% versus 53.2%, p = 0.08), but the differences did not reach statistical significance. For A1C and low-density lipoprotein cholesterol goals, there were no significant differences between the groups. Coronary artery disease was a significant predictor of blood pressure and low-density lipoprotein cholesterol goals.

Conclusions: In patients with poorly controlled type 2 diabetes mellitus, there is not enough evidence to support the use of SNCP instead of with UNC with the aim of helping patients to achieve their ABC goals. However, the use of SNCP is associated with a clear trend of a achievement of diastolic blood pressure goals.

Keywords: Patient care planning, Diabetes mellitus type 2, Prospective studies, Outcome assessment, NANDA, NIC

* Correspondence: juan.cardenas@salud.madrid.org
[1]Dirección Técnica de Sistemas de Información, Gerencia Asistencial de Atención Primaria, Servicio Madrileño de Salud, C/ San Martín de Porres, 6, 28035 Madrid, Spain
[2]Universidad Alfonso X el Sabio, Villanueva de la Cañada, Madrid, Spain
Full list of author information is available at the end of the article

Background

In Spain, approximately 6 million people have diabetes mellitus (DM) [1], and this number is increasing annually [2]. DM represents a major public health problem because it is a well-known risk factor for stroke [3], coronary artery disease (CAD) [4] and cardiovascular disease [5].

Poor control of blood pressure (BP), lipids, and glycosylated hemoglobin (A1C) is strongly associated with adverse outcomes in patients with type 2 DM (T2DM) [6]. The American Diabetes Association (ADA) recommends that patients with DM achieve their ABC goals, namely, A1C < 7%, BP < 130/80 mmHg, and low density lipoprotein cholesterol (LDL-C < 100 mg/dl [7]. However, at least one-third of patients with T2DM [8] fail to achieve their ABC goals.

The responsibility for the care of patients with T2DM in Spain has shifted to multidisciplinary teams based in primary health care (PHC) settings that are composed mainly of family doctors and nurses.

Achieving ABC goals for T2DM patients depends on several factors, such as physical activity levels [9], stress reduction [10], medication adherence [11], and meal plans [12]. These targets form the basis of wide range of interventions implemented by nurses and aimed at improving diabetes care and achieving metabolic control [13].

In the last decade, there has been a considerable improvement in Standardized languages in Nursing Care Plans (SNCP) with NANDA-International [14] Nursing Diagnoses and Interventions (NIC) [15]. Since 1998, these taxonomies have been progressively incorporated into clinical practice and computerized clinical records (CCR) in Madrid (Spain). However they are still not used by 100% of nursing staff [16].

Our group recently established the effectiveness of SNCP for improving health outcomes for T2DM patients [17]. However, to our knowledge, no studies have measured the role of nursing care plans in patients with poorly controlled T2DM. Accordingly, we hypothesize that SNCP may be effective in helping patients with poorly controlled T2DM to achieve their ABC goals. We also consider that it is necessary to know the magnitude of the effect of SNCP and to compare it with that of other therapeutic strategies.

Our study had two objectives. First, we evaluated the effectiveness of SNCP as a component of CCR registration for helping patients with poorly controlled T2DM at baseline (A1C ≥7%, blood pressure ≥ 130/80 mmHg, and LDL-C ≥ 100 mg/dl) to achieve their ABC goals and compared our findings with those of Usual Nursing Care (UNC), provided by dedicated trained nurses in PHC settings, second, we evaluated the factors associated with meeting ABC goals.

Methods

This study was conducted as part of a broader research project which is described in detail elsewhere [17, 18]. A prospective cohort follow-up study was carried out between March 2008 and February 2012 in T2DM patients attending follow-up appointments with a nurse at PHC centers.

The two types of nursing care plans implemented: SNCP (n = 2105) and UNC (n = 2105) were delivered by registered nurses trained in diagnostic reasoning based on NANDA-I and NIC taxonomies and working in 31 PHC centers in the northeastern area of the city of Madrid, Spain.

Eligibility criteria for patients were: age ≥ 30 years with at least two records in the CCR during the previous year and an International Classification of Primary Care [19] code indicating T2DM (T90). Patients were not selected if they met any of the following exclusion criteria: gestational diabetes, being homebound, and a life expectancy of less than 1 year (according to the physician's clinical judgment).

The number of patients selected for this study was lower than in the our previous study [17], as we preferred to restrict our analysis to patients from the SNCP group with at least two A1C values (baseline and end of study) over the four-year follow-up (n = 2105) Therefore, we decided to select a random sample of an equal size in the UNC group (n = 2105).

Figure 1 provide details of the study procedure, patients recruitment and exclusion, and patients without baseline and final A1C, LDL cholesterol and BP values Only those with poor diabetes control were finally included.

The sample size was calculated taking into account a UNC: SNCP ratio of 1:1.10 (estimated a proportion of 30% patients with A1C < 7% in the UNC group, alpha risk of 0.05 and a beta risk of 0.20 in a two-sided test). A sample size of 873 UNC patients and 1029 SNCP patients is necessary to recognise a statistically significant relative risk of good glycemic control (A1C < 7%) of ≥1.22 in the UNC vs. the SNCP group. A drop-out rate of 0.05 was anticipated.

We only analyzed patients who did not meet their ABC goals at baseline: A1C ≥7% (n = 1916; 881 with UNC and 1035 with SNCP), systolic blood pressure (SBP) ≥130 mmHg (n = 2471; 1204 with UNC and 1267 with SNCP), diastolic blood pressure (DBP) ≥80 mmHg (n = 1170; 618 with UNC and 552 with SNCP) and LDL-C ≥ 100 mg/dl (n = 2473; 1257 with UNC and 1216 with SNCP).

Measures

Data were collected under routine clinical practice conditions from CCR at PHC centers in the Madrid Health Service and processed using OMI-AP software., The CCR was previously validated for patients with a diagnosis of T2DM [20].

SNCP was identified based on the following three criteria:

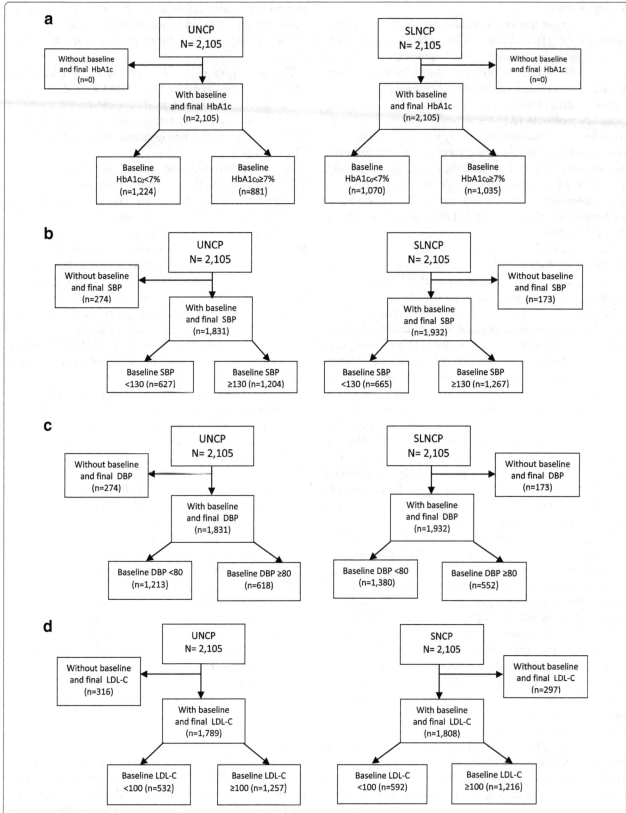

Fig. 1 Procedure and patients included in the study, stratified by ABC goal. ABC goals: (**a**) HbA1c < 7%, (**b**) SBP < 130 mmHg, (**c**) DBP < 80 mmHg and (**d**) LDL-C < 100 mg/dl; UNCP: Usual Nursing Care; SNCP: Standardized languages in Nursing Care Plans; HbA1c: glycosylated hemoglobin; DBP: diastolic blood pressure; SBP: systolic blood pressure; LDL-C: low-density lipoprotein-cholesterol

- Criterion 1. The patient has a CCR code that corresponds to Gordon's functional health patterns [21] in at least one of the following areas: activity and exercise; nutritional and metabolic; and health perception and health management.
- Criterion 2. The problems identified were described using nursing diagnosis statement codes based on the NANDA-I taxonomy, which is used in T2DM patients. A nursing diagnosis based on NANDA-I taxonomy is defined as a clinical judgment concerning a human response to a health condition/life process, or a vulnerability in that response, by an individual, family, group, or community and provides the basis for selection of nursing interventions to achieve outcomes for which the nurse has accountability [14].
- Criterion 3. The nursing intervention carried out was registered according to the NIC taxonomy codes, which used in T2DM patients [15].

The nurses who applied SNCP used the following domains: nutrition, coping/stress tolerance, life principles, health promotion, self-perception, perception/cognition, activity/rest and safety/protection. The main nursing diagnoses were Imbalanced nutrition: more than body requirements (00001), Non-compliance (00079), Ineffective self-health management (00078), Ineffective family therapeutic régimen management (00080), Health-seeking behaviors: Management DM (00084), Deficient knowledge (00126), Sedentary lifestyle (00168) and Impaired skin integrity (00046). The same nurses also delivered UNC to the control group.

UNC was defined as the treatment and monitoring of T2DM including control of blood sugar, control of cardiovascular risk factors, adherence to drug therapy, health education, change in lifestyle and self-management according to local guidelines [22].

The following variables were recorded: sociodemographic characteristics (gender, age), clinical variables (diabetes over time), personal health habits sucha as smoking (cigarettes/day) and drinking (alcohol units/week), physical activity (measured in hours per week with any exercise or activity outside of the patients' regular job being considered, and recoded as vigorous-intensity, moderate-intensity, sedentary), associated morbidity (dyslipidemia, hypertension, coronary heart disease), complications of diabetes mellitus (retinopathy, nephropathy, neuropathy), and the type of treatment prescribed (dietary and pharmacological). Biochemical–biological parameters were also collected, as follows: body mass index (BMI), SBP, DBP, total cholesterol, LDL-C, high-density lipoprotein cholesterol (HDL-C), triglycerides, and A1C.

Blood pressure was measured according to the recommendations of the Seventh Report of the Joint National Committee on Prevention, Detection, Evaluation, and Treatment of High Blood Pressure [23]; these recommendations were current at the start of this study.

Cholesterol and triglycerides were determined using enzyme assays. LDL-C was calculated according to the Friedewald formula [LDL-C = total cholesterol (HDL-C + trigycerides/5)] in participants with triglycerides below 400 mg/dL. HDL-C was measured after precipitation of apoB lipoproteins. A1C was measured using a high-performance liquid chromatography.

Statistical analysis

A descriptive analysis was carried out for each variable included in this study; quantitative variables were expressed as the mean and standard deviation and qualitative variables as. The chi-square test was used to compare the percentage of patients who achieved their ABC goals. The t-test was used for quantitative data. Multiple logistic regression analysis was used to identify the variables associated with each goal (A1C < 7%, DBP < 80 mmHg, SBP < 130 mmHg, and LDL cholesterol < 100 mg/dl) and the relationship between each ABC goal and selected predictor variables was examined. In addition, each logistic regression model was adjusted for all potential confounders, including the variables for which differences between the groups were observed at baseline.

In all instances, the accepted level of significance was 0.05 or less. The 95% confidence interval was reported. All analyses were carried out on an intention-to-treat (ITT) principle. With the analyses were performed using SPSS (SPSS for Windows, V.19.0; IBM Corp, Armonk, New York, USA).

Results

The demographic and clinical characteristics of patients with poorly controlled T2DM at baseline, stratified by SNCP and UNC groups are shown in Table 1. Among patients with A1C ≥7% at baseline, those in the SNCP group were older, had lived with DM for longer, and had received less treatment with diuretics than patients from the UNC group.

Among patients with SBP ≥130 mmHg a statistically significant increased use of oral antidiabetic drugs (OAD) and insulin was found in those in the SNCP group. Similar findings were seen in patients with DBP ≥80 mmHg at baseline. Finally, patients with LDL cholesterol ≥100 mg/dl at baseline who were followed in the SNCP group had lived with DM for longer, had retinopathy, and a more frequently used OADs than those in the UNC group.

Overall, the patients in the SNCP group had a higher prevalence of poor personal health habits, older age, a larger number of complications related to T2DM, and had more frequently received treatment for DM (OAD, insulin) and lipid-lowering drugs (statins).

Table 1 Demographic and clinical characteristics of patients with poorly controlled T2DM at baseline, stratified by SNCP and UNC

	A1C ≥7% (n = 1916)			DBP ≥80 mmHg (n = 1170)			SBP ≥ 130 mmHg (n = 2471)			LDL Chol ≥100 mg/dl (n = 2473)		
	SNCP (n = 1035)	UNC (n = 881)	p value	SNCP (n = 552)	UNC (n = 618)	p value	SNCP (n = 1267)	UNC (n = 1204)	p value	SNCP (n = 1216)	UNC (n = 1257)	p value
Gender female n (%)	581 (56.2)	473 (53.7)	0.27	299 (54.2)	337 (54.5)	0.90	741 (58.5)	677 (56.2)	0.25	684 (56.3)	711 (56.6)	0.89
Age mean (sd)	70 (10)	67.7 (11)	0.00	67.5 (10)	66.3 (10)	0.05	71.5 (8.7)	70.2 (9.3)	0.00	70 (10)	67.9 (10.2)	0.00
Tobacco n (%)	205 (19.8)	190 (21.6)	0.34	120 (21.7)	122 (19.7)	0.40	221 (17.4)	208 (17.3)	0.91	218 (17.9)	238 (18.9)	0.52
CAD n (%)	159 (15.4)	115 (13.1)	0.15	39 (7.1)	49 (7.9)	0.58	151 (11.9)	123 (10.2)	0.18	103 (8.5)	102 (8.1)	0.75
Dyslipidemia n (%)	571 (55.2)	451 (51.2)	0.08	293 (53.1)	323 (52.3)	0.78	684 (54)	616 (51.2)	0.16	682 (56.1)	658 (52.3)	0.06
Retinopathy n (%)	60 (5.8)	53 (6)	0.84	20 (3.6)	16 (2.6)	0.31	60 (4.7)	43 (3.6)	0.15	57 (4.7)	38 (3)	0.03
Nephropathy n (%)	58 (5.6)	47 (5.3)	0.80	28 (5.1)	31 (5)	0.97	78 (6.2)	68 (5.6)	0.59	57 (4.7)	65 (5.2)	0.58
Neuropathy n (%)	21 (2)	24 (2.7)	0.32	7 (1.3)	8 (1.3)	0.97	19 (1.5)	21 (1.7)	0.63	19 (1.6)	19 (1.5)	0.92
Hypertension n (%)	705 (68.1)	624 (70.8)	0.20	429 (77.7)	510 (82.5)	0.04	997 (78.7)	975 (81)	0.16	838 (68.9)	871 (69.3)	0.84
OAD n (%)	885 (85.5)	743 (84.3)	0.48	430 (77.9)	452 (73.1)	0.06	1008 (80)	902 (74.9)	0.00	924 (76)	884 (70.3)	0.00
Insulin n (%)	344 (33.2)	282 (32)	0.57	104 (18.8)	73 (11.8)	0.00	279 (22)	207 (17.2)	0.00	208 (17.1)	187 (14.9)	0.13
OAD + Insulin n (%)	233 (22.5)	184 (20.9)	0.39	76 (13.8)	49 (7.9)	0.00	201 (15.9)	140 (11.6)	0.00	142 (11.7)	122 (9.7)	0.11
Statins n (%)	665 (64.3)	529 (60)	0.06	306 (55.4)	348 (56.3)	0.76	774 (61.1)	712 (59.1)	0.32	681 (56)	707 (56.2)	0.90
Diuretics n (%)	249 (24.1)	249 (28.3)	0.04	146 (26.4)	186 (30.1)	0.17	361 (28.5)	370 (30.7)	0.22	299 (24.6)	337 (26.8)	0.21
Beta-blocker n (%)	159 (15.4)	158 (17.9)	0.13	87 (15.8)	121 (19.6)	0.09	195 (15.4)	214 (17.8)	0.11	165 (13.6)	201 (16)	0.09
Calcium channel blocker n (%)	243 (23.5)	195 (22.1)	0.49	118 (21.4)	143 (23.1)	0.47	326 (25.7)	291 (24.2)	0.37	244 (20.1)	249 (19.8)	0.87
ACE n (%)	407 (39.3)	378 (42.9)	0.11	245 (44.4)	281 (45.5)	0.71	559 (44.1)	561 (46.6)	0.22	461 (37.9)	484 (38.5)	0.76
ARB n (%)	288 (27.8)	231 (26.2)	0.43	169 (30.6)	178 (28.8)	0.50	398 (31.4)	347 (28.8)	0.16	307 (25.2)	283 (22.5)	0.11
Antiplatelet n (%)	742 (71.7)	612 (69.5)	0.29	358 (64.9)	401 (64.9)	0.99	891 (70.3)	827 (68.7)	0.38	796 (65.5)	808 (64.3)	0.54

CAD Coronary arterie disease, *OAD* Oral antidiabetes drug, *ACE* Angiotensin converting enzyme inhibitor, *ARB* Angiotensin receptor blocker

A high percentage of participants – 94.4%- did not achieve all of their ABC goals. No differences were seen between patients aged < 75 years and those aged ≥75 years, although there were differences between genders (males 93.2% vs. females 95.4%, p = 0.003). The BP goal (< 130/80 mmHg) was not achieved in 69.2% patients, with statistically significant differences between age groups (68.2% in < 75 years vs. 71.3% in ≥75 years, p = 0.045) and genders (66.8% in males vs. 71.4% in females, p = 0.001).

A1C ≥7% was recorded in 45.51% of 4210 participants at baseline (n = 1916). Of the 881 participants in the UNC group who had A1C ≥7% at baseline, 275 (31.2%) achieved A1C < 7% after 4 years of follow-up vs. 315 of the 1035 participants in the SNCP group with A1C ≥7% at baseline (30.4%). This difference was not statistically significant (p = 0.713).

The predictors of achieving A1C < 7% after multivariable analysis are shown in Table 2. SNCP did not show any effect with this goal (OR = 0.97; 95% CI, 0.79–1.19). However, the only variables that was directly and significantly associated was: age (OR = 1.02; 95% CI, 1.01–1.03).

The factors that were inversely associated with achievement of A1C < 7% were: duration of DM (OR = 0.98, 95% CI, 0.96–0.99), use of Insulin (OR = 0.27, 95% CI, 0.15–0.49), and use of insulin combined with OAD (OR = 0.31; 95% CI, 0.62–0.98).

Table 2 Predictors of A1C < 7%, Among 1916 Patients Who Did Not Achieve A1C Goals at Baseline after Four-year follow-up (Multivariable Logistic Regression)

Variables	aOR	OR 95% CI	p value
Nursing Care Plans (SNCP/ UNC)	0.97	0.79–1.19	0.761
Gender (male/female)	1.20	0.96–1.50	0.102
Age (years)	1.02	1.01–1.03	0.001
Duration of diabetes mellitus (years)	0.98	0.96–0.99	0.005
OAD (yes/no)	0.73	0.45–1.17	0.190
Insulin (yes/no)	0.27	0.15–0.49	0.000
OAD + insulin (yes/no)	0.31	0.19–0.53	0.000
BMI < 30 kg/m^2 (yes/ no)	0.78	0.62–0.98	0.030

Adjusting for diuretics, statins, ACE inhibitors, beta-blockers, calcium antagonists, smoking, arterial hypertension, dyslipidemia, and CAD

With respect to the goal of SBP < 130 mmHg, 274 (13%) participants in the UNC group and 173 participants (8.2%) in the SNCP group were excluded for not having a BP measurement at baseline and at the end of follow-up. Of the 1204 participants in the UNC group who had SBP ≥130 mmHg at baseline, 345 (28.7%) achieved SBP < 130 mmHg at the final visit vs. 372 from 1267 participants (29.4%) in the SNCP group with SBP ≥130 at baseline. This small difference in favor of the SNCP group did not reach statistical significance (p = 0.699). The main variables associated with SBP < 130 mmHg after 4 years of follow-up were: BMI < 30 kg/m^2 (OR = 1.36; 95% CI, 1.12–1.66), and CAD (OR = 1.38; 1.02–1.87). In addition, an inverse correlation was found between use of calcium antagonists or use of insulin combined with OAD and SBP < 130 mmHg (Table 3) .

Of the 618 participants in the UNC group who had DBP ≥80 mmHg at baseline, 329 (53.2%) achieved DBP < 80 mmHg at the end of follow-up vs. 322 out of 552 patients (58.3%) in the SNCP group who started with DBP ≥80 mmHg. This increase of five percentage points in favor of the SNCP group did not reach statistical significance (p = 0.08).

Table 3 shows that BMI < 30 kg/m^2 is associated with optimal control of DBP (OR = 1.42; 95% CI, 1.08–1.87). However, CAD showed a positive trend for optimal DBP but was notstatistically significant (OR = 1.43; 95% CI, 0.87–2.38). Use of insulin was shown to be a strong predictor of DBP < 80 mmHg (OR = 2.13; 95% CI, 1.06–4.27).

Finally, of the 1257 participants in the UNC group who had LDL-C ≥ 100 mg/dl at baseline, 508 (40.4%) achieved LDL-C < 100 mg/dl at the end of follow-up vs. 472 (38.8%) out of 1216 patients in the SNCP group who started with LDL ≥100 mg/dl. This disadvantage of SNCP did not reach statistical significance (p = 0.417).

The predictor factors for LDL-C < 100 mg/dl after 4 years of follow-up are shown in Table 4. The use of statins (OR = 1.66; 95% CI, 1.36–2.03), treatment of DM with OAD (OR = 1.71; 95% CI, 1.38–2.13), treatment of DM with insulin combined with OAD (OR = 1.91; 95% CI, 1.38–2.64), male sex (OR = 1.49; 95% CI, 1.24–1.78) and having a history of CAD (OR = 1.47; 95% CI, 1.06–2.02) were directly and significantly associated with good control of LDL-C.

Discussion

The present study shows that T2DM patients who were poorly controlled at baseline did not achieve their ABC goals if they were in the SNCP group compared with the UNC group. However, we did observe a trend toward achieving DBP < 80 mmHg in the SNCP group compared with the UNC group.

Early findings from this research project showed that patients in the SNCP group achieved a persistent and significant reduction in DBP, but not in SBP, compared with patients in the UNC group [18]. This improvement in DBP values but not in SBP values reflects the greater difficulty in controlling SBP than DBP, which is highlighted in other studies [24]. In addition, health professionals frequently consider older patients to have good BP control if they reach the DBP goal (< 80 mmHg) even if SBP is above 130 mmHg [25].

In Spain, a similar PHC-based study assessing the outcomes reached over 9 years [26] showed better outcome indicators in chronically ill patients assigned to nurses who implemented care plans than in patients assigned to nurses who did not implement care plans. Specifically, patients in the first group showed higher levels of A1C ≤7% (66.7% vs. 60.3%), BP < 140/90 mmHg (53.3% vs. 50.6%), and total-cholesterol ≤200 mg/dl (39.4% vs. 35.6%; p < 0.05) than the second group. A potential

Table 3 Predictor Factors for SBP < 130 mmHg and DBP < 80 mmHg, among T2DM patients did not achieve BP goal at baseline after four-year follow-up (Multivariable Logistic Regression)

Variables	SBP < 130 mmHg (n = 2147)			DBP < 80 mmHg (n = 1170)		
	aOR	OR 95% CI	p value	aOR	OR 95% CI	p value
Nursing Care Plans (SNCP/ UNCP)	1.03	0.86–1.23	0.783	1.12	0.88–1.43	0.357
Gender (male/female)	1.07	0.88–1.30	0.492	1.08	0.83–1.40	0.557
Age (years)	1.01	0.99–1.02	0.106	1.05	1.03–1.06	0.000
Duration of Diabetes Mellitus (years)	1.01	0.99–1.02	0.883	1.01	0.99–1.03	0.500
OAD (yes/no)	0.81	0.64–1.03	0.082	1.04	0.76–1.41	0.818
Insulin (yes/no)	0.86	0.56–1.32	0.482	2.13	1.06–4.27	0.033
OAD + Insulin (yes/no)	0.60	0.43–0.85	0.004	0.96	0.59–1.56	0.879
BMI < 30 Kg/m^2 (yes/ no)	1.36	1.12–1.66	0.002	1.42	1.08–1.87	0.012
Calcium antagonists (yes/no)	0.70	0.56–0.87	0.002	1.01	0.75–1.36	0.947
CAD (yes/no)	1.38	1.02–1.87	0.035	1.43	0.87–2.38	0.162

Adjusting for diuretics, statins, ACE, beta-blocker, tobacco, arterial hypertension, and dyslipidemia

Table 4 Predictors of LDL-C < 100, Among 2473 Patients Who Did Not Achieve their LDL-C goal at Baseline after Four-year Follow-up (Multivariable Logistic Regression)

Variables	aOR	OR 95% CI	p value
Nursing Care Plans (SNCP/ UNCP)	0.90	0.76–1.06	0.217
Gender (male/female)	1.49	1.24–1.78	0.000
Age (years)	1.01	0.99–1.02	0.728
Duration of diabetes mellitus (years)	1.01	0.99–1.02	0.386
OAD (yes/no)	1.71	1.38–2.13	0.000
Insulin (yes/no)	1.51	0.99–2.30	0.053
OAD + Insulin (yes/no)	1.91	1.38–2.64	0.000
BMI < 30 Kg/m^2 (yes/ no)	0.92	0.77–1.11	0.393
Statins (yes/no)	1.66	1.36–2.03	0.000
Arterial hypertension (yes/no)	1.21	0.98–1.50	0.077
Diuretics (yes/no)	1.18	0.96–1.44	0.111
CAD (yes/no)	1.47	1.06–2.02	0.019

Adjusting for calcium antagonists, ACE inhibitors, beta-blockers, smoking, and dyslipidemia

explanation for the discrepancy between these findings and ours are the different clinical indicators used to define good control and the inclusion criteria (only patients with poor control in the current study vs. all patients in the study by Pérez Rivas et al.) [26].

At baseline, 94.4% of T2DM patients did not meet all three ABC goals. This figure is similar to that found in other studies such as the National Health and Nutrition Examinatin Survey (NHANES) [27] in 1999–2002 and an Israel cohort study [28]. However, more recently, in NHANES 2007–2010 the percentage of patients who did not meet all of their ABC fell to 81.2% [27].

Non-optimal baseline control of A1C (≥7%) was recorded in 45.1% of participants, consistent with other national studies [29] and international studies [30, 31]. Among people with A1C ≥ 7%, both groups showed improvement in control of A1C from baseline, although the differences were not significant. In both groups a third of patients achieved A1C < 7% after 4 years of follow-up. This improvement is particularly hard to achieve, because the longer a patient has lived with T2DM the more difficult it is to achieve glycemic control [32–34].

The predictive factors for attaining A1C < 7% are concordant with results from previous studies showing that patients who have been treated with insulin (alone or combined with OADs) for longer periods showed poor control of A1C [35]. In contrast with other studies [36], we found that BMI < 30 kg/m^2 was not a predictior of optimal glycemic control. Baseline control of SBP was non-optimal (≥130 mmHg) in 69.2% of cases; that of DBP was non-optimal in 32% of cases (≥80 mmHg). An controlled BP (≥130/80 mmHg) was recorded in 69.2%

of participants. These percentage are higher than those found in NHANES 2007–2010, NHANES 2003–2006, and NHANES 1999–2002. A possible explanation is that the mean age of the patients included in these studies was below 60 years whereas in our study it was 69.2 years. On the other hand, our data are similar to those from the NHANES 1988–1994 study [27] and from the National Diabetes Health Promotion Centers survey in Taiwan [31], where participants were aged over 60 years. This finding is consistent with the known inverse relationship between older age and control of arterial hypertension [37, 38].

Optimal control of SBP at the end of the follow-up was achieved by 29.4% patients in the SNCP group vs. 28.7% in the UNC group. This difference was not statistically significant.

The strongest predictive factor for SBP < 130 mmHg was history of CAD, followed by BMI < 30 kg/m^2. A recent clinical-epidemiological study of 55,518 primary care patients in Germany [39] found that previous CAD was a significant predictor of adequate BP control (adjusted OR = 1.52; 95% CI, 1.13–1.39). The benefits of weight loss on control of BP, regardless of drug treatment, are well known [40]. The Trial of Hypertension Prevention (TOHP) [41] showed that an average weight loss of 2 kg. was associated with a drop in SBP/ DBP of 3.7/2.7 mmHg. The SNCP group worked on weight reduction, which had no effect on control of SBP possibly because weight loss requires intense interventions (low-calorie diet plus regular physical activity and, in some cases, behavior therapy) as highlighted in the NIC collection [42].

With respect to patients with non-optimal control of DBP at baseline, adequate control was achieved by 58.3% patients in the SNCP group vs. 53.2% in the UNC group. While not statistically significant, this difference seems clinically relevant.

As with SBP, a history of CAD and BMI < 30 kg/m^2 are shown to be independent predictors of adequate control of DBP. Older age was also positively associated with good control. This finding was previously reported in patients who were of normal weight or overweight [43], although it is not common [44, 45] because older age is usually associated with increased morbidity and poorer control of BP [46].

The percentage of T2DM patients who reached LDL-C < 100 mg/dl was not better in the SNCP group than in the UNC group. Stronger predictors for achieving the LDL-C goal were the administration of statins, treatment with OAD, treatment with insulin combined with OAD, male sex and having a history of CAD. The persistent strength of CAD as a predictor of control of BP and achievement of LDL-C goals could be explained by a self-perception of illness that is more serious and linked to higher medication adherence [47]. It is also possible that patients with previous CAD may have been managed more aggressively [38] than patients without myocardial ischemia.

Long cohort studies typically have high rates of loss to follow-up that potentially affects their validity [48]. Our study had only 15% losses to follow-up, because only patients with at least two HbA1c values during the follow-up period were selected. These patients usually receive better quality care and are more likely to have a second LDL-C than the general population with T2DM.

Our study is subject to a series of limitations. First, the sample was composed of T2DM patients who regularly visited PHC centers and may therefore not be representative of the entire T2DM patient community. However, as we mentioned above, the proportion of T2DM patients in our study who met their ABC goals is similar to that reported elsewhere, and it seems that the potential for selection bias is low. Second, since the quality of evidence from cohort studies is lower than that from clinical trials, our results should be interpreted with caution. Third, the fact that SNCP has been implemented progressively in recent years [26], could reasonably affect our results. Therefore, we carried out an ITT analysis to determine the effect of SNCP; this analysis might have influenced the weaker effect seen in the SNCP group than in the UNC group. However, ITT is the most appropriate study design for this context and is considered standard practice by CONSORT (Consolidated Standards of Reporting Trials). Fourth, we did not control the time the patient remained in each of the study groups. There may have been some crossover that reduced the differences between groups, because there has been significant movement between nursing teams in recent years in Madrid. Furthermore, given the economic recession, nursing teams have become smaller, resulting in nurses having less time with their patients. Fifth, the fact that nursing staff do not receive incentives to improve patient health outcomes could result in less motivation from staff.

Finally, to our knowledge, no studies that have evaluated the effectiveness of SNCP in reaching ABC goals in patients with poorly controlled T2DM at baseline. For this reason, our study is not comparable to other studies with similar efficacy. Further research in this area should be carried out.

Conclusions

We conclude that there is not enough evidence to favor SNCP over UNC with the aim of helping patients with poorly controlled T2DM at baseline to achieve their ABC goals However, SNCP shows a clear trend to improving the proportion of patients who achieve DBP goals.

Abbreviations
A1C: Glycosylated hemoglobin; ADA: The American Diabetes Association; BMI: Body mass index; BP: Blood pressure; CAD: Coronary artery disease; CCR: Computerized Clinical Records; DBP: Diastolic blood pressure; DM: Diabetes mellitus; HDL: High-density lipoprotein; LDL: Low-density lipoprotein; NANDA: NANDA-International; NIC: Nursing interventions classification; OAD: Oral antidiabetic drug; PHC: Primary health care; SBP: Systolic blood pressure; SNCP: Standardized languages in Nursing Care Plans; T2DM: Type 2 diabetes mellitus; TOHP: Trial of Hypertension Prevention; UNC: Usual Nursing Care

Acknowledgements
This article was supported by the Fondo de Investigación Sanitaria, Instituto de Salud Carlos III (PI07/0865). We thank the members of the Madrid Nurse Diagnosis Study Group, who collaborated in the study: Rosa Arnal-Selfa, Luis Sánchez-Perruca, José María Mena-Mateo, Asunción Cañada-Dorado, Inmaculada García-Ferradal and María del Carmen Mustieles-Moreno.

Funding
This article has been supported by the Sanitary Research Fund of the Carlos III Health Institute (ISCIII) (PI07/0865) and the Foundation for Biomedical Research and Innovation of Primary Care FIIBAP through the call for aid for publications 2016. The funders had no role in study design, data collection and analysis, decision to publish, or preparation of the manuscript.

Authors' contributions
JCV had the original idea for the study and prepared the first draft of the manuscript and coordinated responses from the authors. JCV, MASF and PGC got funding. CBL, RJG and FJSAR developed the data collection databases. JCV, MASF, CBL, PGC and MJDD contributed to the study design and analysis methods. ALA, CBL, PGC, RJG, MJDD and JCV designed the case report form and the investigator's brochure. All authors participated in interpreting the data, revising the paper for critically important intellectual content and gave final approval of the submitted version.

Competing interests
The authors declare that they have no competing interests.

Author details
[1]Dirección Técnica de Sistemas de Información, Gerencia Asistencial de Atención Primaria, Servicio Madrileño de Salud, C/ San Martín de Porres, 6, 28035 Madrid, Spain. [2]Universidad Alfonso X el Sabio, Villanueva de la Cañada, Madrid, Spain. [3]Aging and Fragility in the Elderly Group, Hospital La Paz Institute for Health Research (IdiPAZ), Madrid, Spain. [4]MADIABETES Research Group, Madrid, Spain. [5]Facultad de Ciencias de la Salud, Universidad Rey Juan Carlos, Alcorcón, Madrid, Spain. [6]Jefatura de Estudios del Grado en Enfermería, Universidad Alfonso X el Sabio, Villanueva de la Cañada, Madrid, Spain. [7]Innate Immunity Group, Hospital La Paz Institute for Health Research (IdiPAZ), La Paz University Hospital, Madrid, Spain. [8]University Centre of Health Sciences San Rafael-Nebrija, Antonio de Nebrija University, Madrid, Spain. [9]Dirección General de Salud Pública, Subdirección de Promoción, Prevención y Educación de la Salud, Consejería de Sanidad, Madrid, Spain. [10]Red de Investigación en Servicios de Salud en Enfermedades

Crónicas (REDISSEC), Madrid, Spain. [11]Centro de Salud Las Calesas, Madrid, Spain. [12]Centro de Salud Monóvar, Madrid, Spain. [13]Subdirección General de Investigación. Consejería de Sanidad, Madrid, Spain.

References

1. Soriguer F, Goday A, Bosch-Comas A, Bordiú E, Calle-Pascual A, Carmena R, Casamitjana R, Castaño L, Castell C, Catalá M, Delgado E, Franch J, Gaztambide S, Girbés J, Gomis R, Gutiérrez G, López-Alba A, Martínez-Larrad MT, Menéndez E, Mora-Peces I, Ortega E, Pascual-Manich G, Rojo-Martínez G, Serrano-Rios M, Valdés S, Vázquez JA, Vendrell J. Prevalence of diabetes mellitus and impaired glucose regulation in Spain: the Di@bet.es study. Diabetologia. 2012;55:88–93.
2. Valdés S, Rojo-Martínez G, Soriguer F. Evolution of prevalence of type 2 diabetes in adult Spanish population. Med Clin (Barc). 2007;129:352–5.
3. Janghorbani M, Hu FB, Willett WC, Li TY, Manson JE, Logroscino G, Rexrode KM. Prospective study of type 1 and type 2 diabetes and risk of stroke subtypes: the Nurses' health study. Diabetes Care. 2007;30:1730–5.
4. Haffner SM, Lehto S, Rönnemaa T, Pyörälä K, Laakso M. Mortality from coronary heart disease in subjects with type 2 diabetes and in nondiabetic subjects with and without prior myocardial infarction. N Engl J Med. 1998; 339:229–34.
5. Zhang Y, Hu G, Yuan Z, Chen L. Glycosylated hemoglobin in relationship to cardiovascular outcomes and death in patients with type 2 diabetes: a systematic review and meta-analysis. PLoS One. 2012;7(8):e42551.
6. Sowers JR. Diabetes mellitus and vascular disease. Hypertension. 2013;61(5):943–7.
7. Basevi V, Di Mario S, Morciano C, Nonino F, Magrini N. Comment on: American Diabetes Association. Standards of medical care in diabetes-2011. Diabetes Care. 2011;34:S11–61.
8. López-Simarro F, Brotons C, Moral I, Cols-Sagarra C, Selva A, Aguado-Jodar A, Miravet-Jiménez S. Inertia and treatment compliance in patients with type 2 diabetes in primary careMed Clin (Barc). 2012;138:377–84.
9. Marwick TH, Hordern MD, Miller T, Chyun DA, Bertoni AG, Blumenthal RS, Philippides G, Rocchini A. Council on clinical cardiology, American Heart Association exercise, cardiac rehabilitation, and prevention committee; council on cardiovascular disease in the young; council on cardiovascular nursing; council on nutrition, physical activity, and metabolism; interdisciplinary council on quality of care and outcomes research. Exercise training for type 2 diabetes mellitus: impact on cardiovascular risk: a scientific statement from the American Heart Association. Circulation. 2009;119:3244–62.
10. Hartmann M, Kopf S, Kircher C, Faude-Lang V, Djuric Z, Augstein F, Friederich HC, Kieser M, Bierhaus A, Humpert PM, Herzog W, Nawroth PP. Sustained effects of a mindfulness-based stress-reduction intervention in type 2 diabetic patients: design and first results of a randomized controlled trial (the Heidelberger diabetes and stress-study). Diabetes Care. 2012;35:945–7.
11. Tan E, Yang W, Pang B, Dai M, Loh FE, Hogan P. Geographic variation in antidiabetic agent adherence and glycemic control among patients with type 2 diabetes. J Manag Care Spec Pharm. 2015;21:1195–202.
12. Rezabek KM. Medical nutrition therapy in type 2 diabetes. Nurs Clin North Am. 2001;36:203–16.
13. Si D, Bailie R, Weeramanthri T. Effectiveness of chronic care model-oriented interventions to improve quality of diabetes care: a systematic review. Prim Health Care Res Dev. 2008;9(1):25–40.
14. Herdman TH & Kamitsuru S, editors. Nursing diagnoses 2015–17: definitions and classification. 10 th ed. Oxford: Wiley Blackwell; 2014.
15. Bulecheck GM, Butcher H, Dochterman JM, Wagner C. Nursing Interventions Classification (NIC). 6 th ed. St. Louis: Elsevier Health Sciences; 2013.
16. González-Jurado MA. Normalización de la práctica enfermera como contribución a la salud, la calidad asistencial y la seguridad clínica de las personas. Evaluación en los cuidados del paciente neumológico. Tesis. Madrid: Universidad Complutense de Madrid. Facultad de Medicina; 2006.
17. Cárdenas-Valladolid J, Salinero-Fort MA, Gómez-Campelo P, de Burgos-Lunar C, Abánades-Herranz JC, Arnal-Selfa R, Andrés AL. Effectiveness of standardized nursing care plans in health outcomes in patients with type 2 diabetes mellitus: a two-year prospective follow-up study. PLoS One. 2012;7: e43870.
18. Cárdenas-Valladolid J, Salinero-Fort MA, Gómez-Campelo P, López-Andrés A. Standardized nursing care plans in patients with type 2 diabetes mellitus: are they effective in the long-term? Aten Primaria. 2015;47:186–9.
19. The International Classification of Primary Care in the European Community. (With a sixteen language disk of ICPC). H lamberts, M wood, IM Hofmans-Okkes. Oxford: Oxford University Press; 1993.
20. de Burgos-Lunar C, Salinero-Fort MA, Cárdenas-Valladolid J, Soto-Díaz S, Fuentes-Rodríguez CY, Abánades-Herranz JC, del Cura-González I. Validation of diabetes mellitus and hypertension diagnosis in computerized medical records in primary health care. BMC Med Res Methodol. 2011;11:146.
21. Gordon M. Manual of nursing diagnosis. 12 th ed. Ontario: Jones Bartlett Learning; 2010.
22. Grupo de trabajo de la Guía de Práctica Clínica sobre Diabetes tipo 2. Guía de Práctica Clínica sobre Diabetes tipo 2. Madrid: Plan Nacional para el SNS del MSC. Agencia de Evaluación de Tecnologías Sanitarias del País Vasco. Guías de Práctica Clínica en el SNS: OSTEBA N° 2006/08 OSASUN SAILA DEPARTAMENTO DE SANIDAD; 2008.
23. Chobanian AV, Bakris GL, Black HR, Cushman WC, Green LA, Izzo JL Jr, Jones DW, Materson BJ, Oparil S, Wright JT Jr, Roccella EJ. Joint National Committee on prevention, detection, evaluation, and treatment of high blood pressure. National Heart, Lung, and Blood Institute; National High Blood Pressure Education Program Coordinating Committee. Seventh report of the joint National Committee on prevention, detection, evaluation, and treatment of high blood pressure. Hypertension. 2003;42:1206–52.
24. Lloyd-Jones DM, Evans JC, Larson MG, O'Donnell CJ, Roccella EJ, Levy D. Differential control of systolic and diastolic blood pressure: factors associated with lack of blood pressure control in the community. Hypertension. 2000;36:594–9.
25. Lloyd-Jones DM, Evans JC, Larson MG, Levy D. Treatment and control of hypertension in the community: a prospective analysis. Hypertension. 2000; 40:640–6.
26. Pérez Rivas FJ, Santamaría García JM, Minguet Arenas C, Beamud Lagos M, García López M. Implementation and evaluation of the nursing process in primary health care. Int J Nurs Knowl. 2012;23:18–28.
27. Stark Casagrande S, Fradkin JE, Saydah SH, Rust KF, Cowie CC. The prevalence of meeting A1C, blood pressure, and LDL goals among people with diabetes, 1988-2010. Diabetes Care. 2013;36:2271–9.
28. Rapoport M, Harel N, Shasha Y, Barkan R, Kitaee E, Buchs A, Izhakian S, Aviel-Gadot E. Achievement of partial combined control of major diabetes targets in primary care correlates with development of chronic complications in T2DM patients-a real life data. Prim Care Diabetes. 2015;9:412–7.
29. Barrot-de la Puente J, Mata-Cases M, Franch-Nadal J, Mundet-Tudurí X, Casellas A, Fernandez-Real JM, Mauricio D. Older type 2 diabetic patients are more likely to achieve glycaemic and cardiovascular risk factors targets than younger patients: analysis of a primary care database. Int J Clin Pract. 2015; 69:1486–95.
30. Vouri SM, Shaw RF, Waterbury NV, Egge JA, Alexander B. Prevalence of achievement of A1c, blood pressure, and cholesterol (ABC) goal in veterans with diabetes. J Manag Care Pharm. 2011;17:304–12.
31. Yu NC, Su HY, Tsai ST, Lin BJ, Shiu RS, Hsieh YC, Sheu WH. ABC control of diabetes: survey data from National Diabetes Health Promotion Centers in Taiwan. Diabetes Res Clin Pract. 2009;84:194–200.
32. Franch-Nadal J, Roura-Olmeda P, Benito-Badorrey B, Rodríguez-Poncelas A, Coll-de-Tuero G, Mata-Cases M, GEDAPS (Primary care Group for the study of Diabetes). Metabolic control and cardiovascular risk factors in type 2 diabetes mellitus according to diabetes duration. Fam Pract. 2015;32:27–34.
33. Chan JC, Gagliardino JJ, Baik SH, Chantelot JM, Ferreira SR, Hancu N, Ilkova H, Ramachandran A, Aschner P, Investigators IDMPS. Multifaceted determinants for achieving glycemic control: the international diabetes management practice study (IDMPS). Diabetes Care. 2009;32:227–33.
34. Lopez Stewart G, Tambascia M, Rosas Guzmán J, Etchegoyen F, Ortega Carrión J, Artemenko S. Control of type 2 diabetes mellitus among general practitioners in private practice in nine countries of Latin America. Rev Panam Salud Publica. 2007;22:12–20.
35. Fox KM, Gerber Pharmd RA, Bolinder B, Chen J, Kumar S. Prevalence of inadequate glycemic control among patients with type 2 diabetes in the United Kingdom general practice research database: a series of retrospective analyses of data from 1998 through 2002. Clin Ther. 2006;28:388–95.
36. Hoerger TJ, Segel JE, Gregg EW, Saaddine JB. Is glycemic control improving in U.S. adults? Diabetes Care. 2008;31:81–6.
37. Barquilla García A, Llisterri Caro JL, Prieto Díaz MA, Alonso Moreno FJ, García Matarín L, Galgo Nafría A. Blood pressure control in a population of hypertensive diabetic patients treated in primary care: PRESCAP-diabetes study 2010. SEMERGEN. 2015;41:13–23.

38. Duggirala MK, Cuddihy RM, Cuddihy MT, Naessens JM, Cha SS, Mandrekar JN, Leibson CL. Predictors of blood pressure control in patients with diabetes and hypertension seen in primary care clinics. Am J Hypertens. 2005;18:833–8.

39. Labeit AM, Klotsche J, Pieper L, Pittrow D, Einsle F, Stalla GK, Lehnert H, Silber S, Zeiher AM, März W, Wehling M, Wittchen HU. Changes in the prevalence, treatment and control of hypertension in Germany? A clinical-epidemiological study of 50.000 primary care patients. PLoS One. 2012;7:e52229.

40. Whelton PK, Appel LJ, Espeland MA, Applegate WB, Ettinger WH Jr, Kostis JB, Kumanyika S, Lacy CR, Johnson KC, Folmar S, Cutler JA. Sodium reduction and weight loss in the treatment of hypertension in older persons: a randomized controlled trial of nonpharmacologic interventions in the elderly (TONE). TONE Collaborative Research Group. JAMA. 1998;279:839–46.

41. Whelton PK, Appel L, Charleston J, et al. The effects of nonpharmacologic interventions on blood pressure of persons with high normal levels. Results of the trials of hypertension prevention, phase I. JAMA. 1992;267:1213–20.

42. National Institutes of Health. Clinical guidelines on the identification, evaluation, and treatment of overweight and obesity in adults–the evidence report. Obes Res. 1998;6:51S–209S.

43. Chopra I, Kamal KM. Factors associated with therapeutic goal attainment in patients with concomitant hypertension and dyslipidemia. Hosp Pract (1995). 2014;42:77–88.

44. Ben-Hamouda-Chihaoui M, Kanoun F, Ftouhi B, Lamine-Chtioui F, Kamoun M, Slimane H. Evaluation of blood pressure control by ambulatory blood pressure monitoring and study of factors associated with poor blood pressure control in 300 treated hypertensive type 2 diabetic patients. Ann Cardiol Angeiol (Paris). 2011;60:71–6.

45. Coca A, Dalfó A, Esmatjes E, Llisterri JL, Ordóñez J, Gomis R, González-Juanatey JR, Martín-Zurro A, Grupo PREVENCAT. Treatment and control of cardiovascular risk in primary care in Spain. The PREVENCAT study. Med Clin(Barc). 2006;126:201–5.

46. Wong MC, Wang HH, Cheung CS, Tong EL, Sek AC, Cheung NT, Yan BP, Yu CM, Griffiths SM, Coats AJ. Factors associated with multimorbidity and its link with poor blood pressure control among 223,286 hypertensive patients. Int J Cardiol. 2014;177:202–8.

47. Rajpura J, Nayak R. Medication adherence in a sample of elderly suffering from hypertension: evaluating the influence of illness perceptions, treatment beliefs, and illness burden. J Manag Care Pharm. 2014;20:58–65.

48. Kristman V, Manno M, Côté P. Loss to follow-up in cohort studies: how much is too much? Eur J Epidemiol. 2004;19:751–60.

10

Development, modelling, and pilot testing of a complex intervention to support end-of-life care provided by Danish general practitioners

Anna Kirstine Winthereik[1,4]* ⓘ, Mette Asbjoern Neergaard[2], Anders Bonde Jensen[1] and Peter Vedsted[3]

Abstract

Background: Most patients in end-of-life with life-threatening diseases prefer to be cared for and die at home. Nevertheless, the majority die in hospitals. GPs have a pivotal role in providing end-of-life care at patients' home, and their involvement in the palliative trajectory enhances the patient's possibility to stay at home. The aim of this study was to develop and pilot-test an intervention consisting of continuing medical education (CME) and electronic decision support (EDS) to support end-of-life care in general practice.

Methods: We developed an intervention in line with the first phases of the guidelines for complex interventions drawn up by the Medical Research Council. Phase 1 involved the development of the intervention including identification of key barriers to provision of end-of-life care for GPs and of facilitators of change. Furthermore the actual modelling of two components: CME meeting and EDS. Phase 2 focused on pilot-testing and intervention assessment by process evaluation.

Results: In phase 1 lack of identification of patients at the end of life and limited palliative knowledge among GPs were identified as barriers. The CME meeting and the EDS were developed. The CME meeting was a four-hour educational meeting performed by GPs and specialists in palliative care. The EDS consisted of two parts: a pop-up window for each patient with palliative needs and a list of all patients with palliative needs in the practice. The pilot testing in phase 2 showed that the CME meeting was performed as intended and 120 (14%) of the GPs in the region attended. The EDS was integrated in existing electronic records but was shut down early for external reasons; 50 (5%) GPs signed up. The pilot-testing demonstrated a need to strengthen the implementation as attending rate was low in the current set-up.

Conclusion: We developed a complex intervention to support GPs in providing end-of-life care. The pilot-test showed general acceptance of the CME meetings. The EDS was shut down early and needs further evaluation before examining the whole intervention in a larger study, where evaluation could be based on patient-related outcomes and impact on end-of-life care.

Keywords: Continuing medical education, Clinical decision support systems, Palliative care, End-of-life care, COPD, Cancer, General practice, Complex intervention, Denmark

* Correspondence: akwi@oncology.au.dk
[1]Department of Oncology, Aarhus University Hospital, Noerrebrogade 44, 8000 Aarhus C, Denmark
[4]Department of Clinical Medicine, Aarhus University, Noerrebrogade 44, 8000 Aarhus C, Denmark
Full list of author information is available at the end of the article

Background

The general practitioner (GP) has a pivotal role in palliative care in most western countries. In particular, when the patient is at home, the GP is the key physician [1] and optimally ensures all aspects of continuity in the illness trajectory [2]. The GP often acts as gatekeeper to specialist treatment [3] and thus has the potential to assume a coordinating role for patients with cancer and other life-threatening disease.

Most patients with terminal illnesses prefer to be cared for and die at home [4, 5]. Nevertheless, the majority of patients in Denmark and many other western countries end up dying in hospitals [4–6]. Involvement of the GP in the palliative trajectory seems to enhance the patient's possibility to stay and die at home [7–9], but a need for optimising the end-of-life care has been identified among Danish GPs [10]. Furthermore, previous studies have found that cancer patients were more likely to receive palliative care compared to patients suffering from non-malignancies (e.g. COPD and heart failure) [11–13].

Therefore, it is crucial to support and optimise the end-of-life care provided by GPs to both cancer patients and patients suffering from non-malignant diseases. End-of-life refers to the part of the disease trajectory where patients are likely to die within 12 months [14].

No single strategy has so far proven superior in optimising palliative care in general practice [15, 16]. A revised Danish guideline on palliative care in general practice was published in 2014 [17], but a guideline in itself does not change the clinical practice [18]. Continuing medical education (CME) meetings have shown to have a positive effect on changing the GPs' attitudes concerning palliative care, but they seem to have little impact on the actual provision of care [15]. Electronic decision support (EDS) has improved guideline adherence in other areas (e.g. prescription of antibiotics) and changed clinical outcomes [18–23]. However, a Scottish study showed that GPs were reluctant to use EDS in end-of-life care as the term "palliative" was hard to apply to electronically identified patients because of the association with death [24]. Still, it is unknown whether a combination of CME and EDS could optimise end-of-life care provision among GPs.

The aim of this study was to develop and pilot-test an intervention consisting of a CME meeting and EDS to support the end-of-life care in general practice for patients with cancer or COPD.

Methods

This study describes the development of a complex intervention in general practice based on the recommendations of the Medical Research Council (MRC). The MRC guidelines included both recommendations for conducting the study and for reporting the results [25, 26]. The MRC framework suggests four phases in the development of a complex intervention. This study focuses on the first two phases; phase 1 focus on development of the intervention and includes evidence-based identification of *barriers* to GP provision of end-of-life care and perceived *facilitators* to change the clinical practice and the modelling of the intervention. Phase 2 is pilot-testing of the intervention.

To reduce the complexity of the intervention the overall phases in the MRC guideline and how we planned the steps will be presented in the method section. The result section will specify the content and the results of the different steps.

Phase 1: development of the intervention

First part of the development was to *identify* barriers to end-of-life care and facilitators to clinical change in general practice. This was done using three different strategies.

Two narrative literature searches were performed: one focused barriers to end-of-life care and another on facilitators. The following medical databases were searched: biblioteket.dk, SweMed, PubMed, Embase, Cochrane Library, Cinahl and PsyhINFO.

Search terms

1. General practice OR General practitioners OR family practice OR family doctor AND palliative care OR palliative medicine OR end-of-life care OR terminal care
2. General practice OR general practitioners OR family practice OR family doctor AND clinical practice OR change of clinical practice OR intervention study OR continuing medical education

Reference lists were subsequently scrutinised for additional studies, and relevant articles were selected after reading the abstracts.

Secondly, AKW performed unstructured individual interviews with three GPs with a special interest in end-of-life care. The aim of these interviews was not to achieve saturation of data but to test and culturally adapt the established knowledge on barriers and facilitators from the literature to a Danish clinical setting to help choosing the right focus.

Thirdly, the findings were discussed within the research group (constituted of the authors) drawing on own research and clinical experiences.

Second part of the development phase was the *modelling* of the intervention.

Based on the identified evidence base, the research group selected a number of barriers to address from a perspective of importance and barriers possible to address. Furthermore, facilitators to increase the effect of the intervention were selected. A multifaceted approach with a tailored intervention was chosen [27, 28] with two components, which complemented each other: a CME meeting and an EDS. The CME meeting was a one-time event allowing time to reflect and engage with colleagues, whereas the EDS continuously provided contextually relevant evidence-based information without interaction with peers.

Hence, two working groups, including stakeholders with CME experience in general practice, were appointed to assist in designing the components. The group developing the CME meeting comprised of seven participants: the research group (including an oncologist, two researchers with special interest in general practice and a palliative care specialist), one GP responsible for a regional CME, and two academic coordinators for CMEs targeting GPs in the region.

The EDS working group comprised of two GPs, the research group, and medical and technical staff from the Danish Quality Unit of General Practice (DAK-E). Two successive meetings were held during the development with participation from the GPs engaging in CME, administrative staff from all regions in Denmark, and a member of the research group (AKW). The technical development was carried out by DAK-E. The EDS was made using existing technology to ensure compatibility with all electronic patient record (EPR) systems in Danish general practices [3, 29].

Phase 2: pilot-testing

In the pilot-testing, we adapted ideas and terms from the MRC guideline [26] and the process evaluation described by Grol et al. [18]. The purpose of process evaluation is to systematically assess the components in the intervention that could have an impact on the outcome of a pilot study. There is no standard process evaluation, but assessment is suggested to include: 1) the fidelity, 2) the quality and 3) the context of the intervention [18, 26]. We assessed the CME meeting and the EDS separately.

Degree of adherence to the blueprint and the reach of the intervention assessed the *fidelity*.

Adherence to the blueprint examines the extent to which the intervention components were delivered as intended, including whether development of the components succeeded and how well the components were implemented. To ensure adherence to blueprint in the CME meeting and delivery of similar content in each CME meeting, a test run was performed. All persons engaged in teaching at the CME meeting were present and received a copy of a detailed plan.

The implementation plan primarily included using existing newsletters which were sent to all GPs from two different senders. The Quality Unit for Cancer care in

general practice in Central Region Denmark invited and reminded the GPs to participate in a CME meeting (free of charge) in their catchment area. The GPs were informed about the EDS through the regular DAK-E newsletter. Furthermore, the EDS was demonstrated at the CME meetings and briefly presented in a trade journal for Danish GPs [30].

The reach of the intervention was assessed by number of GPs attending CME meetings or signed up for the EDS compared to those who did either one or none of them. Background characteristics were retrieved for all GPs in the region to allow comparisons and to clarify if the intervention targeted specific subgroups of GPs i.e. younger GPs, urban GPs or female.

The *quality* of the CME meeting was investigated by using the attending GPs' experiences of the meeting and the impact of the meeting on provision of end-of-life care. GPs' experiences were assessed by using a mixed-methods approach carried out by an external evaluation unit in the Central Denmark Region [31]. The evaluation was done using questionnaires and interviews. After each meeting, a questionnaire was handed out to all participating GPs for themselves to fill in. The questionnaire consisted of seven items concerning benefits of attending the CME meeting, applied teaching methods, suggestions for improvements and if/how the CME meeting might affect their approach to end-of-life care in the future. Two of the items were answered on a 5-point Likert scale ranging from one to five and the remaining five questions were answered by free text comments (see Additional file 1 to see the questionnaire).

In addition to the questionnaire, three group interviews with fixed questions were conducted. Each interview was performed with a group of three GPs and carried out immediately after three of the six CME meetings (i.e. a total of nine interviewed GPs). The interviews focused on three topics: teaching methods, benefits from the CME meeting and possible improvements for future educational meetings. Each interview took approximately 15 min.

The short-term impact of the CME meeting on the GPs' attitude was assessed by an email sent three months after the CME meeting to all participating GPs. They were asked: Have you changed anything in your approach to palliative care since the CME? (If yes: then what?; if no: then why not?).

To assess participants' experience with the EDS, a postal questionnaire was planned to be send one year after the implementation to the GPs. The questionnaire contained items about relevance and functionality of the EDS. Furthermore, the specific function of the EDS that identified patients with potential palliative needs (more details are available in the results section), was to be adjusted retrospectively by using register-based data on deceased patients to possibly adjust the criterions for identification. These register-based data were also to be compared to how often the GPs ticked the pop-up window as irrelevant. Finally, as a proxy for usage of the EDS, data on how many times a pop-up was opened by the individual GP were to be retrieved.

The impact of the intervention on provision of end-of-life care was to be fully assessed after one year. The assessment would focus on patient-related outcomes on practice level, e.g. number of terminal declarations (a declaration releasing medical reimbursement for end-of-life care), frequency of prescription of anticipatory medication used in the terminal phase and number of home deaths. These data were to be retrieved from national registers using the unique identification number of every Danish citizens and their exact linkage to a general practice. The figures were to be compared before and after the intervention.

Finally, the *context* of the intervention was assessed by focusing on elements that could facilitate or hamper the effect of the intervention.

The overall context was the Danish health care system, which is tax financed and provides free access for all residents to health care services. More than 98% of the Danes are registered with a specific general practice, and the GPs are responsible for the health care provision to their listed patients [3]. If symptom relief or problem solving is too complex or not possible in primary care, the GPs can get advice from specialists or refer to specialist treatment [3]. The GPs are remunerated by Danish Regions according to a nationally negotiated scheme. Continuing medical education (CME) was not compulsory for Danish GPs until 2015, but they could receive remuneration for five days a year to cover education expenses and loss of earnings [32]. This study was performed in the spring 2014 in the Central Denmark Region with 843 GPs organized in 407 practices covering a population of approx. 1.3 million inhabitants.

Data collection
Concerning the CME meeting, all participating GPs were registered (provider number, qualified GP/trainee/other, municipality, place of participation) upon arrival at the meeting for evaluation of the implementation of the CME meeting. GP characteristics (provider number, gender, number of GPs in different areas) were retrieved from the Central Denmark Region to compare participating and non-participating GPs. The external evaluator, who carried out the evaluation of the CME meeting, registered the answers on a Likert scale and collected the answers to the open questions in full wording for each topic and each meeting separately. The interviews were recorded and summarized in themes grouped according to the three overall topics (teaching methods, benefits from the CME meeting and possible

improvements of the meeting) for each of the three interviews and the points were illustrated with typical statements from the interviewed GPs.

Data about EDS sign-up were retrieved from the DAK-E database. The patient-related data we had planned to use to fully assess the intervention was to be retrieved from national registers and DAK-E database.

Analysis
Descriptive analysis regarding the attending GPs and their answers to the questionnaires were made. The Likert Scale answers were presented as percentages. The remaining five items with open answers were described qualitatively on the basis of trends and frequency of issues within each topic. Excel® was used for the descriptive statistics. As the analysis of the interview data were performed by an external evaluator no further information can be provided.

Results
Phase 1: the development phase
The barriers chosen to address by the research group based on the evidence base, unstructured interviews and experience were
Firstly, lack of identification of patients in end-of-life phase, especially for patients with non-malignant diseases [10]. Most clinicians tend to overestimate the remaining life span [33–35], which may compromise timely provision of end-of-life care. Different disease trajectories create different challenges for the GPs in the recognition of end-of-life issues. This could be one reason why patients with COPD tend to get less end-of-life care although their symptoms and prognosis are comparable to those of patients with lung cancer [11, 36, 37]. Secondly, variation in skills and knowledge among GPs concerning the provision of end-of-life care [38–40]. One issue is that some GPs tend to avoid confronting patients and relatives with end-of-life issues, whereas patients and relatives expect the GPs to take such initiatives, to be proactive, and assume the keyworker role in palliative care [40–42].

The facilitors chosen, by the research group, to be used in the intervention to emphasize the effect of the different components are listed in Table 1.

The modelling
The framing of the CME meeting was based on adult learning theory with a problem-based approach to emphasise the relevance to clinical work [28]. The framing paid attention to the independent way in which most GPs work and their preferences for guidance [43, 44]. The content of the CME meeting was supported by research findings on GPs and end-of-life care, and an updated national guideline on palliative care for general

Table 1 Facilitators supporting the effect of a CME meeting

Case-based teaching [23]

Guidance rather than orders [43]

Educational meetings in small groups [13]

Engaging with peers [13, 23, 43, 44]

Active participation [13, 23, 43, 44]

Sharing experiences with end–of-life care [13, 23, 43, 44]

Involving opinion leaders [13]

Encounters with specialist [13, 43]

practice published by the Danish College of General Practitioners (Table 2) [17].

The case-based teaching alternated between lectures and discussions. Three short films were produced for the meetings based on research findings to cover the topics in the meetings (Table 2). The films were used to facilitate the discussions between the GPs. Engaging with peers, participating actively and sharing own experiences with end-of-life care all aimed at increasing the effect of a CME meeting [18, 28, 44, 45]. GPs with special interest in end-of-life care were teaching together with a local palliative care specialist. Six identical CME meetings were held throughout the region based on the catchment area of the specialist palliative care teams.

The final EDS consisted of two connected parts: i) a pop-up window in the patient's medical record (Fig. 1: *The EDS pop-up window generated in the medical records to be filled in by GP*) and ii) a list of patients with end-of-life needs and key elements in their care (Fig. 2: *The list of all patients with palliative needs in the practice divided into patients with cancer and COPD, respectively*).

Table 2 Programme and content of the CME meeting about palliative care

Time	Curriculum covered in each meeting
4.30–5.10 pm	What is palliative care? - Definition and changes in the understanding of palliative care. Focus on end- of-life care - Disease trajectories and the challenges in identifying when end-of-life care is needed - Discussion of patient case: (short film)
5.25–6.00 pm	What are the patients' palliative needs? - Results from a Danish survey among palliative patients - Discussion of two patient cases (short films)
6.30–6.45 pm	Presentation of the local palliative team by the palliative physician
6.45–7.35 pm	Medical skills and practicalities - Prescription of just-in-case[a] box, terminal declaration[b], use of EDS, etc.
7.45–8.00 pm	Local support to patients and relatives - Which alternatives does the GP have? Who else can help and support?

[a]anticipatory medicine

[b]declaration releasing medical reimbursement for end-of-life care

The pop-up window in the patient's medical record had four functions: an identifier of the patient's potential end-of-life needs, a reminder to the GP of the patients and actions to take, a provider of medical advice, and a checklist of palliative tasks to consider during the end-of-life trajectory (Fig. 1).

To serve as an identifier, the pop-up window was triggered on the first time the GP opened the patient's medical record if at least one of the following codes were registered in the electronic patient record (EPR): diagnosis of malignancy, palliative diagnosis or COPD with either MRC dyspnoea scale = 5 [46], body mass index < 18 or forced expiratory volume in 1 s < 30 (see Additional file 2 for exact list of diagnosis). The trigger diagnoses were chosen from existing identification tools [47–49] and available patient information in the EPR. The aim was to identify patients with an estimated remaining life span of 12 months or less. The GP was asked to confirm if the patient was in the end-of-life phase. Additionally, the GP had to indicate the subsequent trigger: either next time the patient would be present in the GP practice or a specific date. This procedure was chosen so that the pop-up could work as a reminder, thereby making it easier for the GP to assume a proactive approach.

The pop-up window provided symptom-specific medical suggestions based on the recommendations from the national clinical guideline [17]. This function of the pop-up was integrated into the medicine module in the EPR to allow quick comparison between medical recommendations and prescribed medications. This easy access to medical advice was made to counterbalance any inadequate medical skills or doubts concerning end-of-life care among the GPs.

The checklist functionality in the pop-up window showed important issues to consider at some point of the palliative trajectory, e.g. making a terminal declaration, prescription of "in-case" box (anticipatory medicine), or registering performance status (Fig. 1). The checklist was linked directly to printable forms and assessment tools to minimize the time spent on administration and paper work. The checklists were also linked directly to the corresponding section in the online version of the national clinical guideline [17], where each issue was explained in detail.

The other part of the EDS was the list of the all patients identified by the GP as being in the end-of-life phase; this list was designed to help organise the care and promote a proactive approach. Two entries into the list were possible: either if the GP filled in anything in the pop-up (apart from 'irrelevant') or registered the patient as being in end of life by applying the International Classification of Primary Care diagnosis code "A99" in the EPR. The list showed key elements in end-of-life care (e.g. receiving specialised palliative care, palliative

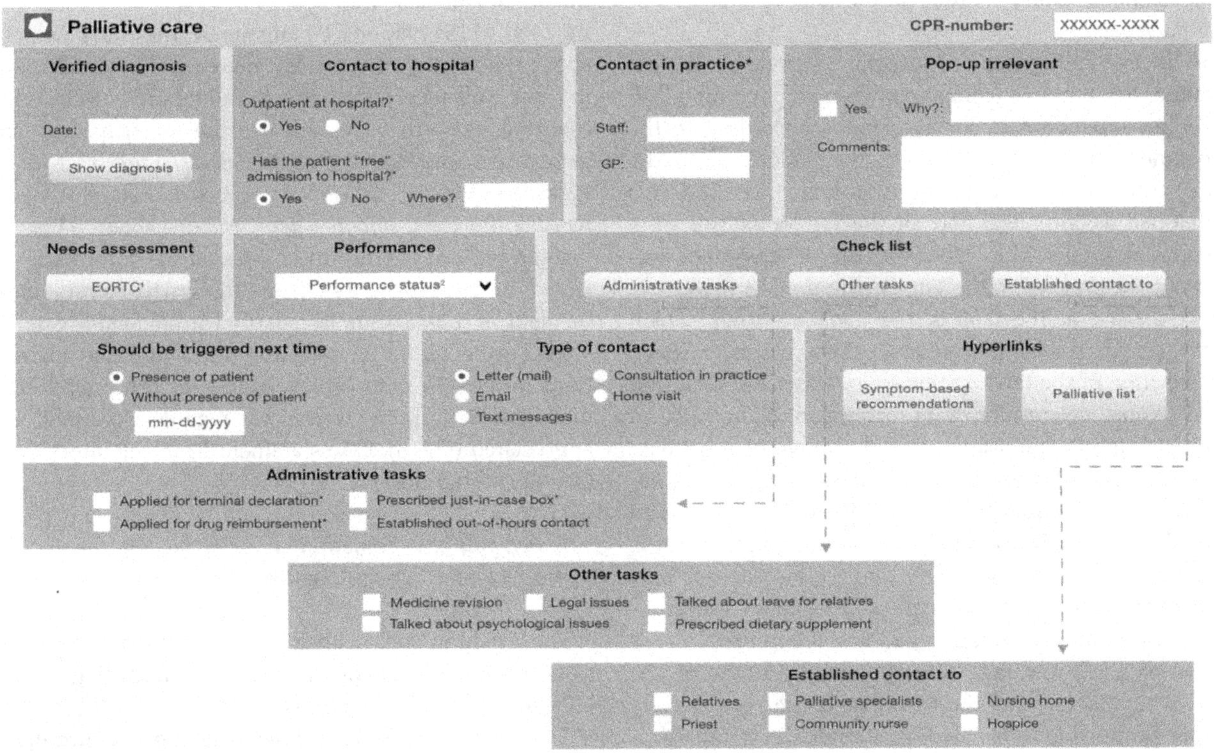

Fig. 1 The EDS pop-up window generated in the medical records to be filled in by GP. 1: Directly linked to the EORTC QLQ-C15-PAL [55] in the palliative guideline [17]: ready to print and hand out to the patient. 2: ECOG Performance Status [56]. * The information is automatically transferred to the palliative list

phase, date for next contact) for each patient listed (Fig. 2). If the GP was uncertain about a heading, the cursor could be dragged to the heading and an explanation would appear.

The information about key elements was automatically retrieved from data in the pop-up window and shown on the list using colour codes and simple explanations. The list was divided into two tabs to allow different information for different patient groups: one for cancer, one for COPD (Fig. 2). Another use of the list was to support the GPs in monitoring the clinical work. Additional suggestions as to how to use the data for this purpose were available for the GPs at the homepage of DAK-E [29].

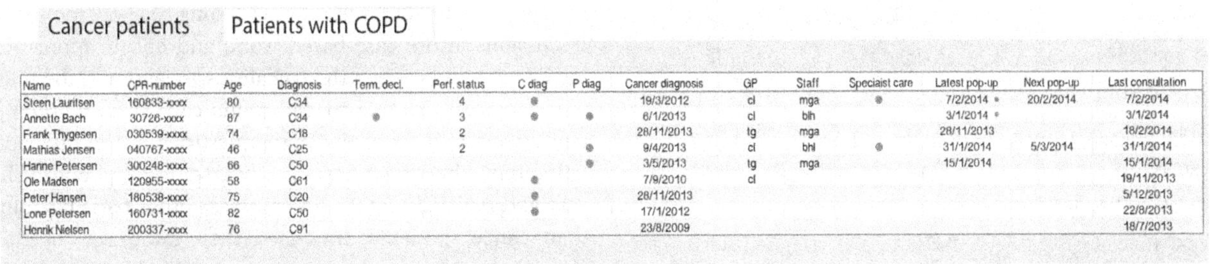
Cancer patients | Patients with COPD

Name	CPR-number	Age	Diagnosis	Term. decl.	Perf. status	C diag	P diag	Cancer diagnosis	GP	Staff	Speciaist care	Latest pop-up	Next pop-up	Last consultation
Steen Lauritsen	160833-xxxx	80	C34		4	•		19/3/2012	cl	mga	•	7/2/2014 •	20/2/2014	7/2/2014
Annette Bach	30726-xxxx	87	C34	•	3	•	•	6/1/2013	cl	blh		3/1/2014 •		3/1/2014
Frank Thygesen	030539-xxxx	74	C18		2			28/11/2013	tg	mga		28/11/2013		18/2/2014
Mathias Jensen	040767-xxxx	46	C25		2		•	9/4/2013	cl	bhl	•	31/1/2014	5/3/2014	31/1/2014
Hanne Petersen	300248-xxxx	66	C50				•	3/5/2013	tg	mga		15/1/2014		15/1/2014
Ole Madsen	120955-xxxx	58	C61			•		7/9/2010	cl					19/11/2013
Peter Hansen	180538-xxxx	75	C20			•		28/11/2013						5/12/2013
Lone Petersen	160731-xxxx	82	C50			•		17/1/2012						22/8/2013
Henrik Nielsen	200337-xxxx	76	C91					23/8/2009						18/7/2013

Fig. 2 The list of all patients with palliative needs in the practice divided into patients with cancer and COPD, respectively. The tab for COPD contains additional information on smoking status, number of exacerbations within the last year and MRC breathlessness score. All information shown in the figure is made up for the figure and not based on real data. CPR number: Personal identification number allocated to every Danish citizen. Diagnosis: The cancer diagnosis (ICD 10). When the cursor marks the diagnosis, it is written in words. Term.decl: Terminal declaration. Data retrieved from the pop-up window. Perf. Status: ECOG performance status [56]. Data retrieved from the pop-up window. C and P diag: Comorbidities and psychiatric comorbidities; a dot means that the patient is registered with comorbidity (written in text when the cursor is dragged to the dot). Data retrieved automatically from the EPR. GP/staff: The patient's contact GP/staff in the practice(s). Data retrieved from the pop-up window. Specialist care: The patient receives specialist palliative care. Data retrieved from the pop-up window. Latest pop-up window: A marker indicates that a note has been left by the GP/staff in the pop-up window (can be read when the cursor is dragged to the dot)

Phase 2: pilot-testing of intervention
The fidelity

The fidelity (adherence to blueprint and reach) was examined for the two components separately. All CME meetings were carried out as planned according to the schedule and the script. Hence, the adherence to the blueprint of the CME meeting was high. The EDS was developed as intended, and all the functionalities were integrated in the EPR. However, the development was delayed with regard to the implementation, as it was not ready for use at the time of the CME meetings, which may have decreased the possibility of synergistic effect. At the time of the intervention there was a discussion of legal issues concerning data collection from GPs in Denmark in general leading to a shutdown of most data collection from GPs in Denmark. Despite this was a national issue unrelated to the present project, we had to shut down the EDS untimely, as it was based on these data. Hence, the EDS was only running for a short time. The functionality showed high adherence to the blueprint but the implementation had low adherence.

The six CME meetings were attended by a total of 120 GPs, which is 14.2% of the 843 invited GPs. A relatively higher proportion of female GPs attended in comparison with the gender distribution among all GPs in the Central Denmark Region (Table 3).

The EDS reached fewer of the 843 invited GPs as only 50 GPs (5.9%) signed up. We could not retrieve information about the GPs who signed up for the EDS due to the above-mentioned untimely shutdown of the system. The overall reach of the intervention was low, which compromises the fidelity.

Table 3 Characteristics of the CME-attending GPs and all GPs in the Central Denmark Region

	Participants[a]	GPs in the Central Denmark Region
GPs (n(%))	120 (100)	843 (100.0)
Age, (median iqr), years	54 (15)	54 (14.4)
Gender, (n(%))		
Male	43 (35.8)	434 (51.5)
Female	77 (64.2)	409 (48.5)
Place of meeting, (n,(%))		
Viborg	8 (6.6)	84 (10.0)
Horsens	18 (15.0)	136 (16.1)
Silkeborg	15 (12.5)	67 (8.0)
Herning	25 (20.8)	185 (22.0)
Randers	25 (20.8)	144 (17.1)
Aarhus	29 (24.2)	223 (26.5)
Unknown	–	4 (0.5)

[a] Additional 19 persons participated: 15 GP trainees, 3 nurses, or 2 other health care persons

Quality of CME meeting

In total, 115 (95%) GPs answered the questionnaire about the quality of the CME meeting. The CME meeting was well received by the attending GPs; overall they reported that they benefited from participating and gained new knowledge (Fig. 3: *The distribution (% of responses (n = 115)) of GPs' self-reported usefulness of attending the CME and the demonstrated tools*). This was further explored in the interviews as the informants all stated to have benefited from the participation, independent of pre-existing familiarity with palliative care.

The presentation of palliative tools and the instructions on how to complete a request for drug reimbursement due to terminal illness was regarded as useful and appreciated (Fig. 3). One statement from the interviewed GPs illustrated this:

"Then you have something to bring back to the practice and show to the others".

The teaching style with a mix of lectures and discussion in smaller groups worked well according to the GPs' questionnaire responses.

The interviewed GPs rated the content of the meeting to be at a high level and found that the teachers were updated in the field of palliative medicine. They also emphasised that teaching by alternating persons and the mix of lectures and discussions with peers worked well. Illustrated by another statement from one of the interviewed GPs:

"You sit and start thinking, and then it is nice to have the opportunity to share the thoughts with people around you".

Potential improvements suggested both by the interviewed GPs and at the open questions in the questionnaire was: to give higher priority to demonstration of the practical skills, extend the duration of the meeting to allow more peer discussions, more case-based work, and ensure more time for interaction between the palliative specialist and the GPs.

Three areas relating to end-of-life care also emerged as new to the GPs from the open questions in the questionnaire: they obtained a broader understanding of end-of-life care and realized that it also embraces other patient groups than cancer patients, increased their awareness of their proactive role, and directed more attention towards patients with potential palliative needs. Furthermore, the importance of using a more systematic approach and organising end-of-life care at practice level was highlighted.

The same points were made by the interviewed illustrated by this statement:

"We might need to enter the playing field and not wait for the patients to come to us, right?"

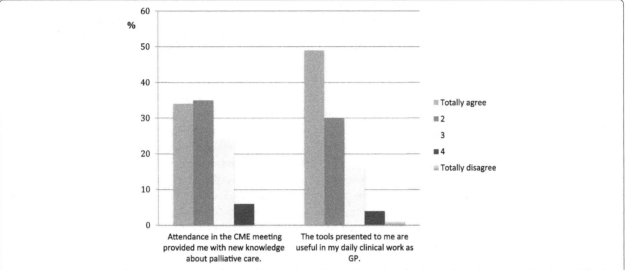

Fig. 3 The distribution (% of responses (n = 115)) of GPs' self-reported usefulness of attending the CME and the demonstrated tools. Made by the Committee for Quality Improvement and Continuing Medical Education in the Central Denmark Region [31] as a part of the evaluation of the CME sessions

The CME meeting succeeded in addressing the main barriers. Yet, several issues that were raised at the CME meetings (e.g. awareness of the relatives' needs and the importance of symptom screening) were not brought up as new insight in either the questionnaire of the interviews as new areas of awareness.

Impact of CME meeting

In total, 29 (25%) GPs participated in the three-month questionnaire evaluation. A fourth of the GPs stated specifically that they had adapted a more proactive approach to end-of-life care. Furthermore, they reported to have obtained increased awareness about palliative needs among patients with non-malignant diseases. Three of the 29 GPs (10%) stated that they had no patients with palliative needs after the CME meeting.

Impact of EDS

Due to the early shutdown of the EDS, we could not evaluate its impact. As the EDS was demonstrated on the CME meeting, many GPs made unprompted positive comments about the EDS in both the questionnaire and the interview. The GPs stated that they looked forward to using the EDS, and their immediate impression was that it would be a helpful tool, illustrated by this interviewed GP:

"I will look forward to using the EDS which is on its way – it seems very applicable".

The context of the intervention

One specific event could in the context have hampered the effect. At the time of the implementation of the

intervention, there was a nationwide disagreement between the GPs and Danish Regions. This might have made some GPs reluctant to participate as the regional administration, i.e. the Central Denmark Region, was involved in establishing the CME meeting. This connection was unintended as the staffs from the Central Denmark Region were involved exclusively to ensure high quality of the CME. The CME meeting was approved by the Public Health and Quality Improvement in the Central Denmark Region to allow remuneration of the attending GPs.

Discussion
Main findings

It was possible to model the intervention to address identified barriers to end-of-life care in general practice and integrated facilitators to enhance the effect of the intervention. Although the participation rate was only 15%, the pilot-testing showed that the CME meeting was well received among the attending GPs. The meeting had an immediate impact on the GPs and addressed the identified barriers, which suggests high quality. Evaluation of the EDS could not be performed due to early shutdown. The process evaluation of the pilot-test revealed a need to look further into how the intervention in full scale could be designed to reach more GPs.

Comparison with other studies

One barrier we intended to address in both the CME meeting and the EDS was identification of patients with palliative needs [33, 50, 51]. A Dutch intervention by Thoosen et al. found that patients with palliative needs identified by their GP had more contact with their GP, less hospital admissions, and were more likely to die at home than not identified patients [52]. These findings underline the importance of the GP's awareness and identification of patients with palliative needs. In the study by Thoosen et al., the GPs had to apply an identification tool (RADPAC) by going through their patients manually. Hence, the identification was still dependent on the GP's awareness of palliative needs. Mason et al. made a computerised tool to identify patients with deteriorating health due to advanced conditions [24]. They found that some GPs were reluctant to register the computer-identified patients as "palliative" due to associations to death. The resistance against using the term "palliative care" earlier in the disease trajectory compromised the effect of the tool. This underlines the need for a change in attitude alongside the implementation of an EDS.

The attendance rate in the CME meeting was low in our study compared to other Danish studies. A disease management programme in 2010 in the same region had an attendance rate of 69% [53]. However, these GPs were remunerated for participating, and the programme formed part of a regional initiative aiming to prioritise and optimise chronic care management. Another Danish study with 1-h CME meetings in 2012 focusing on lung cancer diagnosis had an attendance rate of 49% [54]. The low attendance rate in this study could have several explanations: lack of interest, no need for education in end-of-life care, bad timing of the intervention, or poor implementation of the CME meeting.

The low attendance rate in our study is unlikely to reflect a lack of need for education in end-of-life care. A prior Danish study identified a need of improvement of palliative care skills and a lack of confidence in providing end-of-life care among GPs [10, 38]. Furthermore, a British study reported that most GPs wanted training focusing on different care issues when asked about their educational preferences in palliative care [39]. The timing of the intervention may have adversely affected the attendance rate due to the disagreement between Danish Regions and the GPs. Finally, despite that the newsletter is the common way to invite GPs to participate in continuing medical education, we do not know if they actually read the invitation. Hence, the effect of different methods of inviting the GPs should be investigated in future studies.

Clinical implications and future perspectives
The increased longevity in the population may result in rising incidence of cancer and more terminally ill patients with non-malignant disease. Most of these patients wish to be cared for at home. Hence, there is a growing need for GPs who are skilled and confident in providing palliative care.

The evaluation of the intervention revealed increased awareness among GPs of potential palliative needs in other patient groups than cancer patients. The findings also suggest that the GPs should take a more proactive role and organise the care. Although the participating GPs suggested higher prioritisation of demonstration of practical skills in general in the CME, we recommend maintaining the current balance between practice and theory. The reason for this is increased awareness and broadening of understanding of end-of-life care together with improved skills are prerequisites for optimising care, which would benefit all groups of patients.

As the CME meeting was well received by the GPs and addressed the main barriers to end-of-life care, it is ready to be used in a full-scale study assessing the effect of the intervention on patient-related outcomes. However, the EDS needs to be evaluated before used in full-scale study. Furthermore, it could be beneficial to assess the implementation itself, as the participation rate was low in the set-up tested in this study.

Strengths within the study
One of the strengths of the study was the systematic development of the complex intervention in accordance with the MRC guideline [46], which facilitated integration of evaluation in the design. This allowed analyses of the different steps and elements of the complex intervention and enabled us to investigate if the different components in the intervention worked as intended. This approach generally improves the applicability of tailored interventions to other settings as it makes it easier to adapt relevant components.

Another strength of the study was the inclusion of stakeholders from an early stage of the modelling of the intervention; this increased the applicability and facilitated the implementation. The reach of the intervention was evaluated using register data, which allowed comparisons between attending GPs and all GPs in the region. The external evaluation carried out in the CME meeting reduced the risk of bias, especially with regard to the interviews after the meetings. On the other hand important information might be lost from the interviews as the data was interpreted by an external evaluator. However, the external evaluator had participated in a meeting prior to the evaluation to ensure appropriate focus. The use of questionnaires for evaluation of the CME allowed us to assess both the immediate and the three-month self-perceived effect of the CME meeting on the GPs. However, the low participation in the follow-up compromised the generalisability of the three-month effect.

Limitations within the study
The use of narrative literature search to identify the barriers to end-of-life care introduced a risk of missing

information, as the search was not exhaustive However, as the aim with the literature search only was to investigate barriers this was not a methodological concern in this study.

A limitation of using the guideline was the lack of standard process evaluation [18].

For the impact of the intervention the early shutdown of the EDS was a major limitation. This prevented evaluation of the reach, the participants' experience, and the quality and of the EDS. Another limitation of the study was the low attendance rate at the CME meetings and the lack of possibility to examine attendance further in the current design.

Conclusion

A complex intervention consisting of CME meetings and EDS to aid GPs provide better end-of-life care was developed using MRC guidelines and current evidence. The evaluation of the pilot-test showed overall appreciation of the CME meetings, which addressed identified barriers to providing care. The EDS was shut down early and needs further evaluation before examining the whole intervention in a larger study, where evaluation could be based on patient-related outcomes and the impact on end-of-life care.

Abbreviations

AKW: Anna Kirstine Winthereik (part of research group); CME: Continuing Medical Education; COPD: Chronic Obstructive Pulmonary Disease; EDS: Electronic decision support; EPR: Electronic patient records; GP(s): General practitioner(s); ICD-10: International Classification of Diseases, version 10; MRC: Medical Research Council

Acknowledgements
We wish to thank all the participating GPs in Central Denmark Region. We want to thank the Quality Unit for Cancer Care in general practice for their help with designing and carrying out the CME meeting, especially GP Rikke Pilegaard Hansen, PhD and academic coordinator Gry Stie. Furthermore, we wish to thank the Danish Quality Unit of General Practice for making the EDS, especially GP Berit Lassen, the IT developers, and the administrative staff. Additionally, we want to thank data manager Kaare Rud Flarup, Research Centre for Cancer Diagnosis in Primary Care, Research Unit for General Practice, Aarhus University, Denmark for setting up the questionnaires and Lone Niedziella for linguistic support. Finally, we wish to thank Emil Christian Gram for graphical assistance.

Funding
The Danish Cancer Society and the Danish foundation TrygFonden supported the study through the joint grant 'Safety in Palliative Care' [*Tryghed i palliative forløb*]. The funding body did not have a role in either the design of the study, the data collection, analysis and interpretation of data nor in the writing of the manuscript.

Authors' contributions
AKW, MAN, AB, and PV conceived the idea of the study. All authors were involved in the design of study. AKW took an active part in the shaping of the EDS and the CME meeting. MAN, AB, and PV took part in the design of the CME meeting. AKW acquired, analysed and interpreted the data, and drafted the manuscript. MAN, AB, and PV took part in the interpretation of the data and revised the manuscript. All authors have read and approved the final manuscript.

Competing interests
The authors declare that they have no competing interests.

Author details
[1]Department of Oncology, Aarhus University Hospital, Noerrebrogade 44, 8000 Aarhus C, Denmark. [2]Palliative Care Team, Department of Oncology, Aarhus University Hospital, Noerrebrogade 44, 8000 Aarhus, Denmark. [3]Research Unit for General Practice, Department of Public Health, Aarhus University, Bartholins Allé 2, 8000 Aarhus, Denmark. [4]Department of Clinical Medicine, Aarhus University, Noerrebrogade 44, 8000 Aarhus C, Denmark.

References
1. Definition of General Practice, EURACT (short version, 2011). [http://www.woncaeurope.org/sites/default/files/documents/Definition EURACTshort version revised 2011.pdf] 28 March 2014.
2. Michiels E, Deschepper R, Van Der Kelen G, Bernheim JL, Mortier F, Vander Stichele R, Deliens L. The role of general practitioners in continuity of care at the end of life: a qualitative study of terminally ill patients and their next of kin. Palliat Med. 2007;21(5):409–15.
3. Pedersen KM, Andersen JS, Sondergaard J. General practice and primary health care in Denmark. J Am Board Fam Med. 2012;25(Suppl 1):S34–8.
4. Neergaard MA, Bonde Jensen A, Sondergaard J, Sokolowski I, Olesen F, Vedsted P. Preference for place-of-death among terminally ill cancer patients in Denmark. Scand J Caring Sci. 2011;25(4):627–36.
5. Brogaard T, Neergaard MA, Sokolowski I, Olesen F, Jensen AB. Congruence between preferred and actual place of care and death among Danish cancer patients. Palliat Med. 2012;27(2):155–64.
6. Dødsårsagsregisteret (The Danish Register of Causes of Deaths). [https://sundhedsdatastyrelsen.dk/dar]. Accessed 29 May 2018.
7. Neergaard MA, Vedsted P, Olesen F, Sokolowski I, Jensen AB, Sondergaard J. Associations between home death and GP involvement in palliative cancer care. Br J Gen Pract. 2009;59(566):671–7.
8. Brazil K, Bedard M, Willison K. Factors associated with home death for individuals who receive home support services: a retrospective cohort study. BMC Palliat Care. 2002;1(1):2.
9. Aabom B, Kragstrup J, Vondeling H, Bakketeig LS, Stovring H. Population-based study of place of death of patients with cancer: implications for GPs. Br J Gen Pract. 2005;55(518):684–9.
10. Winthereik A, Neergaard M, Vedsted P, Jensen A. Danish general practitioners' self-reported competences in end-of-life care. Scand J Prim Health Care. 2016;34(4):420–7.
11. Murray SA, Kendall M, Boyd K, Sheikh A. Illness trajectories and palliative care. BMJ. 2005;330(7498):1007–11.
12. Johnson MJ, Booth S. Palliative and end-of-life care for patients with chronic heart failure and chronic lung disease. Clin Med. 2010;10(3):286–9.
13. McKinley RK, Stokes T, Exley C, Field D. Care of people dying with malignant and cardiorespiratory disease in general practice. Br J Gen Pract. 2004; 54(509):909–13.
14. End of life care for adults [https://www.nice.org.uk/guidance/qs13/chapter/Introduction-and-overview] 28 April 2016.
15. Alvarez MP, Agra Y. Systematic review of educational interventions in palliative care for primary care physicians. Palliat Med. 2006;20(7):673–83.
16. van Riet Paap J, Vernooij-Dassen M, Sommerbakk R, Moyle W, Hjermstad MJ, Leppert W, Vissers K, Engels Y, IMPACT research team: Implementation of

improvement strategies in palliative care: an integrative review. Implement Sci 2015, 10:103–015–0293-2.

17. Klinisk vejledning for almen praksis: Palliation (Clinical guideline for palliative Care in general practice)[http://vejledninger.dsam.dk/palliation/] 10 August 2014.

18. Grol R, Wensing M, Eccles M, Davis D. Improving patient care - the implementation of change in health care. 2nd ed. Oxford: Wiley Blackwell BMJ books; 2013.

19. Toth-Pal E, Wardh I, Strender LE, Nilsson G. Implementing a clinical decision-support system in practice: a qualitative analysis of influencing attitudes and characteristics among general practitioners. Inform Health Soc Care. 2008; 33(1):39–54.

20. Robertson J, Moxey AJ, Newby DA, Gillies MB, Williamson M, Pearson SA. Electronic information and clinical decision support for prescribing: state of play in Australian general practice. Fam Pract. 2011;28(1):93–101.

21. Martens JD, van der Weijden T, Winkens RA, Kester AD, Geerts PJ, Evers SM, Severens JL. Feasibility and acceptability of a computerised system with automated reminders for prescribing behaviour in primary care. Int J Med Inform. 2008;77(3):199–207.

22. McDermott L, Yardley L, Little P, Ashworth M, Gulliford M, eCRT Research Team. Developing a computer delivered, theory based intervention for guideline implementation in general practice. BMC Fam Pract. 2010;11:90.

23. Leslie SJ, Hartswood M, Meurig C, McKee SP, Slack R, Procter R, Denvir MA. Clinical decision support software for management of chronic heart failure: development and evaluation. Comput Biol Med. 2006;36(5):495–506.

24. Mason B, Boyd K, Murray SA, Steyn J, Cormie P, Kendall M, Munday D, Weller D, Fife S, Murchie P, Campbell C. Developing a computerised search to help UK general practices identify more patients for palliative care planning: a feasibility study. BMC Fam Pract. 2015;16:99. 0150312-z

25. Moore GF, Audrey S, Barker M, Bond L, Bonell C, Hardeman W, Moore L, O'Cathain A, Tinati T, Wight D, Baird J. Process evaluation of complex interventions: Medical Research Council guidance. BMJ. 2015;350:h1258.

26. Craig P, Dieppe P, Macintyre S, Michie S, Nazareth I, Petticrew M. Developing and evaluating complex interventions: the new Medical Research Council guidance. Int J Nurs Stud. 2013;50(5):587–92.

27. Cheater F, Baker R, Gillies C, Hearnshaw H, Flottorp S, Robertson N, Ej S, Ad O: Tailored interventions to overcome identified barriers to change: effects on professional practice and health care outcomes. Cochrane Database Syst Rev. 2010;17(3).

28. Grol R, Grimshaw J. From best evidence to best practice: effective implementation of change in patients' care. Lancet. 2003;362(9391):1225–30.

29. Dansk Almenmedicinsk kvalitetsEnhed, DAK-E (Danish Quality Unit of General Practice). [https://www.dak-e.dk/]. Accessed 29 May 2018.

30. "Practicus" Medlemsblad for DSAM - ePracticus (Trade journal for general practitioners published by the College of Danish general practioners) [http://www.practicus.dk/] 14 October 2014.

31. CFK Folkesundhed og Kvalitetsudvikling (Unit for Quality and development in Central Denmark Region) [http://www.cfk.rm.dk/in-english/] 13 December 2015.

32. Remuneration for continuing medical education for GPs in Denmark. [https://www.laeger.dk/PLO/refusion]. Accessed 29 May 2018.

33. Abarshi E, Echteld MA, Van den Block L, Donker GA, Deliens L, Onwuteaka-Philipsen BD. Recognising patients who will die in the near future: a nationwide study via the Dutch sentinel network of GPs. Br J Gen Pract. 2011;61(587):e371–8.

34. Thoonsen B, Groot M, Engels Y, Prins J, Verhagen S, Galesloot C, van Weel C, Vissers K. Early identification of and proactive palliative care for patients in general practice, incentive and methods of a randomized controlled trial. BMC Fam Pract. 2011;12:123.

35. Murray SA, Firth A, Schneider N, Van den Eynden B, Gomez-Batiste X, Brogaard T, Villanueva T, Abela J, Eychmuller S, Mitchell G, Downing J, Sallnow L, van Rijswijk E, Barnard A, Lynch M, Fogen F, Moine S. Promoting palliative care in the community: production of the primary palliative care toolkit by the European Association of Palliative Care Taskforce in primary palliative care. Palliat Med. 2015;29(2):101–11.

36. Heffner JE. Advance care planning in chronic obstructive pulmonary disease: barriers and opportunities. Curr Opin Pulm Med. 2011;17(2):103–9.

37. Murray SA, Pinnock H, Sheikh A. Palliative care for people with COPD: we need to meet the challenge. Prim Care Respir J. 2006;15(6):362–4.

38. Gorlén T, Gorlén TF, Vass M, Neergaard MA: Low confidence among general practitioners in end-of-life care and subcutaneous administration of medicine. Danish Med J. 2012;59(4):A4407.

39. Shipman C, Addington-Hall J, Barclay S, Briggs J, Cox I, Daniels L, Millar D. Educational opportunities in palliative care: what do general practitioners want? Palliat Med. 2001;15(3):191–6.

40. Groot MM, Vernooij-Dassen MJ, Crul BJ, Grol RP. General practitioners (GPs) and palliative care: perceived tasks and barriers in daily practice. Palliat Med. 2005;19(2):111–8.

41. Brogaard T, Bonde Jensen A, Sokolowski I, Olesen F, Neergaard MA. Who is the key worker in palliative home care? Scand J Prim Health Care. 2011; 29(3):150–6.

42. Kendall M, Boyd K, Campbell C, Cormie P, Fife S, Thomas K, Weller D, Murray SA. How do people with cancer wish to be cared for in primary care? Serial discussion groups of patients and carers. Fam Pract. 2006;23(6):644–50.

43. Armstrong D. Clinical autonomy, individual and collective: the problem of changing doctors' behaviour. Soc Sci Med. 2002;55(10):1771–7.

44. Armstrong D, Ogden J. The role of etiquette and experimentation in explaining how doctors change behaviour: a qualitative study. Sociol Health Illn. 2006;28(7):951–68.

45. Brown JM, Patel M, Howard J, Cherry G, Shaw NJ. Changing clinical practice: significant events that influence trainees' learning. Educ Prim Care. 2011; 22(1):25–31.

46. Medical research council (MRC): Dyspnoea scale [https://www.mrc.ac.uk/research/facilities/mrc-scales/mrc-dyspnoea-scale-mrc-breathlessness-scale/] 2 May 2016.

47. The GSF Toolkit from National Gold Standards Framework Centre. [https://www.goldstandardsframework.org.uk/cd-content/uploads/files/General%20Files/Prognostic%20Indicator%20Guidance%20October%202011.pdf]. Accessed 29 May 2018.

48. Thoonsen B, Engels Y, Van Rijswijk E, Verhagen S, Van Weel C, Groot M, Vissers K. Early identification of palliative care patients in general practice: development of RADboud indicators for PAlliative care needs (RADPAC). Br J Gen Pract. 2012;62(602):e625–31.

49. Berman AR. Management of patients with end-stage chronic obstructive pulmonary disease. Prim Care. 2011;38(2):277–97. viii-ix

50. Gadoud A, Kane E, Macleod U, Ansell P, Oliver S, Johnson M. Palliative care among heart failure patients in primary care: a comparison to cancer patients using English family practice data. PLoS One. 2014;9(11):e113188.

51. Claessen SJ, Francke AL, Engels Y, Deliens L. How do GPs identify a need for palliative care in their patients? An interview study. BMC Fam Pract. 2013;14: 42. 229614-42

52. Thoonsen B, Vissers K, Verhagen S, Prins J, Bor H, van Weel C, Groot M, Engels Y: Training general practitioners in early identification and anticipatory palliative care planning: a randomized controlled trial. BMC Fam Pract 2015, 16(1):126-015-0342-6.

53. Ribe AR, Fenger-Gron M, Vedsted P, Bro F, Kaersvang L, Vestergaard M. Several factors influenced general practitioner participation in the implementation of a disease management programme. Dan Med J. 2014; 61(9):A4901.

54. Guldbrandt LM: The effect of direct referral for fast CT scan in early lung Cancer detection in general practice A clinical, cluster-randomised trials Paper IV. Aarhus University, Health; 2014.

55. EORTC QLQ-C15-PAL. http://groups.eortc.be/qol/eortc-qlq-c15-pal, 29 May 2018

56. Oken MM, Creech RH, Tormey DC, et al., Toxicity and response criteria of the Eastern Cooperative Oncology Group. Am J Clin Oncol 1982;5(6):649-55.

11

The diagnostic test accuracy of rectal examination for prostate cancer diagnosis in symptomatic patients

Daniel Jones[1*], Charlotte Friend[1], Andreas Dreher[2], Victoria Allgar[3] and Una Macleod[1]

Abstract

Background: Prostate cancer is the most common cancer in men in the UK. NICE guidelines on recognition and referral of suspected cancer, recommend performing digital rectal examination (DRE) on patients with urinary symptoms and urgently referring if the prostate feels malignant. However, this is based on the results of one case control study, so it is not known if DRE performed in primary care is an accurate method of detecting prostate cancer.

Methods: The aim of this review is to ascertain the sensitivity, specificity, positive and negative predictive value of DRE for the detection of prostate cancer in symptomatic patients in primary care.
CENTRAL, MEDLINE, EMBASE and CINAHL databases were searched in august 2015 for studies in which a DRE was performed in primary care on symptomatic patients and compared against a reference diagnostic procedure.

Results: Four studies were included with a total of 3225 patients. The sensitivity and specificity for DRE as a predictor of prostate cancer in symptomatic patients was 28.6 and 90.7%, respectively. The positive and negative predictive values were 42.3 and 84.2%, respectively.

Conclusion: This review found that DRE performed in general practice is accurate, and supports the UK NICE guidelines that patients with a malignant prostate on examination are referred urgently for suspected prostate cancer. Abnormal DRE carried a 42.3% chance of malignancy, above the 3% risk threshold which NICE guidance suggests warrants an urgent referral. However this review questions the benefit of performing a DRE in primary care in the first instance, suggesting that a patient's risk of prostate cancer based on symptoms alone would warrant urgent referral even if the DRE feels normal.

Keywords: General practice, Digital rectal examination, Prostate Cancer, Primary care, Early diagnosis

Background

Prostate cancer is the most common cancer amongst men with 41,736 cases diagnosed in the UK in 2011. Over the last 35 years, the incidence of prostate cancer has more than tripled, though much of this increase is likely to be due to the increasing use of prostate specific antigen (PSA) blood tests. The mortality rate from prostate cancer in the UK is falling after reaching a peak in the 1990s, but in 2012, over 10,000 men died of prostate

cancer. Survival from prostate cancer is relatively good with a five-year survival rate of 85% [1].

There has been considerable debate about the benefits and harms of early diagnosis of prostate cancer, with much of the discussion focused around the use of PSA. Evidence suggests survival is closely related to stage at diagnosis, with 100% five year survival in patients diagnosed with the earliest stage disease compared to less than 33% five year survival if diagnosed at the latest stage [1]. This suggests that early diagnosis of prostate cancer is important. Certainly once a patient is symptomatic, there seems to be little benefit in delaying the diagnosis.

* Correspondence: ugm4djj@gmail.com
[1]Hull York Medical School, Hertford Building, University of Hull, Cottingham Road, Hull HU6 7RX, UK
Full list of author information is available at the end of the article

Asymptomatic screening using PSA is undertaken, and accepted in some countries, including the US, however the U.S. Preventative Services Task Force recommend a discussion on the potential benefits and harms of PSA screening, stating that screening offers a "small potential benefit of reducing the chance of dying of prostate cancer" but also highlighting that "many men will experience potential harms of screening" [2]. In the UK, screening is not recommended routinely, instead Public Health England runs a 'prostate cancer risk management program' in which patients who are concerned about prostate cancer are able to have a PSA test after a discussion with a GP on the benefits and harms of the test in order to make an informed choice [3]. As a result most prostate cancers in the UK are identified when patients present to general practice with a symptom suspicious of prostate cancer such as nocturia or urinary frequency. It is also worth noting however that there is a diagnostic challenge as both urinary tract infections and benign prostatic hypertrophy often present in similar ways and are much more common diagnoses [4, 5].

The National Institute for Health and Care Excellence (NICE) has recently updated the guidance on recognition and referral of suspected cancer in the UK [6]. The latest NICE guidelines give recommendations on the recognition and referral of prostate cancer. These guidelines state patients should be referred urgently if the prostate feels malignant on digital rectal examination and recommends performing digital rectal examination (DRE) on patients presenting with any lower urinary tract symptoms including nocturia, urinary frequency, hesitancy, urgency or retention [6]. A recommendation supported by Walsh et al. who reviewed DREs undertaken in primary care and urology clinics for the diagnosis of prostate cancer and concluded that DRE is a key part of the assessment [7]. However, the evidence base for DRE in symptomatic patients is poor, with NICE guidelines documenting only one case control study by Hamilton et al. [4]. As a result it is not known if DRE performed in primary care is an accurate method of detecting prostate cancer, or what the risk of prostate cancer is, if the general practitioner deems the prostate to be malignant on examination.

Methods

The aim of this review was to evaluate the effectiveness of DRE performed by general practitioners as a predictor of prostate cancer in symptomatic patients in a primary care setting according to the latest NICE guideline recommendations.

The reporting of this systematic review follows the recommendations of the PRISMA (Preferred Reporting Items for Systematic Reviews and Meta-Analyses) statement [8]. A protocol was developed and registered in the PROSPERO register of systematic reviews (registration number PROSPERO 2015:CRD42015025764) [9].

Search strategy

A search was undertaken for empirical research using MEDLINE, CINAHL, EMBASE and the Cochrane Register of Controlled Trials (CENTRAL). Each database was searched from commencement to August 2015. Grey literature was searched using the OpenGrey database. Citations of all potentially relevant reviews and research papers were hand searched. No date or language restrictions were applied to the database searches.

The following terms were used in the search all databases: prostate cancer, DRE, primary care. The search strategy and protocol and be accessed here http://www.crd.york.ac.uk/PROSPERO/display_record.asp?ID=CRD42015025764. Two reviewers (CF and AD) independently screened the title and abstract of all articles identified by the search to determine eligibility. Full texts were obtained for all potentially relevant articles and these were independently assessed by two authors (CF and AD) to determine eligibility. Final inclusion was determined by agreement between both reviewers. If no consensus was reached, a third study author (DJ) was consulted.

Eligibility criteria

We searched for studies that evaluated the use of DRE in primary care for the detection of prostate cancer. To be included in the review studies had to meet three inclusion criteria: studies should be randomized controlled trials, case control or cohort studies; they needed to include symptomatic patients with any of the symptoms listed in the NICE guidelines for referral of prostate cancer; and they studies needed to be conducted in primary care setting. Studies undertaken in secondary care or screening studies of asymptomatic patients were excluded. As this was a review of a diagnostic procedure the studies should compare DRE to a reference test. The reference for this review was histological diagnosis of prostate cancer. The NICE guidelines do not define an abnormal DRE so definitions from all included studies were considered.

Outcomes

The primary outcomes were the sensitivity, specificity, positive (PPV) and negative predictive value (NPV) of DRE in primary care for the detection of prostate cancer in symptomatic patients. This was calculated using the Meta-DiSc software [10]. Secondary outcomes were cost-effectiveness and adverse effects as a result of the intervention. Heterogeneity is almost always presumed in diagnostic test accuracy systematic reviews, and hence, a random-effects model was used [11].

Data extraction

Two reviewers (CF and AD) independently extracted data from included articles using a pre-defined data extraction form. Disagreements were resolved by discussion between the two reviewers with a third reviewer (DJ) consulted if necessary. Data were extracted on study participants including age, ethnicity, setting and symptoms, the studies inclusion and exclusion criteria, the information on the DRE and gold standard test of the study and study outcomes.

Quality assessment

The Newcastle Ottawa quality assessment scale [12] was used to evaluate the quality of included studies. This scale is recommended by the Cochrane Handbook for assessing methodological quality of non-randomised studies and was chosen as it was highlighted as a simple tool to apply using eight assessment domains [13].

Hamilton [4] was a case control study and was determined to be of high methodological quality. The study adequately defined a case, stating they were identified from the cancer registry at the Royal Devon and Exeter Hospital and controls were selected from the community with no history of disease. The study adequately controlled for age and location. Exposure for both cases and controls was ascertained from the GP and hospital records. All cases and controls were included in the final results with no drop outs.

Three cohort studies [14–16] were included and were judged to be of high methodological quality. All were representative of the average age of men with prostate cancer in the community. Ascertainment of exposure for all studies was determined from a secure patient medical record. Participants with a history of prostate cancer were excluded in all studies. All studies controlled for symptomatic patients, location and performance of DRE. However, it should be noted that none of the cohort studies included documentation of how biopsy was taken and whether the individual performing the biopsy was blinded of symptoms and DRE findings.

Results

Study characteristics

Four studies met the inclusion criteria and were included in the review (see Fig. 1). The characteristics of the included studies are shown in Table 1. Three of the studies were cohort studies [14–16] and one was a case control study [4]. Two of the studies were conducted in the US [14, 15], one was conducted in the UK [4] and one in Spain [16]. A total of 3225 patients were included in the four papers. The largest study had 1297 participants [4] and the smallest had just 82 [16]. The age of participants in included studies ranged from 40 to 89. All studies documented the symptoms suffered by patients with the exception of Issa [14] who used the international prostate symptom score (IPSS). All four papers included patients with at least one of symptoms listed in the NICE cancer guidelines, however these were different in each paper. Three of the studies explicitly defined an 'abnormal DRE' with the exception of Gelabert Mas [16]. The three papers used very similar definitions of an abnormal prostate. Hamilton et al. state that "hard, craggy or nodular glands were classified as malignant" [4], Issa et al. state that "DRE findings were classified as abnormal in the presence of prostate induration and/or nodularity" [14] and Mettlin et al. state that "a suspicious DRE outcome is defined by the presence of significant induration, nodularity or asymmetry" [15].

Diagnostic accuracy of DRE

There were 3225 participants included from 4 different studies. For each of the included studies we were able to calculate a 2 × 2 table for reference test (biopsy / diagnosis of prostate cancer) results versus the diagnostic test (DRE). This data was then combined to give an overall sensitivity, specificity, PPV and NPV. This was calculated using Meta-Disc software. Overall, the pooled sensitivity and specificity for DRE as a predictor of prostate cancer in symptomatic patients was found to be 28.6% (95% CI 25.1–32.3%) and 90.7% (95% CI 89.5–91.8%), respectively. These results are shown in Fig. 2. The pooled PPV and NPV were found to be 42.3 and 84.2%, respectively. There was no relevant data extractable regarding secondary outcomes of adverse events or cost effectiveness.

As three out of the four studies were cohort studies, we performed a sub-analysis of the cohort studies alone. This produced a sensitivity of 42.7% (95% CI 37.8–47.7%), a specificity of 86.7% (95% CI 84.9–88.4%), a PPV of 46.1% and a NPV of 85.1%. Showing that excluding the case control study did not significantly affect the results.

Discussion

To the authors' knowledge, this is the first review to evaluate the specificity, sensitivity, positive and negative predictive value of DRE as a predictor of prostate cancer in symptomatic patients in a primary care setting.

With the release of the new cancer referral guidelines in the UK the threshold of risk for referral for possible cancer was reduced from 5 to 3%. This suggests that all patients with signs and symptoms which carry a risk of cancer greater than 3% should be referred urgently to secondary care. This review found the pooled positive predictive value of DRE to detect prostate cancer was 42.3%. This suggests that if a patient with symptoms suggestive of prostate cancer presents to primary care and has an abnormal feeling prostate examination, then that patients risk of cancer is 42.3%. This clearly warrants an

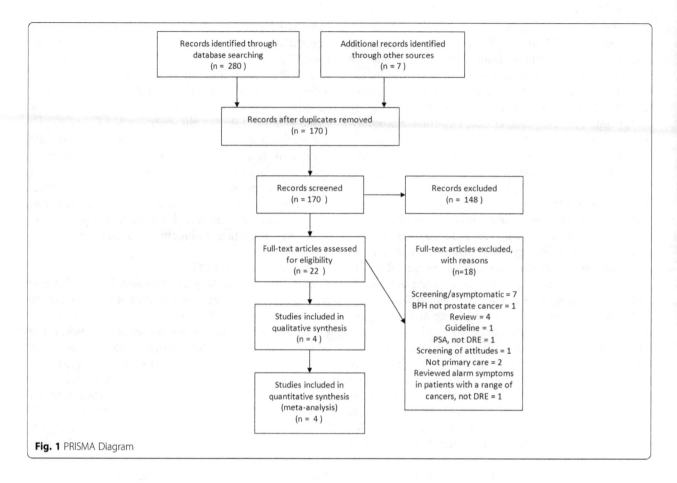

Fig. 1 PRISMA Diagram

urgent referral for suspected cancer and supports the UK NICE guidelines.

However, the pooled sensitivity in this review was low, 28.6% suggesting that many patients diagnosed with prostate cancer do not have an abnormal DRE. In addition to the low sensitivity, the pooled negative predictive value was 84.2%, this suggests that symptomatic patients who present to primary care and have a normal prostate examination still have a risk of cancer of 15.8%, which above the 3% risk threshold suggested by NICE. These findings show that patients in these included studies should be urgently referred for suspected prostate cancer regardless of the DRE result. This suggests

that DRE performed in primary care is an unnecessary investigation, adding little to the decision to refer, which should be made on the basis of symptoms alone. In addition to this, it is possible that DRE may delay the patient in seeking help with some qualitative research finding that the prospect of a DRE may deter some men from seeking medical help for symptoms suggestive of prostate cancer and prostate cancer screening [17–19]. This qualitative research suggests that performing DRE in primary may in fact be delaying the diagnosis of prostate cancer.

The UK NICE guidelines make their recommendations to refer patients with a prostate deemed malignant on

Table 1 Characteristics of included studies

Study ID	Country	Evidence level	Methods	Number of participants	Age range (years)	Index test	Reference	Outcomes
Mettlin 1991	USA	2b	Prospective cohort study	1218	55–70	PSA, DRE and TRUS	Biopsy	Sensitivity, specificity and PPV of DRE, PSA and TRUS.
Gelabert Mas 1997	Spain	2b	Prospective cohort study	82	> 50	PSA/DRE	Biopsy	Sensitivity, specificity, and PPV of DRE and PSA.
Hamilton 2006	UK	4	Case control	1297	≥ 40	PSA/DRE	Diagnosis of prostate cancer	PPV of symptoms, DRE and PSA.
Issa 2006	USA	2b	Retrospective cohort study	628	40–89	PSA/DRE	Biopsy	Sensitivity, specificity, PPV and NPV of DRE and PSA.

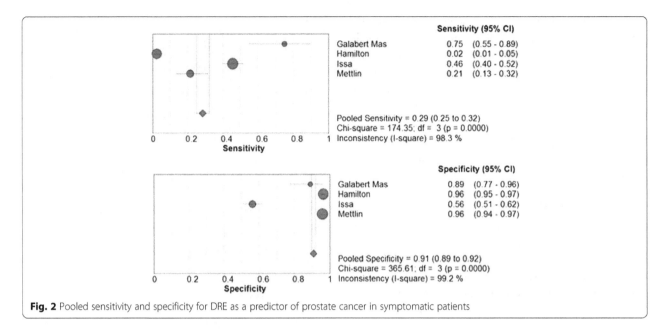

Fig. 2 Pooled sensitivity and specificity for DRE as a predictor of prostate cancer in symptomatic patients

examination on the evidence from just one study. This systematic review includes four studies which consider the effectiveness of DRE for diagnosing prostate cancer in symptomatic patients in primary care and thus provides stronger evidence for performing DRE in these patients. However, the majority of the available literature concentrates on using DRE as a screening test in unselected asymptomatic patients. More research on the effectiveness of DRE in primary care would help to provide further evidence for the NICE guidelines and ensure that DRE is a useful investigation when performed by GPs.

Whilst the included studies were judged to be of high methodological quality it is difficult to draw conclusions based on a small number of studies, all of which were published over ten years ago, are of low impact and are largely heterogeneous. In addition, there are limitations of including case control studies in reviews of diagnostic test accuracy as they tend to overestimate diagnostic accuracy. In addition to this Hamilton et al. included patients diagnosed with prostate cancer by a urologist without having a biopsy which means not all participants in the study received the same index test. Whilst this clinically makes sense and is common in studies in which the reference test is invasive, it is nonetheless a limitation of the study. These limitations were investigated using a sensitivity analysis which excluded the Hamilton et al. study, it was found that excluding the case control study did not significantly affect the results.

To be included in this review the papers had to include patients with at least one of the symptoms suggested by NICE. However, in each paper the combination of symptoms in the patients was different and in some was poorly defined.

Due to the nature of using secondary data, there were some papers in which full information was not available. It was agreed in each study the DRE had been performed in primary care, however it was often not clear who had performed the examination. In addition to this, only three of the four studies adequately defined an abnormal DRE, the forth study did not provide a definition of abnormal or positive DRE.

One of the papers (Issa 2006) caused some difficulty in analysis due to a possible typing error. In the text of the study they state symptoms were classified as mild moderate or severe using IPSS with mild symptoms classified between 1 and 7, however in the results they present mild symptoms as 0–7, this could mean patients with an IPSS score of 0, who may be asymptomatic were included in the results. Clarification was sought from the authors however no response was received.

The vast majority of existing literature focuses on the use of DRE as a screening tool. A Cochrane review on screening for prostate cancer included five studies and found that screening did not significantly decrease prostate cancer-specific mortality [20]. This review supports the recommendations of NICE which suggests that GPs refer patients urgently on the basis of an abnormal DRE. The NICE recommendation was made on the basis of the Hamilton 2006 paper which is included in this review. There is also qualitative literature to suggest that the prospect of a DRE may deter men from presenting to primary care.

Conclusion

The most recent UK NICE guidelines recommend that general practitioners undertake a digital rectal examination on all patients with lower urinary tract symptoms.

The guidelines suggest referring patients under the two week wait referral pathway if the prostate feels malignant. This is the first review to look at the accuracy of digital rectal examination by general practitioners for the diagnosis of prostate cancer in symptomatic patients. We found only four studies on the effectiveness of DRE for the diagnosis of prostate cancer in symptomatic patients in primary care, with much of the available literature focusing on screening. DRE is widely used and recommended for the assessment of patients in primary care. It is a simple, safe and cost-effective diagnostic tool, The findings of the review support the NICE guidelines and recommend urgent referral for suspected cancer in patients with an abnormal DRE, however the review casts doubt on the use of DRE as a diagnostic tool in primary care due to the low sensitivity and negative predictive value. More research is needed to assess its effectiveness in diagnosing prostate cancer in symptomatic patients.

Abbreviations
DRE: Digital rectal examination; NICE: National Institute for Health and Care Excellence; PRISMA: Preferred Reporting Items for Systematic Reviews and Meta-Analyses; PSA: Prostate specific antigen

Acknowledgements
The authors would like to thank Dr. Carla Reigada for her help translating the studies that were in Spanish. We would also like to thank the Haxby Group, Kingswood Health Centre, Hull for allowing AD the time to complete this review.

Authors' contributions
DJ designed the initial project and protocol, performed the searches, acted as a third party for disagreements on inclusion or data extraction, supervised CF and AD and wrote up the manuscript. CF and AD performed the searches at abstract and full text stages, undertook citation and grey literature searches, carried out the data extraction and assessed the methodological quality of the studies as well as contributing to the write up. VA assisted with the analysis and data extraction and contributed to the write up. UM oversaw the project as a whole, provided guidance at the initial planning and design of the project and contributed to the write up. All authors read and approved the final manuscript.

Competing interests
The authors declared that they have no competing interests.

Author details
[1]Hull York Medical School, Hertford Building, University of Hull, Cottingham Road, Hull HU6 7RX, UK. [2]Goethe University Frankfurt, Theodor-W.-Adorno-Platz 1, 60323 Frankfurt am Main, Germany. [3]Faculty of Health Sciences, University of York, Heslington, York YO10 5DD, UK.

References
1. Cancer Research UK. Cancer Statistics for the UK 2015 [cited 2015 27th July].
2. Preventative Services US, Force T. Draft recommendation statement: prostate Cancer. Screening. 2017;
3. Public Health England. Prostate Cancer Risk Management Programme 2015 [cited 2015 27th July].
4. Hamilton W, Sharp DJ, Peters TJ, Round AP. Clinical features of prostate cancer before diagnosis: a population-based, case-control study. The British journal of general practice : the journal of the Royal College of General Practitioners. 2006;56(531):756–62.
5. Frankel S, Smith GD, Donovan J, Neal D. Screening for prostate cancer. Lancet. 2003;361(9363):1122–8.
6. NICE. Suspected cancer: recognition and referral. 2015.
7. Walsh AL, Considine SW, Thomas AZ, Lynch TH, Manecksha RP. Digital rectal examination in primary care is important for early detection of prostate cancer: a retrospective cohort analysis study. The British journal of general practice : the journal of the Royal College of General Practitioners. 2014;64(629):e783–7.
8. Moher D, Liberati A, Tetzlaff J, Altman DG, Group P. Preferred reporting items for systematic reviews and meta-analyses: the PRISMA statement. Open medicine : a peer-reviewed, independent, open-access journal. 2009;3(3):e123–30.
9. Jones D, Dreher A, Friend C, Macleod U. How effective is digital rectal examination for diagnosis of prostate cancer for symptomatic patients in primary care? : PROSPERO international prospective register of. Syst Rev. 2015; Available from: http://www.crd.york.ac.uk/PROSPERO/display_record. asp?ID=CRD42015025764
10. Zamora J, Abraira V, Muriel A, Khan K, Coomarasamy A. Meta-DiSc: a software for meta-analysis of test accuracy data. BMC Med Res Methodol. 2006;6:31.
11. Lee J, Kim KW, Choi SH, Huh J, Park SH. Systematic review and meta-analysis of studies evaluating diagnostic test accuracy: a practical review for clinical researchers-part II. Statistical methods of meta-analysis. Korean J Radiol. 2015;16(6):1188–96.
12. Stang A. Critical evaluation of the Newcastle-Ottawa scale for the assessment of the quality of nonrandomized studies in meta-analyses. Eur J Epidemiol. 2010;25(9):603–5.
13. Higgins JPT, Green S. Cochrane handbook for systematic reviews of interventions Version 5.1.0 2011. Available from: http://training.cochrane.org/handbook.
14. Issa MM, Zasada W, Ward K, Hall JA, Petros JA, Ritenour CW, et al. The value of digital rectal examination as a predictor of prostate cancer diagnosis among United States veterans referred for prostate biopsy. Cancer Detect Prev. 2006;30(3):269–75.
15. Mettlin C, Lee F, Drago J, Murphy GP. The American Cancer Society National Prostate Cancer Detection Project. Findings on the detection of early prostate cancer in 2425 men. Cancer. 1991;67(12):2949–58.
16. Gelabert Mas A, Arango Toro O, Carles Galceran J, Bielsa Gali O, Cortadellas Angel R, Herrero Polo M, et al. Early diagnosis by opportunistic screening in cancer of the prostate. Results of a 1-year protocol. Comparison with historical data. Actas urologicas espanolas. 1997;21(9):835–42.
17. Ferrante JM, Shaw EK, Scott JG. Factors influencing men's decisions regarding prostate cancer screening: a qualitative study. J Community Health. 2011;36(5):839–44.
18. Forrester-Anderson IT. Prostate cancer screening perceptions, knowledge and behaviors among African American men: focus group findings. J Health Care Poor Underserved. 2005;16(4 Suppl A):22–30.
19. Lee DJ, Consedine NS, Spencer BA. Barriers and facilitators to digital rectal examination screening among African-American and African-Caribbean men. Urology. 2011;77(4):891–8.
20. Ilic D, O'Connor D, Green S, Wilt TJ. Screening for prostate cancer: an updated Cochrane systematic review. BJU Int. 2011;107(6):882–91.

12

Challenges in providing maternity care in remote areas and islands for primary care physicians

Ayako Shibata[1][*] [iD], Makoto Kaneko[2,3,4] and Machiko Inoue[4]

Abstract

Background: Maintaining a maternity care system is one of the biggest issues in Japan due to the decreasing number of obstetricians, especially in remote areas and islands. The aim of this qualitative study was to explore the challenges in women's health and maternity care in remote areas and islands for primary care physicians and obstetricians in order to provide an insight necessary to develop a better health care system.

Methods: We conducted semi-structured interviews with 13 primary care physicians and 4 obstetricians practicing maternity care at clinics/hospitals in remote areas and islands across Japan. Interview data were analyzed, using the modified Grounded Theory Approach, to elucidate the challenges primary care physicians faced in their practice.

Results: Primary care physicians who engaged in maternity care recognized the following challenges: low awareness of primary care, lack of training opportunities, unclear goal of the training, lack of certification system, lack of consultation system, and lack of obstetricians to offer support. These six challenges along with the specialty's factors such as sudden changes of patients' condition were considered to result to the provider's hesitation and anxiety to engage in the practice.

Conclusions: This study found six environmental/systemic factors and three specialty's factors as the main challenges for primary care physicians in providing maternity care in remote areas and islands for primary care physicians in Japan. Increasing the awareness of primary care and developing a maternity care training program to certify primary care physicians may enable more primary care physicians to engage in and provide women's health and maternity care in remote areas and islands.

Keywords: Maternity care, Primary care, Qualitative study, Rural medicine, Women's health

Background

The Japanese maternal mortality rate is as low as 4 in 100,000 deliveries; most of those deliveries are covered by obstetricians [1]. However, obstetricians are decreasing in number, creating difficulties in supporting the perinatal care needs of remote areas [2]. The number of new members of the Japan Society of Obstetrics and Gynecology (JSOG) decreased for 3 years straight from 2010 with approximately 24% of members being 65 years old or older [3]. Sixty percent of members aged 30 years old or younger are female physicians [3]. The number of obstetricians working at maternity facilities is expected to decrease going forward. Furthermore, the number of new obstetricians per capita in Japanese prefectures shows marked disparity (expected to increase going forward) between Tokyo (4.51 obstetricians per 100,000 residents) and Fukushima and Ibaraki (0.75 obstetricians per 100,000 residents) [3]. The JSOG has moved forward to concentrate on obstetrics facilities aiming to reduce the burden of obstetricians. This had decreased the number of obstetric hospitals by 20% between 2005 and 2011 [4].

Currently, there are several areas where access from delivery institutions to perinatal medical centers takes 60 min or longer, primarily in Kyushu, Tohoku, Sanyo, Shikoku, and the outer islands, which have keenly experienced the decrease or absence of obstetricians [5]. We

* Correspondence: 3113044@ych.or.jp; sibata700@gmail.com
[1]Department of Obstetrics and Gynecology, Yodogawa Christian Hospital, 1-7-50, Kunijima, Higashiyodogawa-ku, Osaka 533-0024, Japan
Full list of author information is available at the end of the article

must consider how and where to carry out regional maternity care and who will carry out that care.

Some other countries assign primary care physicians (PCPs) to handle low-risk maternity care. Those systems coordinate obstetricians and PCPs especially in areas where obstetricians are scarce. For example, in the U.S., perinatal care, including child delivery, is a required part of specialized training for PCPs (family practitioners). The addition of a one-year obstetrical fellowship allows for PCPs to practice Caesarean section operations. Boston University Municipal Hospital is trying to create a joint maternity care team of obstetricians and PCPs [6]. In Canada, although the percentage of PCPs practicing child delivery has fallen to 11.1%, the percentage of PCPs offering maternity and postpartum care remains high at 50% [7]. Some PCP clinics are trying to focus on perinatal and maternity care [8]. In Australia, a collaborative system called "shared maternity care" was built to coordinate regional PCPs' clinics/maternity centers and high-volume perinatal medical centers handling child delivery [9].

The current training program for Japanese PCPs was accredited by the Japan Primary Care Association (JPCA) [10], which is an academic organization of PCPs established in 2010. It mandated 3 months of pediatric training in addition to 6 months of internal medicine training in 3 years, but training in obstetrics and gynecology (OBGYN) is elective [11]. Currently, places where PCPs offer maternity care are limited to only a handful of remote areas and islands across Japan. Narumoto has surveyed three of these areas where obstetricians and PCPs are collaborating to offer maternity care, showing that the collaboration reduces the burden of the obstetricians and allows them to focus on more specialized care [12]. The JSOG stated the need to consider dividing obstetrician role with primary care physicians in the grand design of renovation of the OBGYN healthcare system (GD2015) [13]. It is possible that Japan will need PCPs to handle some women's health and maternity care in near future. However, the discussion on this issue has not progressed much, and no specific strategies for role sharing have been decided. This qualitative study aimed to clarify the challenges for PCPs and obstetricians in women's health and maternity care in remote areas and islands in order to provide an insight necessary to develop a better health care system.

Methods

We conducted qualitative research using semi-structured interviews. We recruited the participants from the physicians who practiced women's health and maternity care in the remote areas and islands in the member of the JPCA. We included both residency program directors, and residents in order to obtain broader perspectives. We sent e-mails with the research protocol and asked voluntary participation to the study. The first author visited the participants for interview who had agreed to participate. Research participants were 17 doctors (4 obstetricians and 13 PCPs) offering women's health and maternity care in the remote areas and islands: Hokkaido, Tohoku, Ishikawa prefecture, Tokyo, Chiba prefecture, Shizuoka prefecture, Shimane prefecture, and Nagasaki prefecture (Fig. 1).

The interview guide was created through the discussion among the researchers, one of whom had an experience of solo practice in a remote island. Interview questions focused on the following: (1) the types of women's health and maternity care offered by PCPs, (2) the challenges they faced in providing that care, and (3) what would be necessary for PCP–obstetrician collaboration (Appendix 1).

Participants were informed ahead of time of the voluntary nature of survey participation and their freedom to withdraw from participation. Interviews were conducted in private in separate rooms or meeting facilities between April of 2015 and March of 2016. After consent forms were received, interviews were audio-recorded. The interviewer used interview guide along with open-ended questions in order to collect wide range of participants' opinions and feelings. Written consent was obtained from all participants prior to data collection. This research conformed to the provisions of the

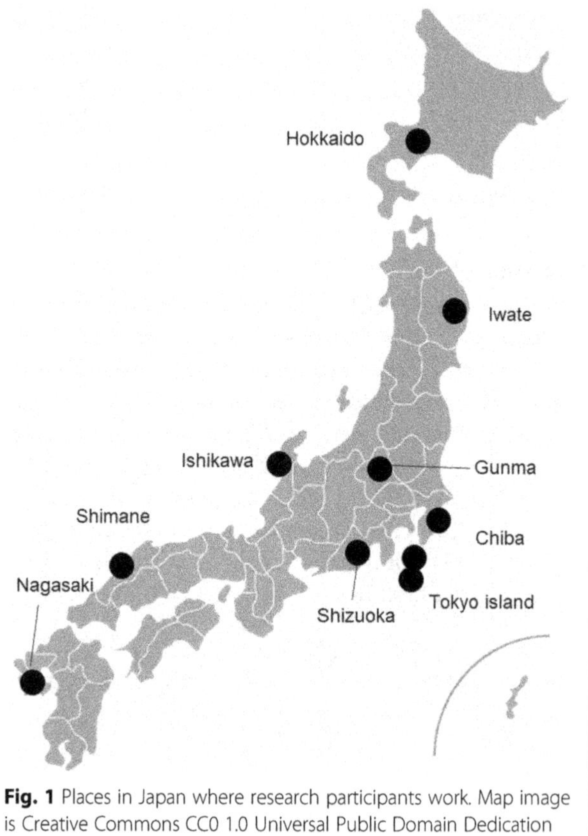

Fig. 1 Places in Japan where research participants work. Map image is Creative Commons CC0 1.0 Universal Public Domain Dedication

Declaration of Helsinki and was approved by the ethics committee of Yodogawa Christian Hospital.

The recordings were transcribed verbatim, and the identifying information was removed. The modified version of Grounded Theory Approach (m-GTA) was used for data analysis [14], which had been developed by Kinoshita on the basis of the grounded theory approach, with following procedure [15]. With m-GTA, the data are not segmented by predefined unit of a word or a sentence as in the grounded theory approach, but by a unit of sentences that allows deeper interpretation of meaning. As we reviewed the transcripts, we extracted concrete examples which reflected the participants' specific views on the challenges they faced, and we shaped concepts derived from these pieces of data by repeatedly interpreting the meaning. Throughout the procedure, we developed an analysis worksheet for each concept with concept name, definition, and concrete examples. We iteratively conducted the analysis and generated new concepts while comparing and examining the examples obtained from new data. We continued the data collection until the point when theoretical saturation was reached where no more new concepts had emerged. Next, we examined the concepts, and by grouping some concepts, deliberated on the categories that represented the challenges PCPs face in providing women's health and maternity care in remote areas and islands. Then, we created a conceptual model by interpreting the interrelationships among the final concepts and categories. All researchers held discussions to agree upon the development of concepts, categories and the conceptual model. We did not use any software for coding.

Results

PCPs in this study included general internists, family practitioners, and senior residents of family practice who engaged in primary care in remote areas and islands. Of the 17 participants, 4 were obstetricians, and 13 were PCPs (with 1 holding obstetrical certification and 2 undergoing obstetrical training); 15 were men, and 2 were women. Six participants were graduates of Jichi Medical School (which requires graduates to work 9 years in remote areas). Four participants are presently offering practice on remote islands; 3 had experience with remote island practice. Participant backgrounds are shown in Table 1. The average interview time was 65 min (ranging from 32 to 101 min).

Three types of women's health and maternity care were offered by the PCPs in Japan. The first type focused on common gynecological disease (office gynecology). The scope of the practice included vaginal discharge, menstrual abnormalities, conception check, menopausal symptoms, cervical cancer screening. The physicians' training period was several weeks in an OBGYN department in addition to the outpatient training at a primary care (PC) clinic. This type of practice was observed in the outer

Table 1 Backgrounds of research participants

No.	Region	Specialty	Position	Training	Sex
1	Gunma	OB/GYN[a]	Attending	Jichi[b]	M
2	Shimane	PCP[c]	Attending	Jichi, Island practice OB/GYN residency training	M
3	Ishikawa	PCP	Resident	OB/GYN residency training	F
4	Ishikawa	OB/GYN	Attending	PC residency training	M
5	Ishikawa	OB/GYN	Attending	OB/GYN attending	M
6	Ishikawa	PCP	Attending	PCP attending	M
7	Nagasaki	PCP	Resident	OB/GYN residency training	M
8	Tokyo island	PCP	Attending	Jichi, Island practice	M
9	Tokyo island	PCP	Resident	Jichi	M
10	Tokyo island	PCP	Resident	Jichi, Island practice	M
11	Tokyo island	PCP	Resident	Jichi, Island practice	M
12	Shizuoka	PCP	Attending	PCP attending	M
13	Shizuoka	PCP	Resident	OB/GYN residency training	F
14	Iwate	OB/GYN	Resident	OB/GYN residency training	M
15	Hokkaido	PCP	Attending	Island practice	M
16	Hokkaido	PCP	Resident	PCP residency training	M
17	Chiba	PCP	Attending	PCP attending	M

[a]OB/GYN Obstetricians/Gynecologist
[b]Jichi A graduate of the Jichi University
[c]PCP Primary care physician

Okinawa islands and PC clinics in the Tohoku area. The second type was office gynecology and prenatal care (not including child delivery). The scope of the practice included common gynecological diseases and prenatal care up to the third trimester. The physicians' training period was 2–3 months outpatient/ward training in an OBGYN department in addition to outpatient training at a PC clinic. This practice was observed in the outer islands and PC clinics in the Kanto area. The third type was comprehensive women's health care including child delivery. The scope of the practice included office gynecology, child delivery, and practice in an OBGYN ward including assistance with C-sections. The physicians' training involved 2–3 months of outpatient/ward training and night duties in an OBGYN department and outpatient training at a PC. This style was observed in PC clinics and hospitals in the Chubu region.

We found following six main challenges faced by PCPs handling women's health and maternity care in Japan (Fig. 2): (1) Low awareness of primary care; (2) Lack of training opportunities; (3) Unclear goal of the training; (4) Lack of certification system; (5) Lack of a consultation system; and (6) Lack of obstetricians to offer support. The six challenges are assembled into three categories; 'Low awareness of primary care', 'Lack of educational system', and 'Lack of support system.' There were also three specialty factors which made difficult for PCPs to engage in maternity care; (1) Sudden changes of patients' condition; (2) Social pressure for safety in perinatal care; and (3) Sensitivity in technical training. 'Low awareness of primary care', 'Lack of educational system', and "Sensitivity in technical training" were considered to result in lack of experiences of PCPs. 'Low awareness of primary care', 'Lack of support system' and lack of experiences were considered to lead to the hesitation and anxiety of the PCPs to engage in handling women's health and maternity

care in remote areas and islands in Japan (Fig. 2). Followings are the explanations of each concept with quotes. Quotes are shown in italics. "PCP" stands for primary care physician, and "OB" stands for obstetrician.

Low awareness of primary care

The awareness of the concept of "primary care" in patients and medical staff (especially in obstetricians) is low. The Japanese society has a poor understanding of the family physicians and general physicians who take care of women's health and pregnancy management.

The majority don't know how much to entrust to PCPs. (15: PCP)

Obstetricians don't know what we (family practitioners) are nor how to utilize us. They don't see our faces and don't know what training we've received. So, they worry about us in managing pregnancies and child deliveries where they know anything could potentially happen. (12: PCP)

We don't know the extent to which family practitioners are seeing pregnant patients. (5: OB)

Patients seem to wonder whether a family practitioner can provide maternity practice, and I don't have time to explain this to them. To refer a patient to the family practitioner, I have to explain what a family practitioner is, which is not a simple task. (5: OB)

Lack of training opportunities

There are few educational programs in which PCPs can acquire skills and experiences in women's health and

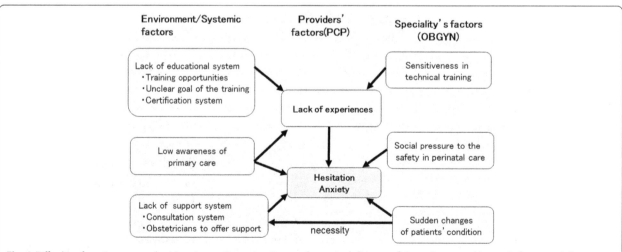

Fig. 2 Difficulties for primary care physicians to practice maternity care Conceptual diagram of six environmental/systemic factors and three specialty's factors faced by primary care physicians handling women's health and maternity care in Japan

maternity care. Insufficient experience leads to hesitation and anxiety of the PCP in the practice.

I do have concerns that something could be overlooked in fetal echo. (3: PCP in obstetricians training)

Unclear goal of the training

In Japan, educational goals for the training for PCPs to learn women's health and maternity care are lacking in primary care training. There is no consistency in the scope and content of the practice offered by family practitioners, family doctors, and primary care doctors in Japan.

Rotating the obstetrics and gynecology department of a big hospital, it tends to be just holding the retractors in the surgery. (16: PCP)

If I extend the scope of my (family medicine) clinic practice too much, I can't imagine what's going to be. (3: PCP)

Lack of certification system

Except for obstetrical board certification, there is no certification system for PCPs to demonstrate their skills and knowledge of women's health and maternity care in Japan. Some PCPs chose to acquire obstetrical board certification, which requires additional 3 years of training.

When thinking about the social pressure for the medical safety, including risks for lawsuits, you must protect yourself in a form to take the obstetrical certification (12: PCP)

Lack of consultation system

When a PCP practices women's health and pregnancy management, a supportive facility is needed that accepts consultations and transportation of serious patients. However, there is no consultation system in which PCPs in remote areas and islands can consult with obstetricians when necessary.

There are some obstetric or gynecological emergencies in a certain probability. We have survived by consulting them to the local obstetric institution. (8: PCP)

I'm wondering what would happen if maternity care were only carried out by a family practitioner. It would be good if we have the mother visit a large hospital for a fetal screening as a risk management, or we can discuss with the midwives and the obstetricians

on several occasions. (13: PCP in obstetricians training)

Lack of obstetricians to offer support

The obstetricians themselves are considered very busy and cannot afford to support PCPs in remote areas.

There are few obstetricians in the remote areas. (4: PCP)

Obstetricians in the university are full of research and their tasks, and it is hard to think of supporting PCPs. (7: OB)

Additionally, we found three specialty's factors affecting why obstetrical practice is difficult and challenging for other medical specialties:

Sudden changes of patients' condition

The patients' condition can change rapidly during child delivery, which sometimes requires rapid consultation and patient transfer.

Some of my patients have become threatened with premature labor or extreme leg edema from preeclampsia. Since there is the possibility of sudden, high-risk fluctuations, we really need the consultation of the obstetricians when taking care of the deliveries. (3: PCP in obstetrical training)

Social pressure for safety in perinatal care

There are liability and lawsuit risks surrounding the perinatal care and child delivery.

I worry about fetal malformations of my patients since we can't provide fetal screening echo. I have few experiences of fetal malformations such as cardiac deformities. (10: PCP)

Sensitivity in technical training

It is considered difficult to teach trainees in the perinatal visit or child delivery, since the patients request not to be seen by trainees.

It is hard to teach while a patient's legs are open. (14: OB)

Teaching by whispering will cause the patient anxiety. (15: OB)

The factors described above (six challenges with three specialty's factors) were considered to result in the provider's hesitation and anxiety to engage in the women's health and maternity care. On the other hand, there were many positive comments on having PCPs in maternity care as follows.

My patients have said, "If my family doctor could deal with gynecological problems, then I'd talk those issues to the doctor." Some patients are reluctant to visit obstetricians because of the hesitation of vaginal exam. We should probably start from this very modest approach. (7: PCP with obstetrical certification)

If we allow PCPs to attend the child delivery, they can also take care of their immunizations later. The mother can also benefit from PCPs, such as annual medical checkup and flu shots. If the mom has any complaints during pregnancy, such as skin issues, asthma, etc., PCPs can take care of it right away without referring her to another doctor. (13: PCP in obstetrical training)

Having a PCP join in our night shifts makes a huge difference in terms of the limited number of obstetricians. (5: OB)

The merits for obstetricians would be easy to ask PCPs to take care of common complains, psychological care, and postpartum care. (3: PCP)

The role of PCPs is to enable specialists to concentrate on the areas their skills are needed in. Hence, the system offers mutual benefits. The patient could have all-around care from the PCPs, and there are cost benefits as well. (7: PCP with obstetrical certification)

Discussion

This research examined the practice styles of PCPs who are offering woman and maternity care and challenges they faced in providing that care. The practice styles include (1) office gynecology (care focusing on common women's health), (2) office gynecology and prenatal care (not including child delivery), and (3) comprehensive women's health care including child delivery. In Japan, practice style (1) and (2) are commonly seen, and few PCP handles child delivery on their own. These practice styles appear to depend on the number of child births in that region and the presence or absence of obstetricians to support PCPs. In regions where PCPs are managing the child delivery, there are collaborative teams of PCPs and obstetricians in the same facility. If we consider PCPs to manage partial obstetrical practice in the remote area, it is necessary to discuss which practice style is desired and to build training programs and goals accordingly.

Three categories of the six environmental/systemic factors for PCPs providing women's health and maternity care were low awareness of primary care, lack of educational system and lack of support system. These three factors impede PCPs from gaining sufficient practice experiences, which leads to their hesitation and anxiety in providing the care. First, the low awareness of primary care is a unique problem for Japan. In Japan, there are many names for "general practitioner": family practitioner, primary care doctor, general practitioner, general internal medicine, hospital generalist, home doctor, and so on. There is no consistency in the definition and content of their practice. There are few people, including patients, obstetricians, and health care professionals, who fully understand the practice offered by each "general practitioner". Hence, obstetricians feel uneasy in referring their patients and need extra time to explain to the patients, which are all obstacles to collaboration. To alleviate these concerns, we must clarify which PCP has the competency to practice women and maternity care through a certification system that verifies the skills and knowledge attained.

The second factor, "lack of educational system" causes the insufficient experiences of PCPs as women's health and maternity care providers. Various foreign countries have handled these challenges by developing systems for PCPs to collaborate with obstetricians. For instance, Boston University has tried including the family medicine residents in their maternity care teams, including rounds, night shifts, and perinatal/post-natal care. Bringing family practitioner residents onto these teams gives them exposure to over 40 deliveries a year and increases their practice experience [6]. These collaborative teams could help PCPs to increase maternity care experiences in a protected learning environment.

The third factor, "lack of support system" such as consulting system to the obstetricians. In our interview, some PCPs mentioned the fear of possibly overlooking abnormalities in fetal echo during perinatal checks. At present, the prenatal care guidelines by the JSOG do not mandate fetal screening echo to detect abnormalities [16], although PCPs desire to secure the quality of care by creating the PCP-obstetrician collaboration system. For instant, Australia has a shared maternity care system in which high-volume perinatal medical centers cooperate with regional facilities (PC clinics and maternity centers). Certified facilities can offer perinatal care (at 7–12, 12–14, 22–26, 33, 38, and 39 weeks) by midwives and family doctors [9]. There are clear guidelines for the practice to be carried out at each gestational week as well as criteria for referrals and transfers, which serve to standardized care. These guidelines could help guarantee the quality of care provided, including care offered through PCP–obstetrician collaboration. Japan also has semi-open/open systems in which obstetrical care centers and local obstetrical clinics and midwifery homes collaborate. There are 43 hub obstetrical facilities and 675 collaborating clinics in Japan [17]. However, there are no open manuals for the semi-open/open system, which makes it hard for PCPs to join the system. In the future, collaboration between PCPs and obstetricians might be needed with expanding these semi-open/open systems to the regional PC clinics.

In addition, there were three specialty factors related to obstetrical practice; "Sudden changes of patients' condition," "Social pressure to the safety in perinatal care," and "Sensitivity in technical training." There are risks of sudden change in condition such as the need for a C-section due to fetal distress or disseminated intravascular coagulation due to postpartum hemorrhage. Therefore, obstetrical care, in contrast to other care, requires a system that allows PCPs to immediately consult with an obstetrician or transfer sick patients to the acute care facilities.

As for social pressure in Japan, there have been multiple cases of medical lawsuits for the accidents in perinatal care, and social pressure is extremely high to ensure the safety of child birth [18]. The Japan Council for Quality Health Care created The Japan Obstetric Compensation System for Cerebral Palsy in 2009 [19]. However, this system is only for the member facilities, which means PCP clinics which do not participate in this system cannot obtain this compensation when medical accidents occur. Recently, the patients have become extremely intent on having the specialist care. The trend is quite strong to request for a specialized physician from the earliest stages of pregnancy and refuse trainee attending. It is getting difficult to provide trainees, including PCPs, with vaginal exam and perineal suture during the training program. From fiscal year 2010, revised residency training systems have started in Japan. Since obstetrical training is not mandatory in 2-year intern training, current residents do not have the opportunity to study child delivery and vaginal exam. To overcome the difficulty of teaching vaginal exam and perineal suture in the clinical settings, we could develop simulations and hands-on training before onsite instruction.

Regardless of these challenges, we have discovered the benefits of involving PCPs in the women and maternity care. Involving PCPs allows the patients to cover various issues all in one place, including perinatal care, infant care, vaccines, cancer screening, blood pressure, and diabetes care after discharge from the delivery ward. Some research reported involving PCPs in maternity care team increases patient satisfaction [6, 20], establishing PCP–obstetrician collaboration could contribute to greater patient satisfaction in Japan, too. Narumoto addressed the benefits of PCP–obstetrician collaboration, explaining that this would ease the burdens on the obstetricians (including inpatients care, outpatient care, and ER walk-ins) and contribute to comprehensive care for the patients [12]. Creating more visibility of those benefits of PCP–obstetrician collaboration should contribute to increase the awareness of primary care in the obstetricians and healthcare professionals.

In the U.S., Brown et al. noted that obstacles to PCP–obstetrician collaboration include trust over sharing care, social pressure over the safety of perinatal care, differences in the culture between specialists and generalists, and patient competition [21]. We revealed six challenges and three specialty factors of difficulties for PCPs to handle the women's health and maternity care in Japan. This is the first research which gathered the on-site opinions who practice women's health and maternity care in the remote areas and islands in Japan. The results would provide useful insights for building better health care delivery system of women's health and maternity care in remote areas and islands.

This study has some limitations. Our research mainly sought the viewpoints of PCPs in Japan to reveal the problems of current health care delivery system. It is necessary to conduct further research on the obstetricians' perspectives to understand a comprehensive picture of the issues and to build a better collaboration system.

In Japan, 95% of childbearing aged women lived within a 30-min distance from the obstetrics facilities in 2011. This ratio would decrease to around 82 to 90% if we concentrated the obstetrics facilities [22]. The JSOG has stated the need of concentrating the obstetrics facilities and PCP–obstetrician collaboration in order to ease the burden of decreasing obstetricians [13]. We must discuss how to reduce the challenges we found in this study for PCPs in practicing women's and maternity care. Since the shape of PCP–obstetrician collaboration varies by the countries, consideration is needed in creating a new system that fits the characteristics of Japan's health care.

Conclusions

This study found six environmental/systemic factors and three specialty's factors as the main challenges for PCPs in providing maternity care in remote areas and islands for primary care physicians in Japan. Low awareness of primary care, lack of educational system, and lack of support system as well as specialty's factors were considered to result in PCP's hesitation and anxiety to engage in the women's health and maternity care. In Japan, increasing the awareness of primary care in the patients as well as the obstetricians and developing a maternity care training program to certify PCPs may enable more physicians to engage in and provide women's health and maternity care in remote areas and islands.

Appendix 1
The semi-structured interview guide

1. Interview introduction

Explanation of the research aim, how the interview data will be used, and voluntary participation rule. Explanation of anonymity and privacy.

2. Background information

Participant's career, training history and current position were asked.

3. Current practice

Could you tell me about your practice in the point of women's health care and maternity care?

- How often do you practice women's health care and maternity care?
- What kind of medical needs do you experience in women's health and maternity care?

4. The challenges they faced in providing the care

Could you tell me about the challenges in providing women's health and maternity care?

- How often and in what situation so you feel those challenges?
- Why do you think those challenges happen?
- Where do you think those challenges come from?

5. About the primary care physicians (PCP) – obstetrician collaboration

Could you talk me about your impression about PCP–obstetrician collaboration in Japan?
Could you talk me about your opinion about PCP–obstetrician collaboration from the perspective of providing women's health and maternity care in remote areas and islands?
What do you think is needed to improve PCP–obstetrician collaboration to provide women's health and maternity care?

6. For a better system

What do you think of women's health and maternity care in the remote areas and islands in Japan?
How do you think women's health and maternity care in the remote areas and islands in Japan can be improved?

What kind of system do you think is needed to improve women's health and maternity care in the remote areas and islands in Japan?

Abbreviations
GD2015: The grand design of renovation of the OBGYN healthcare system; Jichi: A graduate of the Jichi University; JPCA: The Japan Primary Care Association; JSOG: The Japan Society of Obstetrics and Gynecology; OB: Obstetrician; OB/GYN: Obstetricians/Gynecologist; OBGYN: Obstetrics and gynecology; PC: Primary care; PCP: Primary care physicians

Acknowledgements
This research was supported by the research grant of St Luke's International University Center for Clinical Epidemiology.

Funding
This research was supported by the research grant of St Luke's International University Center for Clinical Epidemiology.

Authors' contributions
AS conducted the interview, analyzed the data, and wrote the manuscript. MK contributed to developing the research concept and design and interpreted the data. MI analyzed the data and critically revised the manuscript. All authors read and approved the final manuscript.

Competing interests
The authors declare that they have no competing interests.

Author details
[1]Department of Obstetrics and Gynecology, Yodogawa Christian Hospital, 1-7-50, Kunijima, Higashiyodogawa-ku, Osaka 533-0024, Japan. [2]Musashikoganei Clinic, Japanese Health and Welfare Co-operative Federation, 1-15-9, Honcho, Koganei-shi, Tokyo 184-0004, Japan. [3]Division of Clinical Epidemiology, Jikei University School of Medicine, 3-25-8, Nishishimbashi, Minato-ku, Tokyo 105-8461, Japan. [4]Department of Family and Community Medicine, Hamamatsu University School of Medicine, 1-20-1, Handayama, Higashi-ku, Hamamatsu, Shizuoka 431-3192, Japan.

References
1. Hasegawa J, Sekizawa A. Tanaka H on behalf of the maternal death exploratory Committee in Japan and the Japan Association of Obstetricians and Gynecologists, et al. current status of pregnancy-related maternal mortality in Japan: a report from the maternal death exploratory committee in Japan. BMJ Open. 2016;6(3):e010304.
2. Matsuda H, Nakai A, Adachi T, Tanaka M, Kinoshita K, Terao T. Work environment of obstetricians and gynecologists in Japan. JMAJ. 2010;53(2):91–5.
3. Japan Society of Obstetrics and Gynecology and Japan Association of Obstetricians and Gynecologists. Emergency recommendation for medical reconstruction of obstetrics and gynecology in Japan. 2014 http://www.jsog.or.jp/statement/pdf/kinkyu_teigen_20141213.pdf. Accessed 9 Sept 2017.
4. Matsumoto M, Koike S, Matsubara S, Kashima S, Ide H, Yasunaga H. Selection and concentration of obstetric facilities in Japan: longitudinal study based on national census data. J Obstet Gynaecol Res. 2015;41(6):919–25.
5. Ishikawa M. Nationwide analysis of the travel time from delivery medical institutions to general and regional perinatal medical centers with the use of a geographical information system (analysis of secondary medical districts). J Jpn Assoc Health Care Administrators. 2016;10(1):5–11.

6. Pecci CC, Hines TC, Williams CT, Culpepper L. How we built our team: collaborating with partners to strengthen skills in pregnancy, delivery, and newborn care. J Am Board Fam Med. 2012;25(4):511–21.
7. The College of Family physicians of Canada. Family medicine maternity care: implications for the future. 2009. http://www.cfpc.ca/uploadedFiles/Directories/Committees_List/Family%20Medicine%20Maternity%20Care%20Implications%20for%20the%20Future.pdf. Accessed 9 Sept 2017.
8. Koppula S, Brown JB, Jordan JM. Experiences of family physicians who practice primary care obstetrics in group. J Obstet Gynaecol Can. 2011;33(2):121–6.
9. The Royal Women's Hospital. Guidelines for Shared Maternity Care Affiliates 2015. Mercy Public Hospitals Incorporated and Western Health, Melbourne. 2015. https://www.thewomens.org.au/health-professionals/clinical-resources/shared-maternity-care/shared-care-guidelines#a_downloads. Accessed 9 Sept 2017.
10. the Japan Primary Care Association https://www.primary-care.or.jp/jpca_eng/index.html. Accessed 31 May 2018.
11. Japan Primary Care Association. Training program requirements for family doctors. 2015. http://www.primary-care.or.jp/nintei/pdf/koukikensyusaisoku.pdf. Accessed 9 Sept 2017.
12. Narumoto K. Study on improvement of human resource by collaboration between obstetrician and general clinician. Research report of grant-in-aid by ministry of health, labour and welfare. 2014. http://shusanki.org/reports_page.html?id=67. Accessed 9 Sept 2017.
13. Japan Society of Obstetrics and Gynecology. Grand design 2015 (GD2015) renovation of the obstetrics and gynecology healthcare system in Japan. 2015. http://shusanki.org/theme_page.html?id=282. Accessed 9 Sept 2017.
14. Kinoshita Y. Grounded theory approach no jissen. Tokyo: Koubundou; 2003.
15. The Japanese Society of M-GTA (Modified Grounded Theory Approach). 1999. https://m-gta.jp/en/index.html. Accessed 11 Apr 2018.
16. Minakami H, Maeda T, Fujii T, et al. Guidelines for obstetrical practice in Japan: Japan Society of Obstetrics and Gynecology (JSOG) and Japan Association of Obstetricians and Gynecologists (JAOG) 2014 edition. J Obstet Gynaecol Res. 2014;40(6):1469–99.
17. Japan Association of Obstetricians and Gynecologists. Conference paper: semi-open/open systems. 2012. http://www.jaog.or.jp/sep2012/know/kisyakon/22_090513.pdf. Accessed 9 Sept 2017.
18. Hamasaki T, Hagihara A. A comparison of medical litigation filed against obstetrics and gynecology, internal medicine, and surgery departments. BMC Med Ethics. 2015;16:72.
19. The Japan Council for Quality Health Care. Guide to the Japan obstetric compensation system for cerebral palsy. 2015. http://www.sanka-hp.jcqhc.or.jp/documents/english/pdf/bira_english_color_201501.pdf. Accessed 9 Sept 2017.
20. Yokota M, Tsunawaki S, Narumoto K, Fetters MD. Women's impressions of their inpatient birth care as provided by family physicians in the Shizuoka family medicine training program in Japan. Asia Pac Fam Med. 2013;12(1):1.
21. Brown DR, Cheryl B, Marina K, Lou AL. The phenomenon of collaboration: a Phenomenologic study of collaboration between family medicine and obstetrics and gynecology departments at an Academic Medical Center. Qual Rep. 2014;16(3):657–81.
22. Koike S, Masatoshi M, Ide H, Kashima S, Atarashi H, Yasunaga H. The effect of concentrating obstetrics services in fewer hospitals on patient access: a simulation. Int J Health Geogr. 2016;15:4.

13

Development and validation of the Evidence Based Medicine Questionnaire (EBMQ) to assess doctors' knowledge, practice and barriers regarding the implementation of evidence-based medicine in primary care

Ranita Hisham[1][*], Chirk Jenn Ng[1], Su May Liew[1], Pauline Siew Mei Lai[1], Yook Chin Chia[1,5], Ee Ming Khoo[1], Nik Sherina Hanafi[1], Sajaratulnisah Othman[1], Ping Yein Lee[2], Khatijah Lim Abdullah[3] and Karuthan Chinna[4]

Abstract

Background: Evidence-Based Medicine (EBM) integrates best available evidence from literature and patients' values, which then informs clinical decision making. However, there is a lack of validated instruments to assess the knowledge, practice and barriers of primary care physicians in the implementation of EBM. This study aimed to develop and validate an Evidence-Based Medicine Questionnaire (EBMQ) in Malaysia.

Methods: The EBMQ was developed based on a qualitative study, literature review and an expert panel. Face and content validity was verified by the expert panel and piloted among 10 participants. Primary care physicians with or without EBM training who could understand English were recruited from December 2015 to January 2016. The EBMQ was administered at baseline and two weeks later. A higher score indicates better knowledge, better practice of EBM and less barriers towards the implementation of EBM. We hypothesized that the EBMQ would have three domains: knowledge, practice and barriers.

Results: The final version of the EBMQ consists of 80 items: 62 items were measured on a nominal scale, 22 items were measured on a 5 point Likert-scale. Flesch reading ease was 61.2. A total of 343 participants were approached; of whom 320 agreed to participate (response rate = 93.2%). Factor analysis revealed that the EBMQ had eight domains after 13 items were removed: "EBM websites", "evidence-based journals", "types of studies", "terms related to EBM", "practice", "access", "patient preferences" and "support". Cronbach alpha for the overall EBMQ was 0.909, whilst the Cronbach alpha for the individual domain ranged from 0.657–0.940. The EBMQ was able to discriminate between doctors with and without EBM training for 24 out of 42 items. At test-retest, kappa values ranged from 0.155 to 0.620.

Conclusions: The EBMQ was found to be a valid and reliable instrument to assess the knowledge, practice and barriers towards the implementation of EBM among primary care physicians in Malaysia.

Keywords: Evidence-based medicine, Primary care physicians, Attitudes, Questionnaire

* Correspondence: ranita@um.edu.my
[1]Department of Primary Care Medicine, Faculty of Medicine, University of Malaya, Kuala Lumpur, Malaysia
Full list of author information is available at the end of the article

Background

Evidence-based medicine (EBM) is defined as the integration of best available evidence in a conscientious, explicit and judicious manner from literature and patients' values which then informs clinical decision making [1]. Practicing EBM in clinical practice helps doctors make a proper diagnosis and selects the best treatment available to treat or manage a disease [2]. The use of EBM in clinical setting is thought to provide the best standard of medical care at the lowest cost [3].

Evidence-based medicine has an increasing impact in primary care over recent years [4]. It involves patients in decision making and influences the development of guidelines and quality standards for clinical practice [4]. Primary care physicians are the first person of contact for patients [5]. They have high workload and at the same time they need to uphold the quality of healthcare [6]. Therefore, it is important for them to treat patients based on research evidence, clinical expertise and patient preferences [7]. However, integrating EBM into clinical practice in primary care is challenging as there are variations in team composition, organisational structures, culture and working practices [8].

A search from literature revealed that the international main barriers were lack of time, lack of resources, negative attitudes towards EBM and inadequate EBM skills [9]. A recent qualitative study conducted in 2014 found that the unique barriers in implementing EBM among primary care physicians in Malaysia were lack of awareness and attention toward patient values. Patient values forms a key element of EBM and they still preferred obtaining information from their peers and interestingly, they used WhatsApp—a smart phone messenger [10].

Therefore, we need an instrument to determine the knowledge, practice and barriers of the implementation of EBM among the primary care physicians. It is important to have an instrument to identify the gaps on a larger scale and improve the implementation of EBM in their clinical practice. A systematic review by Shaneyfelt et al. [11] reported that 104 instruments have been developed to evaluate the acquisition of skills by healthcare professionals to practice EBM. These instruments assessed one or more of the following domains on EBM: knowledge, attitude, search strategies, frequency of use of evidence sources, current applications, intended future use and confidence in practice. However, only eight instruments were validated: four instruments assessed the competency in EBM teaching and learning [12–16], whilst four assessed knowledge, attitude and skills [16–19]. However, no instrument has assessed the knowledge, practice and barriers in the implementation of EBM. Therefore, this study aimed to develop and validate the English version of the Evidence-Based Medicine Questionnaire (EBMQ), which was designed to assess knowledge, practice and barriers of primary care physicians regarding the implementation of EBM.

Methods

Development of the evidence-based medicine questionnaire

A literature search was conducted in PubMed; using keywords such as "Evidence-based medicine", "general practioners", "primary care physicians" and "survey/ questionnaire" from this search, nine relevant studies were identified [12–16, 19, 20]. However, only one instrument [20] evaluated the attitude and needs of primary care physicians. Twenty four items from this questionnaire and findings from two previous qualitative studies in rural and urban primary care settings in Malaysia [10, 21] were used to develop the EBMQ (version 1). The EBMQ was developed in English, as English is used in the training of doctors in medical schools and also taught as a second language in all public schools in Malaysia.

Face and content validity of the EBMQ was verified by an expert panel which consisted of nine academicians (a nurse, a pharmacist and seven primary care physicians). Each item was reviewed, and the relevance and appropriateness of each item was discussed (version 2). A pilot test was then conducted on ten medical officers with a minimum of one year working experience wihout any postgraduate qualification. They were asked to evaluate verbally if any items were difficult to understand. Feedback received were that the font was too small and that there was no option for "place of work" for those working in a University hospital. Changes were made based on these comments to produce version 3, which was then pilot tested in another two participants. No difficulties were encountered. Hence, version 3 was used as the final version.

The evidence based medicine questionnaire (EBMQ)

The EBMQ consists of 84 items and 6 sections as shown in Table 1. Only 55 items (33 items in the "knowledge" domain, 9 items in the "practice" domain and 13 items in the "barriers" domain) were measured on a Likert-scale, and could be validated. The final version of the EBMQ is added in Additional file 1. A higher score indicates better knowledge and better practice of EBM and less barriers in practicing EBM.

Participants took 15 to 20 min to complete the EBMQ. We hypothesized that the EBMQ would have 3 domains: knowledge, practice and barriers.

Table 1 The initial version of the Evidence-Based Medicine Questionnaire (version 3)

Section	Description	No. of items	Domain	Type of data	Response options	Response combined for analysis
A	Demographic profile	6	NA	Nominal scale		
B	Frequencies in looking for medical information	20	NA	Nominal scale		
C	Knowledge regarding evidence-based medicine	17	Knowledge regarding information sources	4-point Likert scale[a]	1 = Unaware 2 = Aware but not used in clinical decision making 3 = Have read it but not used in clinical decision making 4 = Read and used in clinical decision making	
		16	Knowledge regarding terms related to EBM	5-point Likert scale[a]	1 = Never heard this term before 2 = Heard of this term but do not understand what this term but would like to 3 = Do not understand this term but would like to 4 = Have some understanding of this term 5 = Understand this term well and able to explain what it means to others	1 = Never heard and do not understand 2 = Do not understand but would like to 3 = Understand
D	Practice of evidence-based medicine	9	Practice	5-point Likert scale[a]	1 = Strongly disagree 2 = Disagree 3 = Neither agree nor disagree 4 = Agree 5 = Strongly agree	1 = Disagree 2 = Neutral 3 = Agree
E	Barriers in practicing evidence-based medicine	13	Barriers	5-point Likert scale[a]	1 = Strongly disagree 2 = Disagree 3 = Neither agree nor disagree 4 = Agree 5 = Strongly agree	1 = Disagree 2 = Neutral 3 = Agree
F	Needs for evidence-based medicine	3	Needs	Nominal scale		
	Total	80				

NA Not applicable
[a]Only items in these domain were tested for construct validity

Validation of the evidence-based medicine questionnaire
Participants
Primary care physicians with or without EBM training, who could understand English and who attended a Diploma in Family Medicine workshop, were recruited from December 2015 to January 2016.

Sample size
Sample size calculation was based on a participant to item ratio of 5:1 to perform factor analysis [22]. There are 55 items in the EBMQ. Hence, the minimum number of participants required was 55*5 = 275.

Procedure
Permission was obtained from the Academy of Family Physicians Malaysia to recruit participants who attended their workshops. For those who agreed, written informed consent was obtained. Participants were then asked to fill in the EBMQ at baseline. Two weeks later, the

EBMQ was mailed to each participant, with a postage-paid return envelope. If a reply was not obtained within a week, participants were contacted via email and/or SMS, and reminded to send in their completed EBMQ form as soon as possible.

Data analysis
Data were analyzed using the Statistical Package for Social Sciences (SPSS) version 22 software (Il, Chicago, USA). Normality could not be assumed, hence non-parametric tests were used. Categorical variables were presented as percentage and frequencies, while continuous variables were presented as median and interquartile range (IQR).

Validity
Flesch reading ease
The readability of the EBMQ was assessed using Flesch reading ease. This was calculated based on the average number of syllables per word and the average number of

words per sentence [23]. An average document should have a score of 60–70 [23].

Exploratory factor analysis

Exploratory factor analysis (EFA) was used to test the underlying structures within the EBMQ. EFA is a type of factor analysis that is utilised to identify the number of latent variables that underlies an entire set of items [24]. EFA was performed to explore the factors appropriateness that can be grouped into specific factors and also to provide information about the validity of each item in each domain. It is important to ensure that the items in each domain of the EBMQ are connected to their basic factors.

Factor loadings were assessed using the Keiser-Meyer-Olkin (KMO) and Bartlett's test of sphericity. The principal components variance with promax variation were used for data reduction purposes, and eigenvalues > 1 was selected to see the variances of the principal components. KMO value of > 0.6, individual factor loadings > 0.5, average variance extracted (AVE) > 0.5 and composite reliability (CR) > 0.7, indicate good structure within the domains [25, 26].

Discriminative validity

To assess discriminative validity, participants were divided into those with or without EBM training. We hypothesized that the knowledge and practice of participants with EBM training would have better knowledge, better practice and less barriers than those without EBM training. The Chi-square test was used to determine if there was any difference between the two groups. A p-value < 0.05 was considered as statistically significant.

Reliability
Internal consistency
Internal consistency was performed to test the consistency of the results and estimates the reliability of the items in the EBMQ. The internal consistency of the EBMQ was assessed using Cronbach's α coefficient. A Cronbach's alpha value of 0.5–0.69 is acceptable, while values of 0.70–0.90 indicate a strong internal consistency [27]. Corrected item-total correlations should be > 0.2 for it to be considered acceptable [28]. If omitting an item increases the Cronbach's α significantly, the item will be excluded.

Test-retest reliability

The test-retest was performed to measure the reliability and stability of the items in the EBMQ over a period of time. It is also important to administer the same test twice to measure the consistency of the answers by the participants. The intra-class correlation coefficient (ICC) was used to assess the total score at test-retest. A ICC agreement value of 0.7 was considered acceptable [29]. ICC values between 0.75 and 1.00 indicate high reliability, 0.60 and 0.74 indicate good reliability, 0.40–0.59 has fair reliability and those below 0.40 indicate low reliability [30].

Results

A total of 343 primary care doctors were approached; of whom 320 agreed to participate (response rate = 93.2%). The majority of them were female (69.4%) with a median age of 32.2 years [IQR = 4.0]. Nearly all (97.2%) were medical officers, working in government health clinics (54.4%) and possessed no postgraduate qualifications after their basic medical degree (78.4%). All participants had heard about EBM, but only 222 (69.7%) had attended an EBM course (Table 2).

Validity

Flesch reading ease of the EBMQ was 61.2. Initially, we hypothesized that the "knowledge" domain would have two factors. However, EFA found that the "knowledge" domain had four factors: ("evidence-based medicine websites", "evidence-based journals", "type of studies" and "terms related to EBM") after 9 items (item C1: "Clinical Practice Guidelines", item C7: "Dynamed", item C11: "InfoPoems", item C4: "Cochrane", item C8: "TRIP database", item C15: "BestBETs", item C9: "MEDLINE", item C17: "Medscape" and item C16: "UpToDate") were removed. This model explained 54.3% of the variation (Table 3).

EFA found that the "practice" domain had only one factor with eight items after one item (item 9: "I prefer to manage patients based on my experience") was removed. This model explained 49.0% of the variation (Table 3).

We hypothesized that the 'barriers' domain would only have one factor. However, EFA revealed that the 'barriers' domain has three factors ("access", "support" and "patient's preferences") after three items were removed (item 7: "I can consult the specialist anytime to answer my queries", item 10: "I have the authority to change the management of patients in my clinic" and item 11: "There are incentives for me to practice EBM"). This model explained 49.9% of the variation (Table 3).

Discriminative validity

In the "knowledge" domain, doctors who had EBM training had significant higher scores in 13 out of 24 items compared to those without training. In the "practice" domain, doctors who had EBM training had significant higher scores in 5 out 8 items compared to those without training. In the "barriers" domain, doctors who had EBM training had significant higher scores in 5 out of 10 items compared to those without training (Table 4).

Table 2 Demographic characteristics of participants

	n (%)
Median age [IQR]	32.2 [4.0]
Female	222 (69.4)
Male	98 (30.6)
No. of participants with postgraduate qualifications	
None	251 (78.4)
Diploma	58 (18.1)
Masters	11 (3.4)
Current designation	
Medical Officer	311 (97.2)
Family Medicine Specialist	9 (2.8)
Current Work Place	
Government health clinics	174 (54.4)
Private clinic	81 (25.3)
Government hospital	42 (13.1)
Others[a]	13 (4.1)
Private hospital	5 (1.6)
University hospital	5 (1.6)
Have heard of the term "evidence-based medicine"	319 (99.7)
Have attended EBM courses	222 (69.7)
Have received formal trainings in literature search	156 (48.8)
Have received formal trainings in questions formulation	121 (37.8)
Have received formal trainings in critical appraisal	111 (34.7)
Have conducted research after graduating from medical school	111 (34.7)
Have published any article in a journal	36 (11.3)

IQR Interquartile range
[a]Others: Military health clinic (n = 6), Private Polyclinic(n = 1), Private University(n = 1), Traditional & Complimentary Medicine Division(n = 1), University Health Clinic(n = 4)

Reliability
Cronbach alpha for the overall EBMQ was 0.909, whilst individual domains ranged from 0.657 to 0.933 (Table 4). All corrected item-total correlation (CITC) values were > 0.2. At retest, 185 participants completed the EBMQ (response rate = 57.85%), as n = 23 (42%) were uncontactable. Thirty items had good and fair correlations (r = 0.418–0.620) while 12 items had low correlations (r = < 0.4). (Table 5).

Discussion
The EBMQ was found to be a valid and reliable instrument to assess the knowledge, practice and barriers of primary care physicians regarding the implementation of EBM. The final EBMQ consists of 42 items with 8

domains after 13 items were removed. The Flesch reading ease was 61.2. This indicates that the EBMQ can be easily understood by 13–15 years old students who study English as a first language [23].

Initially, we hypothesized that there were two factors in the "knowledge" domain: "sources related to EBM" and "terms related to EBM". However, EFA revealed that the EBMQ had four factors: "evidence-based medicine websites", "evidence-based journals", "terms related to EBM" and "type of studies" after 9 items were removed. This was because "sources related to EBM" was further divided into another three factors. It is not surprising because knowledge is a broad concept that can be further recategorized. EFA revealed that the "practice" domain had one factor which concurred with our initial hypothesis. One item (item P9: "I prefer to manage patients based on my experience") was removed as this was regarding doctors'experience rather than their practice. Initially, we hypothesized that there was one factor in the "barriers" domain. However, EFA revealed that there were three factors: 'access to resources', 'patient preferences towards EBM' and 'support from the management' after three items were removed. This may be because instead of one barrier, EFA had re-grouped into three factors that provided a better description of barriers encountered by the primary care physicians. As highlighted in literature [9, 31], there are many barriers to practice EBM and some of it were also categorized according the specific and types of barriers.

The EBMQ was able to discriminate the knowledge, practice and barriers between doctors with and without EBM training. In the knowledge domain, there were significant differences for all items in the "terms related to EBM". This is not surprising as doctors with EBM training would have been exposed to these terms. No differences was found between those with and without EBM training in "information sources related to EBM" as those who did not attend EBM training could still access online information resources. Several studies were found to improve knowledge but did not report in detail which areas on knowledge. Hence, we could not compare their findings to our studies [32–35].

Our findings also showed that doctors with EBM training had better practice of EBM. This differed from several studies which reported changes in practice [32, 36–39] and some reported no changes in practice [35, 40]. However, the authors commented that these findings were not meaningful as it was self-perceived. Other than that, in our findings, doctors who attended EBM training had less barriers regarding the implementation of EBM in their clinical practice. They seemed to have better access to

Table 3 Exploratory factor analysis of the evidence-based medicine questionnaire

Original domains	After EFA was performed	Item No.	Item	Factor 1	Factor 2	Factor 3	KMO	AVE (%)	Bartlett's test	CR
Knowledge	Evidence-based medicine websites (n = 6)	C6	Centre of Evidence-Based Medicine (CEBM)	0.605	–	–	0.834	43.0	< 0.001	0.662
		C10	ACP Journal Club	0.583	–	–				
		C5	Database of abstracts of reviews of effectiveness (DARE)	0.550	–	–				
		C13	InfoClinics	0.545	–	–				
		C2	Bandolier (published in Oxford)	0.495	–	–				
		C14	Centre of Reviews & Dissertation	0.477	–	–				
	Evidence-based journals (n = 2)	C12	BMJ Clinical Evidence	–	0.665	–	0.500	48.9	< 0.001	0.609
		C3	Evidence-Based Medicine (from BMJ publishing group)	–	0.658	–				
	Type of studies (n = 4)	K3	Case-control study	0.654	–	–	0.692	49.7	< 0.001	0.685
		K4	Randomized controlled trial	0.632	–	–				
		K1	Systematic review	0.622	–	–				
		K2	Meta-analysis	0.459	–	–				
	Terms related to EBM (n = 12)	K13	Publication bias	–	0.956	–	0.896	52.0	< 0.001	0.884
		K11	Confidence interval	–	0.817	–				
		K12	Heterogeneity	–	0.745	–				
		K16	Clinical effectiveness	–	0.642	–				
		K7	Odds ratio	–	0.607	–				
		K8	P-value	–	0.589	–				
		K15	Positive predictive value	–	0.569	–				
		K14	Test sensitivity and specificity	–	0.553	–				
		K10	Number needed to treat	–	0.531	–				
		K9	Level of evidence	–	0.524	–				
		K6	Absolute risk	–	0.436	–				
		K5	Relative risk	–	0.416	–				
Practice (n = 9)	Practice (n = 8)	P4	EBM improves my patient care	0.829	–	–	0.892	49.0	< 0.001	0.882
		P7	EBM guides my clinical decision making	0.817	–	–				
		P8	I prefer to manage patients based on EBM	0.759	–	–				
		P3	Reading research papers is important to me	0.739	–	–				
		P6		0.727	–	–				

Latest Findings in Family Medicine

128

Table 3 Exploratory factor analysis of the evidence-based medicine questionnaire (*Continued*)

Original domains	After EFA was performed	Item No.	Item	Factor 1	Factor 2	Factor 3	KMO	AVE (%)	Bartlett's test	CR
			I can implement EBM in my clinical practice							
		P2	I trust the findings from research studies	0.662	–	–				
		P5	EBM reduces my workload	0.521	–	–				
		P1	I support EBM	0.456	–	–				
Barriers (n = 13)	Access (n = 6)	B4	I have time to practise EBM in my clinic	0.686	–	–	0.818	36.8	<0.001	0.774
		B5	My clinic facilities are adequate to support the practice of EBM	0.675	–	–				
		B3	I have time to read research papers	0.633	–	–				
		B6	Research articles are easily available to me	0.632	–	–				
		B1	I am able to assess the quality of research.	0.543	–	–				
		B2	I have access to internet to practice EBM	0.435	–	–				
	Patient preferences (n = 2)	B8	My patients prefers me to practise EBM	–	0.754	–	0.500	56.8	<0.001	0.725
		B9	My patient believes in information that is based on evidence	–	0.754	–				
	Support (n = 2)	B12	My colleagues support the practice of EBM	–	–	0.786	0.500	61.7	<0.001	0.764
		B13	My organization supports the practice of EBM	–	–	0.786				

EBM Evidence-based medicine, *EFA* Exploratory Factor Analysis, *KMO* Keiser-Meyer-Olkin, *AVE* Average Variance Extracted, *CR* Composite Reliability

Table 4 The discriminative validity of the Evidence-Based Medicine Questionnaire

Knowledge Domain (Information sources related to EBM)

Item	Details of item	With EBM training (n = 222) n(%)				Without EBM training (n = 98) n(%)				Chi-square	p-value
		Unaware	Aware but not used in clinical decision making	Have read it but not used in clinical decision making	Read and used in clinical decision making	Unaware	Aware but not used in clinical decision making	Have read it but not used in clinical decision making	Read and used in clinical decision making		
C2	Bandolier	154(69.4)	35(15.8)	19(8.6)	14(6.3)	66(67.3)	13(13.3)	12(12.2)	7(7.1)	1.350	0.717
C5	DARE	155(69.8)	42(18.9)	16(7.2)	9(4.1)	71(72.4)	15(15.3)	12(12.2)	–	6.510	0.089
C6	CEBM	123(56.3)	69(31.1)	17(7.7)	11(5.0)	58(59.2)	22(22.4)	14(14.3)	4(4.1)	5.074	0.166
C10	ACP	147(66.2)	38(17.1)	24(10.8)	13(5.9)	63(64.3)	16(16.3)	14(14.3)	5(5.1)	0.825	0.844
C13	InfoClinics	152(68.5)	44(19.8)	18(8.1)	8(3.6)	63(64.3)	16(16.3)	10(10.2)	9(9.2)	4.946	0.176
C14	CRD	175(78.8)	31(14.0)	15(6.8)	1(0.5)	75(76.5)	12(12.2)	9(9.2)	2(2.0)	2.564	0.464
C3	EBM	10(4.5)	46(20.7)	66(29.7)	100(45.0)	4(4.1)	28(28.6)	24(24.5)	42(42.9)	2.577	0.462
C12	BMJ	26(11.7)	43(19.4)	73(32.9)	80(36.0)	10(10.2)	25(25.5)	22(22.4)	41(41.8)	4.442	0.218

Knowledge Domain (Terms related to EBM)

Item	Details of item	With EBM training (n = 222) n(%)			Without EBM training (n = 98) n(%)			Chi-square	p-value
		Never heard and do not understand	Do not understand but would like to	Understand	Never heard and do not understand	Do not understand but would like to	Understand		
K1	Systematic review	6(2.7)	12(5.4)	204(91.9)	8(8.2)	8(8.2)	82(83.7)	5.975	0.050
K2	Meta-analysis	10(4.5)	14(6.3)	198(89.2)	6(6.1)	14(14.3)	78(79.6)	16.837	≤ 0.001*
K3	Case-control study	4(1.8)	8(3.6)	210(94.6)	5(5.1)	3(3.1)	90(91.8)	2.746	0.253
K4	Randomized controlled trial	4(1.8)	7(3.2)	211(95.0)	4(4.1)	1(1.0)	93(94.9)	2.651	0.266
K5	Relative risk	8(3.6)	25(11.3)	189(85.1)	9(9.2)	16(16.3)	73(74.5)	6.287	0.043*
K6	Absolute risk	8(3.6)	33(14.9)	181(81.5)	10(10.2)	15(15.3)	73(74.5)	5.699	0.058*
K7	Odds ratio	11(5.0)	60(27.0)	151(68.0)	14(14.3)	26(26.5)	58(59.2)	8.395	0.015*
K8	P-value	11(5.0)	38(17.1)	173(77.9)	14(14.3)	19(19.4)	65(66.3)	9.004	0.011*
K9	Level of evidence	7(3.2)	30(13.5)	185(83.3)	9(9.2)	19(19.4)	70(71.4)	7.686	0.021*
K10	Number needed to treat	11(5.0)	41(18.5)	170(76.6)	11(11.2)	20(20.4)	67(68.4)	4.640	0.098*
K11	Confidence interval	17(7.7)	61(27.5)	144(64.9)	21(21.4)	25(25.5)	52(53.1)	12.502	0.002*
K12	Heterogeneity	21(9.5)	74(33.3)	127(57.2)	22(22.4)	35(35.7)	41(41.8)	11.709	0.003*
K13	Publication bias	23(10.4)	65(29.3)	134(60.4)	23(23.5)	30(30.6)	45(45.9)	10.703	0.005*
K14	Test sensitivity and specificity	4(1.8)	25(11.3)	193(86.9)	11(11.2)	13(13.3)	74(75.5)	14.172	≤ 0.001*
K15	Positive predictive value	5(2.3)	36(16.2)	181(81.5)	5(5.1)	36(36.7)	57(58.2)	7.415	0.025*
K16	Clinical effectiveness	10(4.5)	48(21.6)	164(73.9)	16(16.3)	19(19.4)	63(64.3)	12.738	0.002*

Table 4 The discriminative validity of the Evidence-Based Medicine Questionnaire (*Continued*)

		Disagree	Neutral	Agree	Disagree	Neutral	Agree		
Practice Domain									
P1	I support EBM	1(0.5)	8(3.6)	213(95.9)	2(2.0)	6(6.1)	90(91.8)	2.941	0.230
P2	I trust the findings from research studies	1(0.5)	37(16.7)	184(82.9)	3(3.1)	13(13.3)	82(83.7)	4.216	0.121
P3	Reading research papers is important to me	-	25(11.3)	197(88.7)	4(4.1)	20(20.4)	74(75.5)	14.511	0.001*
P4	EBM improves my patient care	-	19(8.6)	203(91.4)	3(3.1)	8(8.2)	87(88.8)	6.862	0.032*
P5	EBM reduces my workload	22(9.9)	87(39.1)	113(50.9)	21(9.4)	39(17.5)	38(17.1)	8.838	0.012*
P6	I can implement EBM in my clinical practice	2(0.9)	23(10.3)	197(88.7)	3(1.3)	16(7.2)	79(35.5)	4.537	0.103
P7	EBM guides my clinical decision making	-	11(5.0)	211(95.0)	3(3.1)	9(9.2)	86(87.8)	9.130	0.010*
P8	I prefer to manage patients based on EBM	2(0.9)	36(16.2)	184(82.9)	3(3.1)	25(25.5)	70(71.4)	6.235	0.044*
Barriers Domain									
B1	I am able to assess the quality of research.	35(15.8)	76(34.2)	111(50.0)	17(17.3)	40(40.8)	41(41.8)	1.871	0.392
B2	I have access to internet to practise EBM	4(1.8)	18(8.1)	200(90.1)	11(11.2)	12(12.2)	75(76.5)	15.573	<0.001*
B3	I have time to read research papers	25(11.3)	93(41.9)	104(46.8)	22(22.4)	39(39.8)	37(37.8)	7.142	0.028*
B4	I have time to practise EBM in my clinic	18(8.1)	60(27.0)	144(64.9)	144(64.9)	17(17.3)	32(32.7)	8.545	0.014*
B5	My clinic facilities are adequate to support the practice of EBM	47(20.2)	85(38.2)	90(40.5)	34(15.3)	34(15.3)	120(54.0)	6.935	0.031*
B6	Research articles are easily available to me	50(22.5)	71(32.0)	101(45.5)	40(40.8)	29(29.6)	29(29.6)	12.447	0.002*
B8	My patients prefers me to practise EBM	28(12.6)	138(62.2)	56(25.2)	15(15.3)	59(60.2)	24(24.5)	0.424	0.809
B9	My patient believes in information that is based on evidence	35(15.8)	95(42.8)	92(41.4)	11(11.2)	47(48.0)	40(40.8)	1.391	0.499
B12	My colleagues support the practice of EBM	13(5.9)	84(37.8)	125(56.3)	12(12.2)	36(36.7)	50(51.0)	3.922	1.141
B13	My organization supports the practice of EBM	12(5.4)	72(32.4)	138(62.2)	8(8.2)	33(33.7)	57(58.2)	1.038	0.595

EBM Evidence-based medicine
*$p \leq 0.05$ is significant

Table 5 The psychometric properties of the Evidence-Based Medicine Questionnaire

No.	Items	Test-Retest Reliability						
		Corrected Item-total Correlation	Cronbach's alpha if items is deleted	Test (n = 320)		Retest (n = 184)		ICC
				Mean (SD)	Median	Mean (SD)	Median	
Knowledge Domain								
C2	Bandolier (Published in Oxford)	0.487	0.811	1.31 (0.650)	1.00	1.68 (1.003)	1.00	0.567
C5	Database of abstracts of reviews of effectiveness(DARE)	0.630	0.778	1.54 (0.916)	1.00	1.67 (0.922)	1.00	0.485
C6	Centre of Evidence-Based Medicine (CEBM)	0.630	0.777	1.44 (0.769)	1.00	1.76 (0.937)	1.00	0.453
C10	ACP Journal Club	0.570	0.791	1.62 (0.844)	1.00	1.55 (0.886)	1.00	0.333
C13	InfoClinics	0.566	0.791	1.58 (0.907)	1.00	1.63 (0.913)	1.00	0.418
C14	Centre of Reviews & Dissertation (CRD)	0.650	0.780	1.52 (0.863)	1.00	1.48 (0.815)	1.00	0.396
C3	Evidence-based medicine (EBM)	0.492	–	1.52 (0.863)	3.00	3.21 (0.881)	3.00	0.416
C12	BMJ Clinical Evidence	0.492	–	3.23 (0.868)	3.00	2.90 (0.997)	3.00	0.379
K1	Systematic review	0.774	0.866	4.19 (0.775)	4.00	4.23(0.814)	4.00	0.421
K2	Meta-analysis	0.718	0.887	2.79(0.516)	3.00	4.10(0.793)	4.00	0.463
K3	Case-control study	0.826	0.848	2.91(0.373)	3.00	4.28(0.681)	4.00	0.497
K4	Randomized controlled trial	0.777	0.866	2.93(0.346)	3.00	4.37(0.686)	4.00	0.522
K5	Relative risk	0.747	0.927	2.77(0.535)	3.00	4.04(0.741)	3.00	0.450
K6	Absolute risk	0.763	0.926	2.74(0.554)	3.00	4.01(0.775)	4.00	0.561
K7	Odds ratio	0.742	0.926	2.58(0.634)	3.00	3.82(0.822)	4.00	0.506
K8	P-value	0.713	0.927	2.67(0.616)	3.00	4.00(0.803)	4.00	0.487
K9	Level of evidence	0.721	0.927	2.75(0.538)	3.00	4.06(0.846)	4.00	0.359
K10	Number needed to treat	0.676	0.929	2.67(0.599)	3.00	3.95(0.943)	4.00	0.528
K11	Confidence interval	0.757	0.926	2.49(0.699)	3.00	3.78(0.882)	4.00	0.529
K12	Heterogeneity	0.663	0.930	2.39(0.713)	3.00	3.54(0.950)	4.00	0.483
K13	Publication bias	0.686	0.929	2.42(0.729)	3.00	3.58(0.997)	4.00	0.580
K14	Test sensitivity and specificity	0.697	0.928	2.79(0.512)	3.00	4.24(0.734)	4.00	0.504
K15	Positive predictive value	0.707	0.928	2.74(0.522)	3.00	4.06(0.861)	4.00	0.503
K16	Clinical effectiveness	0.667	0.929	2.63(0.630)	3.00	2.89(0.938)	4.00	0.570
Practice Domain								
P1	I support EBM	0.417	0.875	2.94 (0.279)	3.00	4.43 (0.648)	4.00	0.605
P2	I trust the findings from research studies	0.618	0.854	4.02 (0.683)	4.00	4.09 (0.611)	4.00	0.323
P3	Reading research papers is important to me	0.684	0.846	4.06 (0.687)	4.00	4.06 (0.679)	4.00	0.477
P4	EBM improves my patient care	0.765	0.838	4.18 (0.642)	4.00	4.27 (0.626)	4.00	0.301
P5	EBM reduces my workload	0.499	0.877	3.44 (0.898)	3.00	3.43 (0.830)	3.00	0.532
P6	I can implement EBM in my clinical practice	0.682	0.846	4.04 (0.661)	4.00	3.90 (0.743)	4.00	0.532
P7	EBM guides my clinical decision making	0.748	0.841	4.18 (0.607)	4.00	4.10 (0.600)	4.00	0.344
P8	I prefer to manage patients based on EBM	0.699	0.844	4.01 (0.713)	4.00	4.02 (0.689)	4.00	0.422

Table 5 The psychometric properties of the Evidence-Based Medicine Questionnaire *(Continued)*

No.	Items	Test-Retest Reliability						
		Corrected Item-total Correlation	Cronbach's alpha if items is deleted	Test (n = 320)		Retest (n = 184)		ICC
				Mean (SD)	Median	Mean (SD)	Median	
Barrier Domain								
B1	I am able to assess the quality of research.	0.472	0.747	2.31 (0.736)	2.00	3.34 (0.808)	3.00	0.475
B2	I have access to internet to practice EBM	0.386	0.767	2.81 (0.497)	3.00	3.83 (0.874)	4.00	0.388
B3	I have time to read research papers	0.546	0.728	3.32 (0.803)	3.00	3.29 (0.795)	3.00	0.494
B4	I have time to practise EBM in my clinic	0.583	0.718	3.55 (0.810)	4.00	3.45 (0.774)	4.00	0.356
B5	My clinic facilities are adequate to support the practice of EBM	0.583	0.718	3.13 (0.894)	3.00	3.30 (2.367)	3.00	0.142
B6	Research articles are easily available to me	0.547	0.731	3.16 (0.982)	3.00	3.06 (0.942)	3.00	0.275
B8	My patients prefers me to practise EBM	0.569	–	3.14 (0.798)	3.00	3.24 (0.690)	3.00	0.323
B9	My patient believes in information that is based on evidence	0.569	–	3.29 (0.853)	3.00	3.41 (0.717)	3.00	0.547
B12	My colleagues support the practice of EBM	0.618	–	3.53 (0.795)	4.00	3.53 (0.752)	4.00	0.620
B13	My organization supports the practice of EBM	0.618	–	3.63 (0.756)	4.00	3.53 (0.771)	4.00	0.471

ICC Intraclass correlation
*Statistically significant at *p* < 0.05

resources, more patients had a positive attitude towards EBM, and better support from management to practice EBM compared to those without EBM training. This could be because doctors with EBM training knew how to overcome problems that would prevent them from practicing EBM. In the systematic review [41], the barriers in the implementation of EBM remains unclear as it was not reported.

The overall Cronbach's alpha as well as the individual domains were > 0.7. This indicates that the EBMQ has adequate psychometric properties, which was similar to previous studies [12, 14–16, 19, 42]. The majority (71.4%) of the items in EBMQ had good and fair correlation at test-retest, which indicates that the EBMQ has achieved adequate reliability. The reliability testing two weeks later did not affect the methodology as the acceptable time interval for test-retest reliability is approximately 2 weeks [28]. The discriminative validity was performed using the baseline data and not after retest which then impact on the methodology.

To our knowledge, this was the first validation study assessed the discriminative validity (i.e. between doctors with and without EBM training) that assessed

their implementation of EBM. One of the limitations of this study was that participants were recruited whilst attending a Family Medicine module workshop. This may mean that participants that were recruited may be more interested in the practice of EBM as they are already interested in furthering their postgraduate studies. This cohort are likely to be more interested with the practice of EBM as they are more incline to further their studies rather than the normal general practitioners. Hence, our result may not be generalizable.

Conclusions

The EBMQ was found to be a valid and reliable instrument to assess the knowledge, practice and barriers of primary care physicians towards EBM in Malaysia. The EBMQ can be used to assess doctors' practices and barriers in the implementation of EBM. Information gathered from the administration of the EBMQ will assist policy makers to identify the level of knowledge, practice and barriers of EBM and to improve its uptake in clinical practice. Although the findings of this study are not generalizable, they may be of interest to primary care physicians in other countries.

Abbreviations
AVE: Average variance extracted; CITC: Corrected item-total correlation; CR: Composite reliability; EBM: Evidence-based medicine; EBMQ: Evidence-based medicine questionnaire; EFA: Exploratory factor analysis; ICC: Intra-correlation coefficient; IQR: Interquartile range; KMO: Kaiser-Meyer-Oklin; SPSS: Statistical Package for Social Sciences

Acknowledgements
We would like to thank the participants of this study.

Funding
This study was funded by University of Malaya Research Grant (RP037A-15HTM).

Authors' contributions
NCJ and LSM conceived the study and CYC, KEM, NSH, SO, LPY, KLA participated in its design and coordination. RH, NCJ, LSM and LSMP contributed to data analysis and interpretation. KC provided statistical advice, data analysis and interpretation. RH drafted the manuscript and all the authors critically revised it and approved the final manuscript.

Competing interests
The authors declare that they have no competing interests.

Author details
[1]Department of Primary Care Medicine, Faculty of Medicine, University of Malaya, Kuala Lumpur, Malaysia. [2]Department of Family Medicine, Faculty of Medicine and Health Sciences, Universiti Putra Malaysia, UPM Serdang, Selangor, Malaysia. [3]Department of Nursing Sciences, Faculty of Medicine, University of Malaya, Kuala Lumpur, Malaysia. [4]Department of Social and Preventive Medicine, Julius Centre University of Malaya, University of Malaya, Kuala Lumpur, Malaysia. [5]Department of Medical Sciences School of Healthcare and Medical Sciences Sunway University, Selangor, Malaysia.

References
1. Sackett DL, Rosenberg WMC, Gray JAM, Haynes RB, Richardson WS. Evidence based medicine: what it is and what it isn't. BMJ. 1996;312:71–2.
2. Saarni SI, Gylling HA. Evidence based medicine guidelines: a solution to rationing or politics disguised as science? J Med Ethics. 2004;30:171–5.
3. Lewis SJ, Orland BI. The importance and impact of evidence-based medicine. J Manag Care Pharm. 2004;10:S3–5.
4. Slowther A, Ford S, Schofield T. Ethics of evidence based medicine in the primary care setting. J Med Ethics. 2004;30:151–5.
5. Kumar R. Empowering primary care physicians in India. J Fam Med Prim Care. 2012;1:1–2.
6. Mohr DC, Benzer JK, Young GJJD. Provider workload and quality of care in primary care settings: moderating role of relational climate. Med Care. 2013;51:108–14.
7. Tracy CS, Dantas GC, Upshur REG. Evidence-based medicine in primary care: qualitative study of family physicians. BMC Fam Prac. 2003;4:6–6.
8. Craig P, Dieppe P, Macintyre S, Michie S, Nazareth I, Petticrew M. Developing and evaluating complex interventions: the new Medical Research Council guidance. BMJ. 2008;337:a1655.
9. Sadeghi-Bazargani H, Tabrizi JS, Azami-Aghdash S. Barriers to evidence-based medicine: a systematic review. J Eval Clin Pract. 2014;20:793–802.
10. Hisham R, Liew SM, Ng CJ, Mohd Nor K, Osman IF, Ho GJ, Hamzah N, Glasziou P. Rural doctors' views on and experiences with evidence-based medicine: the FrEEDoM qualitative study. PLoS One. 2016;11:e0152649.
11. Shaneyfelt T, Baum KD, Bell D, Feldstein D, Houston TK, Kaatz S, Whelan C, Green M. Instruments for evaluating education in evidence-based practice: a systematic review. JAMA. 2006;296:1116–27.
12. Ruzafa-Martinez M, Lopez-Iborra L, Moreno-Casbas T, Madrigal-Torres M. Development and validation of the competence in evidence based practice questionnaire (EBP-COQ) among nursing students. BMC Med Educ. 2013;13:19.
13. Adams S, Barron S. Development and testing of an evidence-based practice questionnaire for school nurses. J Nurs Meas. 2010;18:3–25.
14. Johnston JM, Leung GM, Fielding R, Tin KY, Ho LM. The development and validation of a knowledge, attitude and behaviour questionnaire to assess undergraduate evidence-based practice teaching and learning. Med Educ. 2003;37:992–1000.
15. Fritsche L, Greenhalgh T, Falck-Ytter Y, Neumayer H, Kunz R. Do short courses in evidence based medicine improve knowledge and skills? Validation of berlin questionnaire and before and after study of courses in evidence based medicine. BMJ. 2002;325:1338–41.
16. Ramos KD, Schafer S, Tracz SM. Validation of the Fresno test of competence in evidence based medicine. BMJ. 2003;326:319–21.
17. Rice KHJ, Abrefa-Gyan T, Powell K. Evidence-based practice questionnaire: a confirmatory factor analysis in a social work sample. Adv Soc Work. 2010;11:158–73.
18. Iovu MB, Runcan P. Evidence-based practice: knowledge, attitudes, and beliefs of social workers in Romania. Revista de Cercetare si Interventie Sociala. 2012;38:54–70.
19. Upton D, Upton P. Development of an evidence-based practice questionnaire for nurses. J Adv Nurs. 2006;53:454–8.
20. McColl A, Smith H, White P, Field J. General practitioners' perceptions of the route to evidence based medicine: a questionnaire survey. BMJ. 1998;316:361–5.
21. Blenkinsopp A, Paxton P. Symptoms in the pharmacy: a guide to the management of common illness. 3rd ed. Oxford. Blackwell Science; 1998.
22. Gorsuch RL. Factor analysis. 2nd ed. Lawarence Erlbaum Associates: Hillsdale; 1983.
23. Flesch R. A new readability yardstick. J Appl Psychol. 1948;32:221–33.
24. van der Eijk C, Rose J. Risky business: factor analysis of survey data – assessing the probability of incorrect dimensionalisation. PLoS One. 2015;10:e0118900.
25. Kaiser HF. A second generation little jiffy. Psychometrika. 1970;35:401–15.
26. Hidalgo B, Goodman M. Multivariate or multivariable regression? Am J Pub Health. 2013;103:39–40.
27. Cronbach LJ. Coefficient alpha and the internal structure of tests. Psychometrika. 1951;16:297–334.
28. Streiner DN. G. Health measurement scales: a practical guide to their development and use. 2nd ed. Oxford: Oxford University Press; 1995.
29. Terwee CB, Bot SD, de Boer MR, van der Windt DA, Knol DL, Dekker J, Bouter LM, de Vet HC. Quality criteria were proposed for measurement properties of health status questionnaires. J Clin Epidemiol. 2007;60:34–42.
30. Cicchetti DV. Guidelines, criteria, and rules of thumb for evaluating normed and standardized assessment instruments in psychology. Psychol Assess. 1994;6:284–90.
31. Zwolsman S, te Pas E, Hooft L, Wieringa-de Waard M, van Dijk N. Barriers to GPs' use of evidence-based medicine: a systematic review. Br J Gen Pract. 2012;62:e511–21.
32. Dizon JM, Grimmer-Somers K, Kumar S. Effectiveness of the tailored evidence based practice training program for Filipino physical therapists: a randomized controlled trial. BMC Med Educ. 2014;14:147.
33. Chen FC, Lin MC. Effects of a nursing literature reading course on promoting critical thinking in two-year nursing program students. J Nurs Res. 2003; 11:137–47.
34. Bennett S, Hoffmann T, Arkins M. A multi-professional evidence-based practice course improved allied health students' confidence and knowledge. J Eval Clin Pract. 2011;17:635–9.
35. McCluskey A, Lovarini M. Providing education on evidence-based practice improved knowledge but did not change behaviour: a before and after study. BMC Med Educ. 2005;5:40.
36. Levin RF, Fineout-Overholt E, Melnyk BM, Barnes M, Vetter MJ. Fostering evidence-based practice to improve nurse and cost outcomes in a

community health setting: a pilot test of the advancing research and clinical practice through close collaboration model. Nurs Adm Q. 2011; 35:21–33.

37. Stevenson K, Lewis M, Hay E. Do physiotherapists' attitudes towards evidence-based practice change as a result of an evidence-based educational programme? J Eval Clin Pract. 2004;10:207–17.

38. Kim SC, Brown CE, Ecoff L, Davidson JE, Gallo AM, Klimpel K, Wickline MA. Regional evidence-based practice fellowship program: impact on evidence-based practice implementation and barriers. Clin Nurs Res. 2013;22:51–69.

39. Lizarondo LM, Grimmer-Somers K, Kumar S, Crockett A. Does journal club membership improve research evidence uptake in different allied health disciplines: a pre-post study. BMC Res Notes. 2012;5:588.

40. Yost J, Ciliska D, Dobbins M. Evaluating the impact of an intensive education workshop on evidence-informed decision making knowledge, skills, and behaviours: a mixed methods study. BMC Med Educ. 2014;14:13.

41. Hecht L, Buhse S, Meyer G. Effectiveness of training in evidence-based medicine skills for healthcare professionals: a systematic review. BMC Med Educ. 2016;16:103.

42. Rice K, Hwang J, Abrefa-Gyan T, Powell K. Evidence-based practice questionnaire: a confirmatory factor analysis in a social work sample. Adv Soc Sci. 2010;11:158–73.

14

Preliminary effects of a regional approached multidisciplinary educational program on healthcare utilization in patients with hip or knee osteoarthritis

Aniek A. O. M. Claassen[1*] (iD), Henk J. Schers[2], Sander Koëter[3], Willemijn H. van der Laan[1],
Keetie C. A. L. C. Kremers-van de Hei[3], Joris Botman[4], Vincent J. J. F. Busch[5], Wim H. C. Rijnen[6]
and Cornelia H. M. van den Ende[1,7]

Abstract

Background: Providing relevant information on disease and self-management helps patients to seek timely contact with care providers and become actively involved in their own care process. Therefore, health professionals from primary care, multiple hospitals and health organisations jointly decided to develop an educational program on osteoarthritis (OA). The objective of the present study was to determine preliminary effects of this OA educational program on healthcare utilization and clinical outcomes.

Methods: We developed an educational group-based program consisting of 2 meetings of 1.5 h, provided by a physiotherapist, a general practitioner (GP) and orthopaedic surgeon or specialized nurse. The program included education on OA, (expectations regarding) treatment options and self-management. Patients were recruited through searching the GPs' electronic patients records and advertisements in local newspapers. At baseline and at 3 months follow-up participating OA patients completed questionnaires. Paired-sample t-tests, McNemar's test and Wilcoxon Signed-Rank test were used to estimate the preliminary effects of the program.

Results: A total of 146 participants in 3 districts attended the sessions, of whom 143 agreed to participate in this study; mean age 69.1 years (SD10.2).107 (75%) participants completed both baseline and follow up assessments. The proportion of participants who had visited their GP in the 3 months after the program was lower than 3 months previous to the program (40% versus 25%, *p*-value 0.01). Also, we observed a decrease in proportion of patients who visited the physio- and exercise therapist, (36.1% versus 25.0%, *p*-value 0.02). Both illness perceptions and knowledge on OA and treatment options changed positively (Δ-1.8, 95%CI:0.4–3.4, and Δ2.4, 95%CI:-3.0 - -1.6 respectively). No changes in BMI, pain, functioning and self-efficacy were found. However, a trend towards an increase in physical activity was observed.

Conclusions: Our results show that a multidisciplinary educational program may result in a decrease in healthcare utilization and has a positive effect on illness perceptions and knowledge on OA due to clear and consistent information on OA and it treatment options.

Keywords: Patient education, Hip, Knee, Osteoarthritis, Self-management, Consistent information, Multidisciplinary

* Correspondence: a.claassen@maartenskliniek.nl
[1]Department of Rheumatology, Sint Maartenskliniek, PO Box 9011, 6500, GM,
Nijmegen, The Netherlands
Full list of author information is available at the end of the article

Background

Osteoarthritis (OA) is the most prevalent form of disability of posture and movement worldwide [1]. OA of the hip and knee is characterised by pain and stiffness which can impair daily functioning, and decrease physical activity [2]. This physical and accompanying mental burden influences the quality of life in patients with OA. Although there are no curative treatment options for OA, multiple effective non-surgical and surgical treatment options for reducing pain and improving movement ability and quality of life are available [2, 3].

International guidelines recommend a combination of pharmacological and non-pharmacologic modalities as primary approach for hip or knee OA [2–4]. Non-pharmacological treatment modalities include psycho-educational interventions to improve self-management, physical activity and exercise therapy, and weight reduction. Recommended pharmacological treatment consists of the use of acetaminophen (paracetamol), the use of non-steroidal anti-inflammatory drugs (NSAIDs) or, when the patient is not responding satisfactorily to oral analgesic/anti-inflammatory agents, intra-articular injections [2]. Once non-surgical treatments become unsuccessful, joint replacement surgery is a cost-effective procedure that can be considered for patients with severe symptoms [3]. However, joint replacement surgery is advised to be postponed as long as possible, as the lifespan of prostheses are limited [2] and the results can vary [4].

In recent years the total number of hip and knee replacement surgeries increased with 50 and 196% respectively, especially in the age group of 75–85 years [5]. Possible explanations for this overall increase are ageing of the population and increase in obesity resulting in more people suffering from symptomatic OA. Despite recommendations, conservative treatment modalities in hip or knee OA are underused [6, 7] while timely usage of these treatment modalities is advocated [8] and may prevent untimely surgery.

The underuse of conservative treatment can be caused by healthcare providers related barriers for recommending conservative treatment modalities. Research shows that outcome expectations about conservative treatment options differ widely among healthcare providers and the confidence in competencies of other healthcare providers is low [9–11]. As a result, patients with OA may not receive consistent information about effective, conservative treatment options. Receiving conflicting information is found to be associated with undesirable outcomes like non-adherence to treatment [12, 13]. Therefore, information on treatment options and strategies should be disseminated from a joint perspective of healthcare providers.

In addition, patient related factors might also influence the use of treatment modalities. Some patients are not aware of what they can do themselves and what conservative

treatment options can be offered for their OA [14]. Providing relevant disease-related and self-management related information helps patients to become actively involved in their own care process [15]. Moreover, negative beliefs or unrealistic thoughts about different treatment modalities by patients might also influence the choice of treatment [16]. A recent systematic review showed that OA patients have a negative attitude towards the efficacy of conservative treatment and tend to prefer surgical treatment [17]. This emphasises the importance that patients are aware of benefits as well as possible disadvantages of both conservative and surgical treatment options, in order to have realistic expectations [4].

During a regional conference in the area of Nijmegen, the Netherlands, healthcare providers from different disciplines involved in the care for people with OA decided to develop a patient educational program with a multidisciplinary approach to tackle above outlined barriers for suboptimal care.

The aim of this program was to increase patients' knowledge on OA, to stimulate self-management, to discuss benefits and disadvantages of treatment options, to promote the stepped care approach of treatments [8] and to provide consistent answers to frequently asked questions by patients. The objective of the present study was to determine preliminary effects of this OA educational program on healthcare utilization (HCU) and clinical outcomes.

Methods

Design and setting

An observational pilot study was performed in three districts in the Nijmegen area, the Netherlands, to evaluate a knee and hip OA educational program at baseline, and 3 months after finishing the course. In the period of October 2015 – March 2016, the program was organized 11 times (3–4 times per district). According to the Central Committee on Research involving Human Subjects (CCMO), this type of study does not require approval from an ethics committee in the Netherlands. This study was approved by the local Medical Research Ethics Committee, region Arnhem-Nijmegen (protocol number. 2015–2024).

Study population

Patients were eligible for the program when they were aged 18 years or older and had a clinical diagnosis of OA in the knee or hip (diagnosed by a general practitioner (GP) or medical specialist). Exclusion criteria were inability to read or understand the Dutch language, and previous joint replacement surgery. A maximum of 20 people (including patients and their partner or other significant person) could participate in each of the 11 planned programs, in order to facilitate group interaction. We aimed to include a total of 110–132 patients with knee or hip OA (10–12 patients per program).

Procedure

GPs' and physiotherapists in the three different participating districts and several orthopaedic surgeons in de region were informed about the objectives, background and content of the study. They were asked to offer eligible patients a flyer with information about the knee and hip OA educational program. Additionally, in each district the GPs also invited patients with an already known OA diagnosis by mail. In order to minimize selection bias we selected all patients with a diagnosis code for hip or knee OA in the GP's information system. GPs manually excluded patients who already had undergone joint replacement surgery or were not capable to understand the Dutch language. Moreover, an advertisement was placed in local newsletters and a local newspaper to invite patients. Once registered, a researcher checked eligibility of those patients.

After registration for the program, eligible patients received a letter with information of the study. By filling in a reply-card, patients could sign up for the program in their district. Participants received an additional information letter and an informed consent form, accompanied by a questionnaire on baseline characteristics and outcome parameters by mail, two weeks prior to the start of the course (T0). Three months after finishing the course, participants received a second questionnaire (T1) to assess the outcome parameters again.

Intervention

The organised knee and hip OA educational program consisted of two 1.5-h meetings. The program was led by a physiotherapist and a GP, both working in the district where the program was held. Additionally, an orthopaedic surgeon or orthopaedic nurse practitioner and when available a public health advisor attended the program. One of the healthcare professionals in each of the carried out meetings was part of the research team. They were asked to approach healthcare providers in their own district to help them carrying out the meetings.

The educational program was developed by an expert group working in the field of OA. The expert group consisted of 2 orthopaedic surgeons, 1 rheumatologist, 1 nurse practitioner, 3 physiotherapists, 1 GP and 2 physiotherapist-researchers. First an inventory of frequently asked questions (FAQs) about OA was made among local health professionals. Second, a prioritising exercise was used among OA-patients and health professionals to determine the most important FAQs. Finally, the expert group discussed and formulated answers to the 20 most important FAQs until consensus was reached. A detailed description of the process of inventory and prioritising of FAQs is described in Additional file 1. The content of the program was based on this structured inventory of informational needs and on consensus-based information addressing those needs. The FAQs and answers were incorporated in the course material. In line with current guidelines on education for patients with knee or hip OA [18], the program consisted of information on: OA and its disease course, evidence based tailored conservative treatment in a stepped-care format [8], and surgical treatment options. Moreover, education was given on outcome risks of treatment options and expectation management. This information provided patients with knowledge on where to find the (treatment) help they needed, at the time they needed it, with the appropriate expectations about this treatment. Additionally, the program included information on regional options to enhance self-management and physical activity, tips, practical assignments and mottos on OA.

To support the information given during the course, participants received a booklet consisting of information, monitoring forms, course handouts, the 20 FAQs, a pedometer and a list of useful websites, mobile applications and contact information of organisations.

Data collection

Baseline data

At baseline, patients' characteristics were collected on: age, gender, the number of important comorbidities (ranging from 0 to 15) according to the Dutch Arthritis Impact Measurement Scales [19], living situation (alone / living with partner and/or family), education (low / high), ethnicity (native / foreign), employment (workless/paid work), duration of symptoms (< 1 year / 1–5 years / 5–10 years / > 10 years) and location of OA (hip and/or knee), and number of painful joints (including hip, knee, neck, back, shoulders, elbows, wrists, hands, ankle and feet).

Measurement instruments

Outcome parameters at baseline and 3 months follow-up were HCU, pain medication use, pain and functioning in daily living, illness perceptions, patient activation, knowledge, physical activity and patient satisfaction with the course.

HCU was assessed with a self-developed questionnaire. Patients were asked which healthcare providers they visited in the preceding 3-month period related to their hip or knee symptoms (yes/no) and to indicate the number of visits to these healthcare providers.

In addition, to record the use of pain medication, participants were asked if they used (yes/no) pain medication (paracetamol / non-steroidal anti-inflammatory drugs (NSAID) / other (i.e. tramadol, morphine)) in the past 3 months regarding their hip or knee OA.

To calculate BMI (weight/height^2) weight and height were self-collected.

Two subscales of the Western Ontario McMaster University Index of osteoarthritis (WOMAC) were used to assess pain and limitations in functional activities. The WOMAC is a 24-item questionnaire, subdivided in 3 subscales: pain, stiffness and physical functioning [20]. WOMAC pain and physical functioning subscales were calculated and presented as normalized scores (0 to 100, with higher scores indicating less pain and better functioning).

Participants were asked to fill out the Dutch General Self-efficacy Scale (GSES) to measure self-efficacy [21]. The GSES has 10 items of which a total score can be calculated ranging from 10 to 40. With higher scores indicating higher self-efficacy.

The Brief illness perception questionnaire (IPQ) is a 8-item scale and was used to measure illness perceptions [22]. It measures patient's cognitive and emotional perceptions with respect to their OA. The maximum score on the Brief IPQ is 80, with higher scores reflecting more threatening view of the OA.

To assess patient activation, defined as patients' knowledge, skill, and confidence for self-management, the Patient Activation Measure (PAM-13) was used [23]. A total score can be calculated ranging from 13 (low confidence for managing own health and healthcare) to 52 (high confidence for managing own health and healthcare).

Physical activity was measured using the Short Questionnaire to Asses physical activity (SQUASH) [24]. The SQUASH consists of three main questions (days per week, average time per day and intensity) per activity-category (i.e. commuting activities, leisure-time and sports activities, household activities, and activities at work and school). A total activity score in min/week was calculated.

For the WOMAC, GSES, IPQ, PAM-13 and SQUASH a change of 20% was considered clinically relevant.

Based on identified frequently asked questions on OA in a previous study and consensus-based answers to those questions, 22 statements were formulated to test knowledge of participants on OA (and treatment). Each statement could be scored as: "I totally disagree", "Disagree", "Agree", "Totally agree" or "I don't know". A total score with a maximum of 22 could be calculated by awarding each correct response with 1 point. Each incorrect or undecided ("I don't know") answer was scored as 0 points.

Patient satisfaction was measured directly after finishing the course. Patients were asked how they overall rated the course on a scale from 1 to 10.

Statistical analyses

Baseline descriptive statistics were calculated as mean and standard deviation (SD), numbers with percentages (%) or median and Interquartile range (IQR). Changes over time in contacts with different healthcare providers were analysed using the exact McNemar's test and Wilcoxon Signed-Rank test. Difference between baseline and follow-up in secondary outcomes were analysed using the exact McNemar's test or Paired sample t-tests (two-sided). For all analyses a significance level of $p \leq 0.05$ was assumed.

Results

Patient characteristics

In total 146 patients with knee or hip OA and 54 of their partners participated in the educational program. Overall mean rating of satisfaction with the program was 8.0 (range 1–10). A total of 143 patients agreed to participate in the present study, 107 (75%) participants filled out both questionnaires, 4 were considered drop-outs, as they did not come to the intervention and did not want to continue with the study. Two participants had undergone surgery during the follow-up period and did not feel like to continue. One did have knee OA, but as symptoms of her hand OA were more severe, she did not feel like filling out another questionnaire. All other 29 participants were lost to follow-up without providing a reason. We found no differences on baseline characteristics between drop-out/loss to follow-up and those who completed follow-up questionnaires. Despite the exclusion criteria, 17 participants reported to have had previous joint replacement. Sensitivity analyses showed no differences on HCU regarding surgical visits. Therefore, these participants were not excluded from analysis.

The average age of participants was 69.1 years (SD 10.2), with the majority being female (62.9%). Fifty-six percent of the participants had experienced their OA symptoms for less than 5 years. Patient characteristics are presented in Table 1.

Healthcare utilization

Table 2 shows the HCU during the 3 months before baseline and during 3-months follow-up. Most common were visits to a physio- or exercise therapist, GP and orthopaedic surgeon regarding knee or hip OA. A significant decrease in proportion of patients who visited the physio- or exercise therapist and GP in the previous 3 months was observed. Although no changes in median number of contacts were seen, the total number of contacts increased. Small but non-significant changes in proportion of patients who visited a medical specialist were found. However, median number of visits to a medical specialist showed a small decrease, which was also seen in the total number of contacts in secondary care.

Secondary outcomes

Changes in secondary outcomes are shown in Table 3. Illness perceptions changed positively (Δ-1.8; 95% CI: 0.4–3.4), and knowledge on OA and treatment options improved (Δ2.4 95% CI: -3.0 - -1.6). No changes in BMI, pain, functioning, self-efficacy and patient activation

Table 1 Baseline demographic and clinical characteristics of participants ($n = 143$)

Social-demographic characteristics	
Gender, n (%)	
Female	90 (62.9)
Age *(years)*, mean ± SD	69.1 ± 10.2
Ethnicity, n (%)	
Native	131 (91.6)
Living situation, n (%)	
Living together with partner and/or family	102 (71.8)
Level of Education, n (%)	
Low (< 12 years)	90 (64.3)
Work, n (%)	
Paid work	28 (19.7)
District	
1	44 (30.8)
2	44 (30.8)
3	55 (38.5)
Clinical characteristics	
Location, n (%)	
Hip	77 (53.9)
Knee	103 (72.0)
Number of painful joints (range 0–10); median (IQR)	3 (2–4)
Duration of symptoms, n (%)	
< 1 years	13 (9.2)
1–5 years	66 (46.8)
5–10 years	32 (22.7)
> 10 years	30 (21.3)
Number of comorbidities (range 0–15); median (IQR)	1 (0–3)

were found. However, a trend towards an increase in physical activity was seen.

Discussion

Results of the present study show a decreased HCU, the proportion of patients having contact with a physio- or exercise therapist, or general practitioner decreased after following the educational program. We found an increase in knowledge on OA and patients' perceptions towards their OA changed positively after the course. No significant changes were found in BMI, pain and functioning, physical activity, patient activation and self-efficacy.

Overall, our results are in line with the Cochrane review on self-management programs of Kroon el al. [25]; we also did not find any changes on self-efficacy, pain and functioning. This review however, did not evaluate the effect of self-management programs on illness perceptions, OA knowledge and HCU. We believe that the changes in these

parameters are relevant to patients. This is in line with a recent randomized controlled trial, evaluating the effect of a patient decision aid for patients considering joint replacement, (including patient education on treatment options, benefits and risks) that reported positive results on knowledge and illness perceptions [26]. This is important to ensure realistic expectations of treatment outcomes in patients with hip or knee OA, and ultimately, to support self-management in the long-term.

The primary outcome in the evaluation of educational and self-management interventions is under debate [27–29]. In the review by Newman et al. (2004) some included studies used outcomes that are not specifically targeted at the intervention. They concluded that this may decrease the overall effectiveness of educational self-management programs [27]. Similarly, Nolte et al. (2013) argue to critically choose outcome measures which are linked to those targeted for in the intervention, in order to prevent incorrect interpretation of effectiveness [28, 29]. However, in general, multiple outcome dimensions are targeted in self-management interventions. As a result across studies a wide variety of outcome measures is used to evaluate self-management interventions. Usually, pain and/or physical functioning are the primary outcome measures [25]. However, it is questionable whether changes can be expected in these outcomes, when self-management programs are aimed at providing individuals with skills how to cope with symptoms, manage their disease in daily living and navigate the healthcare system [29]. Knowledge on disease management is not the same as changing your behaviour into actually doing it yourself. Therefore, knowledge is often used as a process outcome, and seems more appropriate as secondary outcome. In contrast, HCU is more a measure for behaviour. Based on previous observations that self-management interventions can result in changes in healthcare utilization [29–31] and the assumption that effective self-management ultimately impacts healthcare consumption our choice to explore HCU as primary outcome seems to be appropriate.

In our program we educated patients on what they can do for themselves, when to seek guidance for conservative treatment options and helped them to form realistic thoughts on the expected results of surgical treatment. Following this perspective, changes in HCU patterns could be expected. Our results showed a decrease in patients visiting primary care providers. However, only small non-significant changes in number of patients visiting secondary care specialists were found. Both observations may be explained by the short-term follow-up and small sample of our study. First, as we educated patients on what they can do for themselves (i.e. lifestyle advice on exercise, weight reduction and medication use), some patients may not have felt the need to visit a primary care healthcare provider on short-term, because they directly can put into practice what they have learned during

Table 2 Changes in proportion of patients visiting different healthcare providers and total number of contacts with healthcare providers between baseline and 3 months follow-up (n = 107)

	Baseline	Follow-up	
	Contacted in last 3 months n (%)	Contacted in last 3 months n (%)	p-value[a]
Primary care			
General practitioner	43 (40.2)	27 (25.2)	0.01*
Physio- or exercise therapist	39 (36.5)	26 (24.3)	0.02*
Dietician	3 (2.8)	3 (2.8)	1.00
Occupational therapist	2 (1.9)	–	–
Psychologist	1 (0.9)	–	–
Nurse (in GP practice)	6 (5.6)	5 (4.7)	1.00
District nurse/home care	1 (0.9)	2 (1.9)	–
Total number of contacts Median (IQR)	258 1 (0–2)	327 0 (0–3)	0.48[b]
Secondary care			
Rheumatologist	6 (5.6)	3 (2.8)	0.25
Orthopaedic surgeon	20 (18.7)	15 (14.0)	0.30
Physician assistant / nurse practitioner	3 (2.8)	2 (1.9)	1.00
Multidisciplinary team care / pain clinic	1 (0.9)	–	–
Total number of contacts Median (IQR)	46 0 (0–0)	24 0 (0–0)	0.02[b]*

[a]Exact McNemar significance probability
[b]Wilcoxon Signed-Rank test
*Significant for p-value ≤0.05

the program [32]. Second, it is possible that patients were already referred to secondary care previous to the intervention, resulting in no short-term changes in secondary care use. Besides, research has shown that education in combination with exercise therapy may postpone surgery in hip OA patients in the long term [33, 34]. This emphasizes the

desirability to study long-term results of our educational program in a larger sample.

Remarkably, the total number of contacts in primary care increased whereas the median number of contacts did not change. This finding may reflect the great variability in HCU between participants and specifically the

Table 3 Differences between baseline and follow-up on secondary outcome measures (n = 107 complete cases)

	Baseline	Follow-up	p-value
BMI (kg/m²), mean (SD)	27.1 (4.4)	26.7 (4.1)	0.16[b] *
WOMAC pain (range 0–100), mean (SD)	66.8 (21.4)	69.7 (20.1)	0.13[b]
WOMAC functioning (range 0–100), mean (SD)	68.3 (19.6)	67.8 (21.2)	0.78[b]
Medication use, n (%)			
Paracetamol	65 (61.9)	62 (59.1)	0.65[a]
NSAIDS	33 (32.4)	25 (24.5)	0.08[a]
Other	14 (13.1)	17 (15.9)	0.45[a]
SQUASH Total activity (min/week), mean (SD)	2128.9 (1023.1)	2349.2 (1246.8)	0.07[b]
IPQ Illness perceptions (range 0–100), mean (SD)	41.3 (10.5)	39.5 (10.5)	0.02[b] *
GSES Self-efficacy (10–40), mean (SD)	32.1 (5.9)	32.2 (5.6)	0.85[b]
PAM-13, patient activation (13–52), mean (SD)	39.3 (0.5)	40.1 (0.5)	0.15[b]
Knowledge on OA (0–22), mean (SD)	10.5 (3.7)	12.9 (3.1)	0.00[b] *

[a]Exact McNemar significance probability
[b]Paired sample t-test, two-sided
*Significant for p-value ≤0.05

difference in treatment between healthcare professionals. For example, patients will visit their GP once or twice for OA within 3 months, whereas they may visit a physiotherapist once or twice a week. This can sum up to a total of 12–24 visits over 3 months. In the present study several patients started physiotherapy treatment 1–2 weeks prior to the intervention (1–4 visits in the previous 3 months) and continued this treatment after the intervention (> 10 visits in the 3 months post-intervention) (data not shown). This may have contributed to the increased number of total visits in our sample. However, the low number of participants and short-term follow-up of the present study do not allow firm conclusions on this aspect of HCU.

We chose a multidisciplinary approach; in both the developmental process as well as in the execution of the program. This approach is based on previous research which argues to focus on the communication between healthcare providers involved in OA treatment to improve prescription of non-surgical treatment options [9]. In the process of achieving consensus on the content of the program and answering frequently asked questions on OA, we targeted differences in beliefs among healthcare providers regarding the efficacy of non-surgical treatments [9, 35] and clarified roles of different healthcare providers in the management of OA-patients [11]. Consequently, this resulted in clear and consistent information that could be disseminated during the course. This could explain the increased knowledge of patients after participating in the program. So far, little research has been done on the impact of consistency of information on self-management skills across settings and across disciplines for patients with osteoarthritis. In our opinion this is an important area for future research.

We chose to adapt the program to local context and patients preferences as it is known that adapting to local context positively influences knowledge translation [32, 36]. We involved local health care providers in the development and the execution of the program to support the role that health care providers have in patients' treatment consideration [37] and offering patients options for local support. This may have contributed to the accessibility of the program and may have resulted that our educational program was highly valued by participants (satisfaction score 8 on a scale 1–10).

An important factor in the set-up of our program was the option for participants to bring their partner or a significant other person. Previous studies that focused on explaining reasons for underuse of conservative treatment, underline the importance of the social environment of patients to be involved their care process [9, 37]. Involving a spouse in an intervention may even enhance self-efficacy and improve coping abilities [38], and improve physical activity levels in in OA patients [39]. Our results showed no improvement in self-efficacy

after the intervention and only a small, but non-significant increase in physical activity. However, only one-third of the patients who participated in the educational program indeed brought their partner. Future improvements of our intervention should focus on ways to better involve patients' social environment [9].

This study has several limitations that should be taken into account when interpreting the results. First, the uncontrolled design of the study and the small sample size urges that conclusions drawn about the effect of the intervention should be taken with caution. In our study we examined short-term preliminary effects of a multidisciplinary educational program. However, a controlled trial with long-term follow-up is needed to further explore effects on HCU behaviour in patients with hip or knee OA. Second, we had a 25% loss to follow up, despite reminder letters. The overall high age of our participants might have contributed to the loss. Last, there may be a matter of selection bias. Although we tried to minimize this in our procedure when inviting patients for our study, we have no data available of patients who did not respond to our invitation to participate in our study.

Conclusions
Our results suggest that a multidisciplinary educational program, may result in changes in HCU and have positive effects on illness perceptions and knowledge in patients with hip or knee OA. These results indicate that patients may better understand and adjust their health seeking behaviour as a result of the program. Especially, the collaboration between health professionals from different disciplines, both in developing and executing the educational program, provides in adequate and consistent information on OA, treatment and self-management options. A randomized controlled trial with long-term follow-up with larger number of patients is needed to confirm these results.

Abbreviations
BMI: body mass index; FAQ: frequently asked question; GP: general practitioner; GSES: General Self-efficacy Scale; HCU: healthcare utilization; IPQ: Illness perceptions questionnaire; NSAID: Non-steroidal anti-inflammatory drug; OA: osteoarthritis; SQUASH: Short Questionnaire to Asses physical activity; WOMAC: Western Ontario McMaster University Index of osteoarthritis

Acknowledgements
We thank Gertie Schouten, Wilma Peters and Heleen Govers (patient representatives) for their contribution to the project group. We thank Tanya Lévy (consultant health innovations, VGZ), Pieter van Haren (manager Innovations, VGZ), Marjolein de Rijk (manager Partnerships, VGZ), Wim Scheurs (orthopaedic surgeon, Radboudumc), Marlies van Pelt (physiotherapist, Fysiotherapie Hatert) and John Reijnen (physiotherapist, Medical Training Malden) for their work in the project group. We thank Bastiaan Plant (GP, De Kroonsteen Beneden), Joris Stoppels (GP, Hatertse

Hoed), Nicole Blijleven (physiotherapist, Thermion) and Mark Loeffen (physiotherapist, Thermion) for their contribution as course leaders.

Funding
This project was funded by the healthcare insurance company Coöperatie VGZ.

Authors' contributions
AAOMC, CHME and HJS participated in the design of the study. All authors participated in the development of the intervention. AAOMC carried out the data collection. All authors were responsible for the analysis and interpretation of the data. AAOMC and CHME were responsible for drafting the article, all other authors critical reviewed the article. Furthermore, all authors approved the final version of the manuscript.

Competing interests
The authors declare that they have no competing interests.

Author details
[1]Department of Rheumatology, Sint Maartenskliniek, PO Box 9011, 6500, GM, Nijmegen, The Netherlands. [2]Department of Primary and Community Care, Radboud University Medical Center, Nijmegen, The Netherlands. [3]Department of Orthopaedic Surgery, Canisius Wilhelmina Hospital, Nijmegen, The Netherlands. [4]Stichting Gezondheidscentrum De Kroonsteen - De Vuursteen, Nijmegen, The Netherlands. [5]Department of Orthopaedic Surgery, Sint Maartenskliniek, Nijmegen, The Netherlands. [6]Department of Orthopaedic Surgery, Radboud University Medical Center, Nijmegen, The Netherlands. [7]Department of Rheumatology, Radboud University Medical Center, Nijmegen, The Netherlands.

References
1. Arden N, Osteoarthritis NMC. epidemiology. Best Pract Res Clin Rheumatol. 2006;20:3–25.
2. Zhang W, Moskowitz RW, Nuki G, Abramson S, Altman RD, Arden N, et al. OARSI recommendations for the management of hip and knee osteoarthritis, part II: OARSI evidence-based, expert consensus guidelines. Osteoarthritis Cartilage. 2008;16:137–62.
3. Rasanen P, Paavolainen P, Sintonen H, Koivisto AM, Blom M, Ryynanen OP, et al. Effectiveness of hip or knee replacement surgery in terms of quality-adjusted life years and costs. Acta Orthop. 2007;78:108–15.
4. Beswick AD, Wylde V, Gooberman-Hill R, Blom A, Dieppe P. What proportion of patients report long-term pain after total hip or knee replacement for osteoarthritis? A systematic review of prospective studies in unselected patients. BMJ Open. 2012;2:e000435.
5. Otten R, van Roermund PM. Picavet HS. [trends in the number of knee and hip arthroplasties: considerably more knee and hip prostheses due to osteoarthritis in 2030]. Ned Tijdschr Geneeskd. 2010;154:A1534.
6. Snijders GF, den Broeder AA, van Riel PL, Straten VH, de Man FH, van den Hoogen FH, et al. Evidence-based tailored conservative treatment of knee and hip osteoarthritis: between knowing and doing. Scand J Rheumatol. 2011;40:225–31.
7. Conrozier T, Marre JP, Payen-Champenois C, Vignon E. National survey on the non-pharmacological modalities prescribed by French general practitioners in the treatment of lower limb (knee and hip) osteoarthritis. Adherence to the EULAR recommendations and factors influencing adherence. Clin Exp Rheumatol. 2008;26:793–8.
8. Smink AJ, van den Ende CH, Vliet Vlieland TP, Swierstra BA, Kortland JH, Bijlsma JW, et al. "beating osteoARThritis": development of a stepped care strategy to optimize utilization and timing of non-surgical treatment modalities for patients with hip or knee osteoarthritis. Clin Rheumatol. 2011; 30:1623–9.
9. Hofstede SN, Marang-van de Mheen PJ, Vliet Vlieland TP, van den Ende CH, Nelissen RG. Van Bodegom-Vos L: barriers and facilitators associated with

non-surgical treatment use for osteoarthritis patients in Orthopaedic practice. PLoS One. 2016;11:e0147406.
10. Smink AJ, Bierma-Zeinstra SM, Dekker J, Vliet Vlieland TP, Bijlsma JW, Swierstra BA, et al. Agreement of general practitioners with the guideline-based stepped-care strategy for patients with osteoarthritis of the hip or knee: a cross-sectional study. BMC Fam Pract. 2013;14:33.
11. Selten EM, Vriezekolk JE, Nijhof MW, Schers HJ. Van der Meulen - Dilling RG, van der Laan WH et al. barriers impeding the use of non-pharmacological, non-surgical care in hip and knee osteoarthritis: the views of general practitioners, physical therapists, and medical specialists. J of Clin Rheumatol. in press
12. Carpenter DM, Elstad EA, Blalock SJ, DeVellis RF. Conflicting medication information: prevalence, sources, and relationship to medication adherence. J Health Commun. 2014;19:67–81.
13. Carpenter DM, DeVellis RF, Fisher EB, DeVellis BM, Hogan SL, Jordan JM. The effect of conflicting medication information and physician support on medication adherence for chronically ill patients. Patient Educ Couns. 2010; 81:169–76.
14. Sanders C, Donovan JL, Dieppe PA. Unmet need for joint replacement: a qualitative investigation of barriers to treatment among individuals with severe pain and disability of the hip and knee. Rheumatology (Oxford). 2004;43:353–7.
15. Novak M, Costantini L, Schneider S, Beanlands H. Approaches to self-management in chronic illness. Semin Dial. 2013;26:188–94.
16. Selten EM, Vriezekolk JE, Geenen R, van der Laan WH, Van der Meulen-Dilling RG, Nijhof MW, et al. \Reasons for treatment choices in knee and hip osteoarthritis: a qualitative study. Arthritis Care Res (Hoboken). 2016;68:1260–7.
17. Smith TO, Purdy R, Lister S, Salter C, Fleetcroft R, Conaghan PG. Attitudes of people with osteoarthritis towards their conservative management: a systematic review and meta-ethnography. Rheumatol Int. 2014;34:299–313.
18. Fernandes L, Hagen KB, Bijlsma JW, Andreassen O, Christensen P, Conaghan PG, et al. EULAR recommendations for the non-pharmacological core management of hip and knee osteoarthritis. Ann Rheum Dis. 2013;72:1125–35.
19. Riemsma RP, Taal E, Rasker JJ, Houtman PM, Van Paassen HC, Wiegman O. Evaluation of a Dutch version of the AIMS2 for patients with rheumatoid arthritis. Br J Rheumatol. 1996;35:755–60.
20. Roorda LD, Jones CA, Waltz M, Lankhorst GJ, Bouter LM, van der Eijken JW, et al. Satisfactory cross cultural equivalence of the Dutch WOMAC in patients with hip osteoarthritis waiting for arthroplasty. Ann Rheum Dis. 2004;63:36–42.
21. Scholz U, Doña BG, Sud S, Schwarzer RI. General self-efficacy a universal construct? Psychometric findings from 25 countries Eur J Psychol Assess. 2002;18:242–51.
22. Broadbent E, Petrie KJ, Main J, Weinman J. The brief illness perception questionnaire. J Psychosom Res. 2006;60:631–7.
23. Rademakers J, Nijman J, van der Hoek L, Heijmans M, Rijken M. Measuring patient activation in the Netherlands: translation and validation of the American short form patient activation measure (PAM13). BMC Public Health. 2012;12:577.
24. Wagenmakers R. Van dA-S, I, Groothoff JW, Zijlstra W, Bulstra SK, Kootstra JW et al. reliability and validity of the short questionnaire to assess health-enhancing physical activity (SQUASH) in patients after total hip arthroplasty. BMC Musculoskelet Disord. 2008;9:141.
25. Kroon FP, van der Burg LR, Buchbinder R, Osborne RH, Johnston RV, Pitt V. Self-management education programmes for osteoarthritis. Cochrane Database Syst Rev. 2014; https://doi.org/10.1002/14651858.CD008963.pub2.
26. Stacey D, Taljaard M, Dervin G, Tugwell P, O'Connor AM, Pomey MP, et al. Impact of patient decision aids on appropriate and timely access to hip or knee arthroplasty for osteoarthritis: a randomized controlled trial. Osteoarthr Cartil. 2016;24:99–107.
27. Newman S, Steed L, Mulligan K. Self-management interventions for chronic illness. Lancet. 2004;364:1523–37.
28. Nolte S, Elsworth GR, Newman S, Osborne RH. Measurement issues in the evaluation of chronic disease self-management programs. Qual Life Res. 2013;22:1655–64.
29. Nolte S, Osborne RH. A systematic review of outcomes of chronic disease self-management interventions. Qual Life Res. 2013;22:1805–16.
30. Cuperus N, van den Hout WB, Hoogeboom TJ, van den Hoogen FH, Vliet Vlieland TP, van den Ende CH. Cost-utility and cost-effectiveness analyses of face-to-face versus telephone-based nonpharmacologic multidisciplinary treatments for patients with generalized osteoarthritis. Arthritis Care Res (Hoboken). 2016;68:502–10.

31. Panagioti M, Richardson G, Small N, Murray E, Rogers A, Kennedy A, et al. Self-management support interventions to reduce health care utilisation without compromising outcomes: a systematic review and meta-analysis. BMC Health Serv Res. 2014;14:356.

32. Thorstensson CA, Garellick G, Rystedt H, Dahlberg LE. Better Management of Patients with osteoarthritis: development and Nationwide implementation of an evidence-based supported osteoarthritis self-management Programme. Musculoskeletal Care. 2014;13:67–75.

33. Svege I, Nordsletten L, Fernandes L, Risberg MA. Exercise therapy may postpone total hip replacement surgery in patients with hip osteoarthritis: a long-term follow-up of a randomised trial. Ann Rheum Dis. 2015;74:164–9.

34. Pisters MF, Veenhof C, de Bakker DH, Schellevis FG, Dekker J. Behavioural graded activity results in better exercise adherence and more physical activity than usual care in people with osteoarthritis: a cluster-randomised trial. J Physiother. 2010;56:41–7.

35. Egerton T, Diamond LE, Buchbinder R, Bennell KL, Slade SCA. Systematic review and evidence synthesis of qualitative studies to identify primary care clinicians' barriers and enablers to the management of osteoarthritis. Osteoarthr Cartil. 2016;25:625–38.

36. Graham ID, Logan J, Harrison MB, Straus SE, Tetroe J, Caswell W, et al. Lost in translation: time for a map? J Contin Educ Heal Prof. 2006;26:13–24.

37. Selten EM, Geenen R, Schers HJ, van den Hoogen FH, van der Dilling m, RG, van der Laan WH, et al. Treatment beliefs underlying intended treatment choices in knee and hip osteoarthritis. Int J Behav Med. 2017; https://doi.org/10.1007/s12529-017-9671-2.

38. Keefe FJ, Caldwell DS, Baucom D, Salley A, Robinson E, Timmons K, et al. Spouse-assisted coping skills training in the management of knee pain in osteoarthritis: long-term followup results. Arthritis Care Res. 1999;12:101–11.

39. Martire LM, Stephens MA, Mogle J, Schulz R, Brach J, Keefe FJ. Daily spousal influence on physical activity in knee osteoarthritis. Ann Behav Med. 2013; 45:213–23.

15

Polypharmacy in older patients with chronic diseases: a cross-sectional analysis of factors associated with excessive polypharmacy

Anja Rieckert[1]* (iD), Ulrike S. Trampisch[2], Renate Klaaßen-Mielke[2], Eva Drewelow[3], Aneez Esmail[4], Tim Johansson[5], Sophie Keller[5], Ilkka Kunnamo[6], Christin Löffler[3], Joonas Mäkinen[6], Giuliano Piccoliori[7], Anna Vögele[7] and Andreas Sönnichsen[1,4]

Abstract

Background: Polypharmacy is common in older people and associated with potential harms. The aim of this study was to analyse the characteristics of an older multimorbid population with polypharmacy and to identify factors contributing to excessive polypharmacy in these patients.

Methods: This cross-sectional analysis is based on the PRIMA-eDS trial, a large randomised controlled multicentre study of polypharmacy in primary care. Patients' baseline data were used for analysis. A number of socioeconomic and medical data as well as SF-12-scores were entered into a generalized linear mixed model to identify variables associated with excessive polypharmacy (taking ≥10 substances daily).

Results: Three thousand nine hundred four participants were recruited. Risk factors significantly associated with excessive polypharmacy were frailty (OR 1.45; 95% CI 1.22–1.71), > 8 diagnoses (OR 2.64; 95% CI 2.24–3.11), BMI ≥30 (OR 1.18; 95% CI 1.02–1.38), a lower SF-12 physical health composite score (OR 1.47; 95% CI 1.26–1.72), and a lower SF-12 mental health composite score (OR 1.33; 95% CI 1.17–1.59) than the median of the study population (≤36.6 and ≤ 48.7, respectively). Age ≥ 85 years (OR 0.83; 95% CI 0.70–0.99) led to a significantly lower risk for excessive polypharmacy. No association with excessive polypharmacy could be found for female sex, low educational level, and smoking. Regarding the study centres, being recruited in the UK led to a significantly higher risk for excessive polypharmacy compared to being recruited in Germany 1/Rostock (OR 1.71; 95% CI 1.27–2.30). Being recruited in Germany 2/Witten led to a slightly significant lower risk for excessive polypharmacy compared to Germany 1/Rostock (OR 0.74; 95% CI 0.56–0.97).

Conclusions: Frailty, multimorbidity, obesity, and decreased physical as well as mental health status are risk factors for excessive polypharmacy. Sex, educational level, and smoking apparently do not seem to be related to excessive polypharmacy. Physicians should especially pay attention to their frail, obese patients who have multiple diagnoses and a decreased health-related quality of life, to check carefully whether all the drugs prescribed are evidence-based, safe, and do not interact in an unfavourable way.

Keywords: Aged, Risk factors, Protective factors, Polypharmacy, Europe, Cross-sectional study, PRIMA-eDS

* Correspondence: Anja.Rieckert@uni-wh.de
[1]Institute of General Practice and Family Medicine, Faculty of Health, Witten/Herdecke University, Alfred-Herrhausen-Str. 50, 58448 Witten, Germany
Full list of author information is available at the end of the article

Background

Older adults (≥65 years) make up an increasing proportion of the European population, particularly the oldest old (≥80 years) [1], and drug use in this age group is common. Depending on setting and age, older adults are prescribed an average of 5.3–6.9 drugs [2–5]. Around 44.2–57.7% of older adults are on ≥5 different drugs, and additional 9.1–23.2% on ≥10 different drugs [4, 6–8]. Concurrent use of multiple medications is known as polypharmacy [9]. However, there is no consensus on the definition of polypharmacy in the literature. Likewise, there is no agreed definition of excessive polypharmacy, though the cut-off point of ≥10 drugs is often used [10].

In some cases, polypharmacy may be inevitable, however, in many patients it appears to be inappropriate [11]. This may be specifically true for older people, as age-related changes in pharmacokinetics and pharmacodynamics increase the risk of adverse drug events [12]. There is some evidence, mostly from observational studies, that polypharmacy in older adults is associated with a number of negative health outcomes such as decreased functional and cognitive health status, increased risk of falls, adverse drug events, hospitalisations, and mortality. However, not all studies found these associations [13]. Risks of adverse drug outcomes increase with an increasing number of medications [14]. Wimmer et al. assessed the association between medication regimen complexity in older people and clinical outcomes, and they concluded that regimen complexity is associated with medication nonadherence and increased rates of hospitalisation [15]. In a retrospective cohort study of adults aged ≥20 years, Payne et al. found an association between unplanned hospital admission and consumption of multiple medications. However, after controlling for multimorbidity only consumption of ≥10 medications was significantly associated with unplanned admissions [16]. Also, the King's Fund has proposed a cut-off of ≥10 medications as a pragmatic approach to identify polypharmacy patients 'at risk', whilst recognising that there is no universal consensus around this [17].

In previous research the association between no-polypharmacy and polypharmacy as well as between no-polypharmacy and excessive polypharmacy was investigated [4, 5, 18–25]. To our knowledge no study so far has analysed possible predictors for excessive polypharmacy in patients consuming multiple drugs. Given the increased risk of adverse health outcomes in older adults taking ≥10 medications it is important to investigate which factors contribute to excessive polypharmacy. We therefore are analysing in this study the independent descriptive variables of the PRIMA-eDS-trial (Polypharmacy in chronic diseases: Reduction of Inappropriate Medication and Adverse drug events in older populations by electronic Decision Support) population to identify possible predictors of excessive polypharmacy (using the cut-off of ≥10 substances as proposed above).

Methods

Study design and population

This cross-sectional study is based on the baseline data of the PRIMA-eDS trial. In 2015, GPs in five study centres (UK/Manchester, Italy/Bolzano, Austria/Salzburg, Germany 1/Rostock, Germany 2/Witten) were enrolled to recruit patients with polypharmacy. Patient eligibility criteria included age ≥ 75 and taking ≥8 medications regularly. Patient data were collected between September 2014 and September 2015. A more detailed description of the PRIMA-eDS trial has been published [26]. These baseline patient data were used in the analysis presented here.

Data collection

At each practice the GP or an authorised staff member collected patient data and entered it into an electronic case report form (eCRF; Additional file 1). In the UK, data was also collected at some practices by a regional Clinical Research Network research nurse working with the practice. Baseline data used for this study included: age, sex, height, weight, all drugs with an Anatomical Therapeutic Chemical (ATC) code (prescribed and over the counter), all diagnoses, smoking status, and frailty according to the clinical frailty scale [27]. A health-related quality of life questionnaire (SF-12v2) [28] was also administered to each patient and entered into the eCRF by staff of the study centres. Educational level was recorded according to ISCED-97 which was filled out by the patient [29].

Outcome and independent variables

According to the King's Fund [17] and the median number of drugs used by all patients participating in the study, we defined the outcome variables as non-excessive polypharmacy (< 10 substances) and excessive polypharmacy (≥10 substances). Drugs were coded using the ATC [30] classification system of the World Health Organisation and updated to correspond with changes in 2016 and 2017. Each substance was recorded separately. We took into consideration all substances at baseline with an ATC code. Diagnoses were recorded using the ICD-10 code [31].

Independent variables used in the analysis were age, sex, educational level, physical and mental health composite scores derived from the SF-12, frailty status, body mass index (BMI), smoking status, study centre, and number of diagnoses.

Statistical analysis

Descriptive statistics were used to describe patient demographics and other variables. Means and standard deviations (SD) were used for continuous variables, and proportions for categorical variables. A multivariable generalized linear mixed model was applied to identify factors associated with excessive polypharmacy, with GP practice as a random effect. For the purposes of this analysis, some independent variables were re-categorised: age (into ≥85 years versus < 85); educational level (low versus medium/high); frailty (frail/terminally ill versus managing well/vulnerable); body mass index (BMI ≥30 kg/m^2 versus BMI < 30 kg/m^2); smoking status (smoker versus non-smoker/ex-smoker). The number of diagnoses was grouped as >median versus ≤median (> 8 vs ≤8 diagnoses). Physical and mental health composite scores were all grouped as ≤median versus >median, which was for the physical health composite score ≤ 36.635 versus > 36.636 and for the mental health composite score ≤ 48.7 versus > 48.8. Lower physical and mental health composite scores, meaning that they are below the median, imply poorer health-related quality of life. As some variables have a high share of missing data, we performed multiple imputations by fully conditional specification. Cramer's V was used to look for bivariate associations. A significance level of $\alpha = 0.05$ was used throughout. Data was analysed using the SAS v9.4 statistical software.

Results

Three hundred fifty nine GPs and 3904 patients were recruited. Baseline characteristics of the study sample are presented in Tables 1, 2 and 3, in Additional files 2 and 3. A few patients did not meet the inclusion criteria for the randomised controlled trial (see Table 1), but were included for this analysis. On average, participants were taking 10.5 substances (±2.4) and had 9.5 diagnoses (±4.9). HMG CoA reductase inhibitors were the most commonly used drug, followed by proton pump inhibitors, selective beta blocking agents, platelet aggregation inhibitors, ACE inhibitors, sulphonamides, and dihydropyridine derivatives. Among the ten most commonly used substances according to ATC 5 level, pantoprazole was considered as inappropriate according to the EU(7)-PIM list, and for acetylsalicylic acid, bisoprolol, and amlodipine the EU(7)-PIM list recommended an alternative [32]. Essential (primary) hypertension was the most common diagnosis, followed by disorders of lipoprotein metabolism, type 2 diabetes mellitus, and arthrosis.

Factors associated with excessive polypharmacy

Table 4 reports the results of the multivariable analysis. Factors were used as described in the methods section. Regarding study centres, Germany 1 as the one having the highest percentage of patients taking ≥10 drugs was chosen as reference for all other centres. Factors significantly associated with excessive polypharmacy were being frail/terminally ill (OR 1.45; 95% CI 1.22–1.71), having more than 8 diagnoses (OR 2.64; 95% CI 2.24–3.11), being obese (OR 1.18; 95% CI 1.02–1.38), having a

lower physical health composite score up to the median (OR 1.47; 95% CI 1.26–1.72), and a lower mental health composite score up to the median (OR 1.33; 95% CI 1.17–1.59). In contrast, being ≥85 years old (OR 0.83; 95% CI 0.70–0.99) was significantly associated with a lower risk for excessive polypharmacy. No association with excessive polypharmacy could be found for being female (OR 1.03; 95% CI 0.89–1.19), having a low educational level (OR 0.95; 95% CI 0.80–1.13), and being a smoker (OR 0.85; 95% CI 0.60–1.21). Regarding the study centres, being recruited in the UK led to a significantly higher risk for excessive polypharmacy compared to being recruited in Germany 1 (OR 1.71; 95% CI 1.27–2.30). Being recruited in Germany 2 led to a slightly significant lower risk for excessive polypharmacy compared to Germany 1 (OR 0.74; 95% CI 0.56–0.97). There were no significant associations between recruitment in Austria and Germany 1 (OR 0.97; 95% CI 0.72–1.31) or Italy and Germany 1 (OR 0.90; 95% CI 0.67–1.21).

Discussion

This cross-sectional study is based on a large sample of older patients with polypharmacy recruited for the European randomised controlled multicentre trial PRIMA-eDS. Results suggest that frailty, multimorbidity, and obesity as well as lower physical and mental health composite scores on the SF-12 are independent risk factors for excessive polypharmacy. Also, in multivariable analysis, the country or even the region plays an important role. Old age alone (≥85 years) does not seem to increase the risk of polypharmacy and may even be associated with lower risk. In our study sample, sex, educational level, and smoking status apparently do not contribute to excessive polypharmacy.

Interpretation and comparison with existing literature

It is easily understandable that > 8 diagnoses contribute to excessive polypharmacy because guideline-adherent treatment of multiple diseases will inevitably lead to a large number of drugs being prescribed. This has also been shown by other studies with no polypharmacy as a comparison to excessive polypharmacy [20, 21, 24].

In our study, being frail/terminally ill is significantly associated with excessive polypharmacy. Saum et al. [33] and Herr et al. [34] showed that taking ≥10 drugs compared to taking ≤4 drugs is significantly associated with frailty [24]. Morley et al. [35] described frailty as a risk factor for a medication increase as physicians lack a concept on how to treat frail old people and thus often start medication. However, the question of causality remains unsettled as polypharmacy may also lead to frailty [36], and polypharmacy as well as frailty may be a result of multimorbidity. Studies suggested that there is a dose-response relationship between the number of drugs taken and the risk of being frail [33, 37].

Table 1 Demographic and clinical characteristics of the population

Characteristics	All subjects (n = 3904)		Polypharmacy 7–10 substances[b] (n = 1644)		Excessive Polypharmacy ≥10 substances (n = 2260)	
	n		n		n	
Sociodemographic data						
Age	3904					
75-85[c] (n, %)	3036	77.8	1270	77.3	1766	78.1
≥ 85 (n, %)	868	22.2	374	22.7	494	21.9
mean ± SD (years)	3904	81.5 ± 4.4	1644	81.6 ± 4.4	2260	81.5 ± 4.4
Sex	3904					
Female, n (%)	2240	57.4	913	55.5	1327	58.7
Male, n (%)	1664	42.6	731	44.5	933	41.3
Educational level, n (%)	3578[a]					
Low	1536	39.3	669	40.7	867	38.4
Medium	1465	37.5	583	35.5	882	39.0
High	577	14.8	239	14.5	338	15.0
Health-related factors	3736[a]					
Smokers, n (%)	154	3.9	72	4.4	82	3.6
BMI, n (%)	3904					
BMI < 18.5	34	0.9	15	0.9	19	0.8
BMI 18.5–24	957	24.5	435	26.5	522	23.1
BMI 25–29	1606	41.1	710	43.2	896	39.7
BMI ≥30	1307	33.5	484	29.4	823	36.4
Frailty level, n (%)	3781[a]					
Managing well	1643	42.1	804	48.9	839	37.1
Vulnerable	868	22.2	358	21.8	510	22.6
Mildly frail	660	16.9	237	14.4	423	18.7
Moderately frail	505	13.0	153	9.3	352	15.6
Severely frail	97	2.5	32	2.0	65	2.9
Very severely frail	8	0.2	2	0.1	6	0.2
Physical health composite score, median (range)	3484[a]	36.6 (10–68)	1454	39.4 (12–68)	2030	34.7 (10–63)
Mental health composite score, median (range)	3483[a]	48.7 (12–76)	1454	50.3 (14–76)	2029	47.4 (12–74)
Study centre, n (%)	3904					
Austria	587	15.0	259	15.8	328	14.5
Germany 1	981	25.1	351	21.3	630	27.9
Germany 2	742	19.0	334	20.3	408	18.1
Italy	901	23.4	439	26.7	462	20.4
UK	693	17.8	261	15.9	432	19.1
Substances, n (mean ± SD)	3904	10.5 ± 2.4	1644	8.5 ± 0.6	2260	12.0 ± 2.2
Diagnoses, n (mean ± SD)	3898[a]	9.5 ± 4.9	1644	8.2 ± 4.2	2260	10.5 ± 5.2

[a]As n differs from 3904, the rest of the patients have missing data regarding the variable
[b]7 patients took < 7 substances
[c]5 patients were < 75 years old
Legend: *BMI* body mass index, *Germany* 1 Rostock, *Germany* 2 = Witten, *SD* Standard deviation

Regarding health-related quality of life, a lower physical and mental health composite score indicating worse functioning within these health domains are significantly associated with excessive polypharmacy. Jyrkka et al. found moderate and poor self-reported health to be risk factors for excessive polypharmacy compared to no polypharmacy [20]. Polypharmacy patients usually suffer from several diseases and we expect them to have a

Table 2 Percentage of the population using substances (ATC level 4) according to polypharmacy status

Substances		All subjects		Polypharmacy < 10 substances		Excessive polypharmacy ≥10 substances	
		n	(%)	n	(%)	n	(%)
C10AA	HMG CoA reductase inhibitors	2479	63.5	999	60.8	1480	65.5
A02BC	Proton pump inhibitors	2328	59.6	837	50.9	1491	66.0
C07AB	Beta blocking agents, selective	2240	57.4	909	55.3	1331	58.9
B01AC	Platelet aggregation inhibitors excl. Heparin	1952	50.0	762	46.4	1190	52.7
C09AA	ACE Inhibitors, plain	1751	44.9	792	48.2	959	42.4
C03CA	Sulfonamides, plain	1715	43.9	569	34.6	1146	50.7
C08CA	Dihydropyridine derivates	1611	41.3	658	40.0	953	42.2
C09CA	Angiotensin II antagonists, plain	1355	34.7	505	30.7	850	37.6
C03AA	Thiazides, plain	1354	34.7	555	33.8	799	35.4
A11CC	Vitamin D and analogues	1120	28.7	345	21.0	775	34.3

reduced health-related quality of life due to illness. Here again, causality may not be easily determined as polypharmacy could also lead to a decrease in health-related quality of life e.g. due to adverse effects of drugs.

It is not surprising that obesity is associated with excessive polypharmacy. Obesity has been shown to lead to an increased use of drugs [38] and can result in chronic diseases especially with advancing age [39]. However, a causal inference cannot be made as chronic diseases caused by obesity may be associated with excessive polypharmacy and it might be that obesity is an intermediate variable or a confounder.

We found that being ≥85 years of age is a protective factor against excessive polypharmacy. This was also found by Kim et al. [21] when comparing older patients with and without polypharmacy, and by Onder et al. [24] who detected an inverse correlation between polypharmacy and increasing age. However, Jyrkka et al. [20] found ≥85 years to be a risk factor for excessive polypharmacy compared to no polypharmacy, and two further studies [19, 25] showed being ≥80 years of age to be a risk factor. One

explanation for the decreased use of drugs might be that due to a limited life expectancy of these very old people preventive medications are stopped in order to improve the patients' current well-being [40]. However, whether this really happens is questionable. Age does not influence patients' priorities in taking preventive medication and reducing adverse events [41], and GPs find deprescribing of preventive medication difficult [42]. Another interpretation could be that excessive polypharmacy patients die earlier and do not reach the very old age.

We did not find that sex was significantly associated with excessive polypharmacy. The literature is conflicting here [19, 20, 24, 25]. In this study there was no significant association between educational level and excessive polypharmacy. In the literature it has been shown that educational level had an impact on health, however, this effect appeared to decrease with age and was not significant anymore in adults ≥51 years [43].

Smoking contributes to the burden of disease. Surprisingly, smoking was not associated with excessive

Table 3 Most common diagnoses of the population according to polypharmacy status

Diagnoses		All subjects		Polypharmacy < 10 substances		Excessive polypharmacy ≥10 substances	
		n	(%)	n	(%)	n	(%)
I10	Essential (primary) hypertension	3428	87.8	1426	86.7	2002	88.6
E78	Disorders of lipoprotein metabolism and other lipidaemias	2078	53.2	814	49.5	1264	55.9
E11	Type 2 diabetes mellitus	1850	47.4	686	41.7	1164	51.5
M19	Osteoarthritis	1752	44.9	683	41.6	1069	47.3
I25	Chronic ischaemic heart disease	1473	37.7	566	34.4	907	40.1
M54	Dorsalgia	1442	36.9	499	30.4	943	41.7
I48	Atrial fibrillation and flutter	1172	30.0	471	28.7	701	31.0
I50	Heart failure	1142	29.3	412	25.1	730	32.3
K21	Gastro-oesophageal reflux disease	982	25.2	369	22.5	613	27.1
F32	Depressive episode	853	21.9	292	17.8	561	24.8

Table 4 Factors associated with excessive polypharmacy (≥10 substances); results from the multivariable generalized linear mixed model

Factors	Univariable		Multivariable	
	OR (95% CI)	p	OR (95% CI)	p
Sex (female vs male)	1.18 (1.03–1.35)	0.0189	1.03 (0.89–1.19)	0.6718
Age group (≥85 vs < 85)	0.96 (0.82–1.13)	0.6388	0.83 (0.70–0.99)	0.0328
Educational level (low vs medium/high/missing)	0.94 (0.81–1.10)	0.4440	0.95 (0.80–1.13)	0.5506
Frailty (frail/terminally ill vs managing well/vulnerable/missing)	1.83 (1.57–2.13)	<.0001	1.45 (1.22–1.71)	<.0001
BMI (≥30 vs < 30)	1.34 (1.16–1.54)	<.0001	1.18 (1.02–1.38)	0.0303
Smoker (smoker vs non-smoker/ex-smoker/missing)	0.83 (0.59–1.16)	0.2763	0.85 (0.60–1.21)	0.3579
Research centre (Austria vs Germany 1)	0.69 (0.52–0.93)	0.0139	0.97 (0.72–1.31)	0.8519
Research centre (Italy vs Germany 1)	0.58 (0.44–0.75)	<.0001	0.90 (0.67–1.21)	0.4950
Research centre (UK vs Germany 1)	0.92 (0.70–1.22)	0.5561	1.71 (1.27–2.30)	0.0004
Research centre (Germany 2 vs Germany1)	0.71 (0.54–0.94)	0.0150	0.74 (0.56–0.97)	0.0303
Number of diagnoses (> 8 vs ≤8)	2.70 (2.32–3.14)	<.0001	2.64 (2.24–3.11)	<.0001
Physical health composite score (≤36.635 vs > 36.636)	1.83 (1.58–2.11)	<.0001	1.47 (1.26–1.72)	<.0001
Mental health composite score (≤48.7 vs > 48.8)	1.53 (1.33–1.76)	<.0001	1.36 (1.17–1.59)	<.0001

Legend: Germany 1 = Rostock, Germany 2 = Witten

polypharmacy in older polypharmacy patients, but there were very few smokers among the patients in our study.

There was a slightly significant association between excessive polypharmacy and the study centre Germany 1 when compared to Germany 2. One possible explanation could be the differences between the two settings. Germany 1 recruited patients in a more rural setting in the former Eastern part of Germany while Germany 2 recruited patients in the large metropolitan area of the highly industrialised Ruhr-region. These differences cannot be explained by the variables recorded in this study and deserve further investigation. The study centre in the UK was significantly associated with excessive polypharmacy compared to the study centre Germany 1 in the multivariable analysis. A sensitivity analysis showed that the UK was significantly associated with excessive polypharmacy compared to all other centres. Interestingly, the univariable analysis showed a slightly divergent result which was not significant (OR 0.92; 95% CI 0.70–1.22).

The patients in Germany 1 seemed to be frailer and had more diagnoses compared to the patients in the UK. In multivariable analysis the UK resulted in having more excessive polypharmacy. A reversal of effect can result due to the adjustment in the multivariable model. A possible explanation could be the "Quality and Outcomes Framework" (QOF) introduced in 2004 in the UK, which set financial incentives for certain performance indicators (pay-for-performance). Among these were indicators that relate to chronic conditions [44], some of them directly naming the prescription of certain drugs while other indicators indirectly entailed drug treatment in order to reach the targets [45]. Studies observed rising prescription rates of drugs indicated by QOF around the time when the framework was implemented, such as

lipid-regulating drugs, renin-angiotensin system drugs [45], ß-blockers or antiplatelet therapy [46].

Implications

Understanding the health characteristics of an aged population taking several drugs, and investigating factors influencing excessive polypharmacy is highly relevant in times when the geriatric population is growing. This study helps to develop targeted strategies to reduce polypharmacy by identifying factors contributing to excessive polypharmacy. Physicians should especially pay attention to their frail, obese patients that have > 8 diagnoses, check whether all medications are necessary, evidence based and appropriate, and whether there are relevant interactions. To do so, GPs should perform medication reviews for their patients with excessive polypharmacy on a regular basis to optimise these patients' medication. They should allocate extra time to care for these complex patients which needs to be reimbursed by the health care system.

Strengths and limitations

The major strength of our study is that we examined a very large sample of older patients representing several different health care settings/countries. We collected various parameters in this geriatric study population which gave us a comprehensive overview of demographic, clinical and functional status, and recorded the frailty level to distinguish between the fitter and the less fit ones. A major limitation of our study is that its cross-sectional design does not allow conclusions on causality. Further limitations are that the health-related quality of life was self-reported and all variables in the eCRF were reported by the GP, by practice staff or by a clinical research nurse. Even though instructions to record patient data were the same throughout all settings, we do not know whether the documentation of variables differs in different settings. True drug consumption is difficult to assess. We instructed the GPs to talk to their patients about all drugs they are taking. However, we were not able to verify drug consumption. Also, in this cross-sectional analysis, only patients were analysed who were recruited according to the inclusion criteria of the PRIMA-eDS trial. We therefore could only investigate patient characteristics associated with excessive polypharmacy in comparison to less excessive polypharmacy as patients without polypharmacy were not included in the trial. Furthermore, external characteristics e.g. of the prescribers could not be taken into account, and we did not judge whether medication intake was appropriate or not.

A further limitation of this study is that multiple relationships between variables exist. Multicollinearity is the cause of conspicuous differences between univariable and multivariable analysis. The interpretation for the affected variables should be regarded with caution. Noticeable correlations were found for the relationship between the research centre and the educational level (Cramer's $V = 0.48$), or the number of diagnoses (Cramer's $V = 0.40$) respectively, as well as between frailty, the two SF-12 scales (physical health composite score Cramer's $V = 0.20$ and mental health composite score Cramer's $V = 0.33$) and age (Cramer's $V = 0.22$).

The physical and the mental health composite scores as well as frailty were identified as risk factors in both univariable and multivariable analysis, but the ORs are smaller in multivariable analysis because of the dependencies. Frailty and health-related quality of life are closely associated [47], still we retained these variables in our analysis as they measure different concepts.

In univariable analysis, age was not significantly related to polypharmacy. It could be that there is a connection of the variable age with information about the condition of the patient, such as frailty, health-related quality of life, and diagnoses. Frailty [48], lower health-related quality of life [49], and a high number of diagnoses [50] are more common in old age. On the other hand, these factors increase the likelihood of excessive polypharmacy regardless of age [33, 50, 51]. Therefore, the positive effect of high age may become more apparent when adjusting for these factors.

Problematic is the variable "research centre", which significantly increases the associations found after adjustment for UK/Manchester. This is mainly attributable to the consideration of the number of diagnoses. After adjustment for this variable, the OR increases from 1.10 to 1.71. We did not want to give up the number of diagnoses as an independent variable, as in the literature this is reported as an important risk factor. The variable "research centre" also

seemed essential for the model, since this variable represents a variety of influences, such as the quality of the data collection, country-specific features and so on. Yet, it must be regarded with caution.

Conclusion

Our data suggest that frailty, multimorbidity, obesity as well as low physical and mental health status may be risk factors for excessive polypharmacy. Very old age appears to be a protective factor. Sex, educational level, and smoking are not associated with excessive polypharmacy. To avoid excessive polypharmacy with its possibly unfavourable effects, physicians should carefully review the appropriateness of medication, especially in multimorbid, obese and frail patients.

Abbreviations
ATC: Anatomical Therapeutic Chemical; BMI: Body mass index; CI: Confidence interval; GP: General practitioner; OR: Odds ratio; PRIMA-eDS: Polypharmacy in chronic diseases: Reduction of Inappropriate Medication and Adverse drug events in older populations by electronic Decision Support; QOF: Quality and Outcomes Framework; SD: Standard deviation; UK: United Kingdom

Acknowledgements
We would like to express our gratitude to all participating GPs and patients. Furthermore, we would like to thank the PRIMA-eDS team for their support in collecting data.

Funding
This study is funded by the 7th framework programme of the European Union, theme Health-2012-Innovation-1-2.2.2-2, grant agreement no. 305388–2.

Authors' contributions
AR and AS conceptualised the study. ED, AE, TJ, SK, CL, IK, JM, GP, AR, and AV were involved in collecting data. RKM and UST performed the analysis. AR drafted the manuscript. ED, AE, TJ, SK, RKM, CL, IK, JM, GP, AS, UST, and AV critically reviewed the manuscript. All authors read and approved the final manuscript.

Ethics approval and consent to participate
The PRIMA-eDS study has been approved by the five local ethics committees: 1. Ethikkomission der Universität Witten/Herdecke, 3 December 2013, ref. 103/2013; 2. NRES Committee North West Greater Manchester East, 6 June 2014, ref. 14/NW/0197; 3. Ethikkommission für das Bundesland Salzburg, 15 September 2013, ref. 08.04.2014 (415-E/1509/20–2014); 4. Ethikkommission der Universitätsmedizin Rostock, 3 February 2014, ref. A 2014–0020; and 5. Comitato etico di Belluno (Azienda ULSS), 19 June 2013, ref. 305,388–2. Furthermore, all participants provided written informed consent.

Competing interests
The authors declare that they have no competing interests.

Author details

[1]Institute of General Practice and Family Medicine, Faculty of Health, Witten/Herdecke University, Alfred-Herrhausen-Str. 50, 58448 Witten, Germany. [2]Department of Medical Informatics, Biometry and Epidemiology, Ruhr University, Universitätsstr. 105, 44789 Bochum, Germany. [3]Institute of General Practice, Rostock University Medical Center, Doberaner Str. 142, 18057 Rostock, Germany. [4]NIHR School of Primary Care Research, University of Manchester, Oxford Road 176, M13 9PL, Manchester, UK. [5]Centre for Primary Care, NIHR School of Primary Care Research, University of Manchester, Oxford Road M13 9PL, Manchester, UK. [6]Duodecim Medical Publications Ltd., Kaivokatu 10 A, 00100 Helsinki, Finland. [7]South Tyrolean Academy of General Practice, Wangergasse 18, 39100 Bolzano, Italy.

References

1. Eurostat. Population structure and ageing. 2016. http://ec.europa.eu/eurostat/statistics-explained/index.php/Population_structure_and_ageing#Further_Eurostat_information.
2. Halvorsen KH, Selbaek G, Ruths S. Trends in potentially inappropriate medication prescribing to nursing home patients: comparison of three cross-sectional studies. Pharmacoepidemiol Drug Saf. 2017;26:192–200. https://doi.org/10.1002/pds.4142 .
3. Tsoi CS, Chow JY, Choi KS, Li H-W, Nie JX, Tracy CS, et al. Medical characteristics of the oldest old: retrospective chart review of patients aged 85+ in an academic primary care Centre. BMC Res Notes. 2014;7:340. https://doi.org/10.1186/1756-0500-7-340 .
4. Wauters M, Elseviers M, Vaes B, Degryse J, Dalleur O, Vander Stichele R, et al. Polypharmacy in a Belgian cohort of community-dwelling oldest old (80+). Acta Clin Belg. 2016;71:158–66. https://doi.org/10.1080/17843286.2016.1148298 .
5. Junius-Walker U, Theile G, Hummers-Pradier E. Prevalence and predictors of polypharmacy among older primary care patients in Germany. Fam Pract. 2007;24:14–9. https://doi.org/10.1093/fampra/cml067.
6. Herr M, Robine J-M, Pinot J, Arvieu J-J, Ankri J. Polypharmacy and frailty: prevalence, relationship, and impact on mortality in a French sample of 2350 old people. Pharmacoepidemiol Drug Saf. 2015;24:637–46. https://doi.org/10.1002/pds.3772 .
7. Hovstadius B, Petersson G, Hellström L, Ericson L. Trends in inappropriate drug therapy prescription in the elderly in Sweden from 2006 to 2013: assessment using national indicators. Drugs Aging. 2014;31:379–86. https://doi.org/10.1007/s40266-014-0165-5 .
8. Guerriero F, Orlando V, Tari DU, Di Giorgio A, Cittadini A, Trifiro G, Menditto E. How healthy is community-dwelling elderly population? Results from Southern Italy Transl Med UniSa. 2015;13:59–64.
9. Bushardt RL, Massey EB, Simpson TW, Ariail JC, Simpson KN. Polypharmacy: misleading, but manageable. Clin Interv Aging. 2008;3:383–9.
10. Masnoon N, Shakib S, Kalisch-Ellett L, Caughey GE. What is polypharmacy? A systematic review of definitions. BMC Geriatr. 2017;17:230. https://doi.org/10.1186/s12877-017-0621-2 .
11. Guthrie B, Makubate B, Hernandez-Santiago V, Dreischulte T. The rising tide of polypharmacy and drug-drug interactions: population database analysis 1995-2010. BMC Med. 2015;13:74. https://doi.org/10.1186/s12916-015-0322-7 .
12. Corsonello A, Pedone C, Incalzi RA. Age-related pharmacokinetic and pharmacodynamic changes and related risk of adverse drug reactions. Curr Med Chem. 2010;17:571–84.
13. Fried TR, O'Leary J, Towle V, Goldstein MK, Trentalange M, Martin DK. Health outcomes associated with polypharmacy in community-dwelling older adults: a systematic review. J Am Geriatr Soc. 2014;62:2261–72. https://doi.org/10.1111/jgs.13153 .
14. Agostini JV, Han L, Tinetti ME. The relationship between number of medications and weight loss or impaired balance in older adults. J Am Geriatr Soc. 2004;52:1719–23. https://doi.org/10.1111/j.1532-5415.2004.52467.x .
15. Wimmer BC, Cross AJ, Jokanovic N, Wiese MD, George J, Johnell K, et al. Clinical outcomes associated with medication regimen complexity in older people: a systematic review. J Am Geriatr Soc. 2017;65:747–53. https://doi.org/10.1111/jgs.14682 .
16. Payne RA, Abel GA, Avery AJ, Mercer SW, Roland MO. Is polypharmacy always hazardous? A retrospective cohort analysis using linked electronic health records from primary and secondary care. Br J Clin Pharmacol. 2014; 77:1073 82. https://doi.org/10.1111/bcp.12292

17. The King's Fund. Polypharmacy and medicines optimisation: Making it safe and sound. 2013.
18. Corsonello A, Pedone C, Corica F, Incalzi RA. On behalf of the Gruppo Italiano di. Polypharmacy in elderly patients at discharge from the acute care hospital. Ther Clin Risk Manag. 2007;3:197–203. https://doi.org/10.2147/tcrm.2007.3.1.197.
19. Haider SI, Johnell K, Weitoft GR, Thorslund M, Fastbom J. The influence of educational level on polypharmacy and inappropriate drug use: a register-based study of more than 600,000 older people. J Am Geriatr Soc. 2009;57:62–9. https://doi.org/10.1111/j.1532-5415.2008.02040.x .
20. Jyrkka J, Enlund H, Korhonen MJ, Sulkava R, Hartikainen S. Patterns of drug use and factors associated with polypharmacy and excessive polypharmacy in elderly persons: results of the Kuopio 75+ study: a cross-sectional analysis. Drugs Aging. 2009;26:493–503. https://doi.org/10.2165/00002512-200926060-00006 .
21. Kim H-A, Shin J-Y, Kim M-H, Park B-J. Prevalence and predictors of polypharmacy among Korean elderly. PLoS One. 2014;9:e98043. https://doi.org/10.1371/journal.pone.0098043 .
22. Mayer S, Osterle A. Socioeconomic determinants of prescribed and non-prescribed medicine consumption in Austria. Eur J Pub Health. 2015;25:597–603. https://doi.org/10.1093/eurpub/cku179 .
23. O'Dwyer M, Peklar J, McCallion P, McCarron M, Henman MC. Factors associated with polypharmacy and excessive polypharmacy in older people with intellectual disability differ from the general population: a cross-sectional observational nationwide study. BMJ Open. 2016;6:e010505. https://doi.org/10.1136/bmjopen-2015-010505 .
24. Onder G, Liperoti R, Fialova D, Topinkova E, Tosato M, Danese P, et al. Polypharmacy in nursing home in Europe: results from the SHELTER study. J Gerontol A Biol Sci Med Sci. 2012;67:698–704. https://doi.org/10.1093/gerona/glr233 .
25. Walckiers D, van der Heyden J, Tafforeau J. Factors associated with excessive polypharmacy in older people. Arch Public Health. 2015;73:50. https://doi.org/10.1186/s13690-015-0095-7 .
26. Sonnichsen A, Trampisch US, Rieckert A, Piccoliori G, Vogele A, Flamm M, et al. Polypharmacy in chronic diseases-reduction of inappropriate medication and adverse drug events in older populations by electronic decision support (PRIMA-eDS): study protocol for a randomized controlled trial. Trials. 2016;17:57. https://doi.org/10.1186/s13063-016-1177-8 .
27. Rockwood K, Song X, MacKnight C, Bergman H, Hogan DB, McDowell I, Mitnitski A. A global clinical measure of fitness and frailty in elderly people. CMAJ. 2005;173:489–95. https://doi.org/10.1503/cmaj.050051 .
28. Maruish MEE. User's manual for the SF-12v2 health survey. 3rd ed. Lincoln, RI: QualityMetric Incorporated; 2012.
29. OECD. Classifying Educational Programmes – Manual for ISCED-97 Implementation in OECD Countries – 1999 Edition. OECD. 1999.
30. World Health Organization. The Anatomical Therapeutic Chemical Classification System with Defined Daily Doses (ATC/DDD). http://www.who.int/classifications/atcddd/en/. Accessed 14 Feb 2018.
31. World Health Organization. Classification of Diseases (ICD). http://www.who.int/classifications/icd/en/. Accessed 14 Feb 2018.
32. Renom-Guiteras A, Meyer G, Thürmann PA. The EU(7)-PIM list: a list of potentially inappropriate medications for older people consented by experts from seven European countries. Eur J Clin Pharmacol. 2015;71:861–75. https://doi.org/10.1007/s00228-015-1860-9 .
33. Herr M, Sirven N, Grondin H, Pichetti S, Sermet C. Frailty, polypharmacy, and potentially inappropriate medications in old people: findings in a representative sample of the French population. Eur J Clin Pharmacol. 2017; https://doi.org/10.1007/s00228-017-2276-5 .
34. Saum K-U, Schöttker B, Meid AD, Holleczek B, Haefeli WE, Hauer K, Brenner HI. Polypharmacy associated with frailty in older people? Results from the ESTHER cohort study. J Am Geriatr Soc. 2017;65:e27–32. https://doi.org/10.1111/jgs.14718.
35. Morley JE. Inappropriate drug prescribing and polypharmacy are major causes of poor outcomes in long-term care. J Am Med Dir Assoc. 2014;15:780–2. https://doi.org/10.1016/j.jamda.2014.09.003 .
36. Morley JE, Vellas B, van Kan GA, Anker SD, Bauer JM, Bernabei R, et al. Frailty consensus: a call to action. J Am Med Dir Assoc. 2013;14:392–7. https://doi.org/10.1016/j.jamda.2013.03.022 .
37. Veronese N, Stubbs B, Noale M, Solmi M, Pilotto A, Vaona A, et al.

Polypharmacy is associated with higher frailty risk in older people: an 8-year longitudinal cohort study. J Am Med Dir Assoc. 2017;18:624–8. https://doi.org/10.1016/j.jamda.2017.02.009 .

38. Counterweight Project Team. The impact of obesity on drug prescribing in primary care. Br J Gen Pract. 2005;55:743–9.

39. Amarya S, Singh K, Sabharwal M. Health consequences of obesity in the elderly. J Clinical Gerontology Geriatrics. 2014;5:63–7. https://doi.org/10.1016/j.jcgg.2014.01.004 .

40. Lee SJ, Leipzig RM, Walter LC. Incorporating lag time to benefit into prevention decisions for older adults. JAMA. 2013;310:2609–10. https://doi.org/10.1001/jama.2013.282612 .

41. Tinetti ME, McAvay GJ, Fried TR, Allore HG, Salmon JC, Foody JM, et al. Health outcome priorities among competing cardiovascular, fall injury, and medication-related symptom outcomes. J Am Geriatr Soc. 2008;56:1409–16. https://doi.org/10.1111/j.1532-5415.2008.01815.x .

42. Schuling J, Gebben H, Veehof LJG, Haaijer-Ruskamp FM. Deprescribing medication in very elderly patients with multimorbidity: the view of Dutch GPs. A qualitative study. BMC Fam Pract. 2012;13:56. https://doi.org/10.1186/1471-2296-13-56 .

43. Baker DP, Leon J, Smith Greenaway EG, Collins J, Movit M. The education effect on population health: a reassessment. Popul Dev Rev. 2011;37:307–32. https://doi.org/10.1111/j.1728-4457.2011.00412.x .

44. Roland M. Linking physicians' pay to the quality of care–a major experiment in the United Kingdom. N Engl J Med. 2004;351:1448–54. https://doi.org/10.1056/NEJMhpr041294 .

45. MacBride-Stewart SP, Elton R, Walley T. Do quality incentives change prescribing patterns in primary care? An observational study in Scotland. Fam Pract. 2008;25:27–32. https://doi.org/10.1093/fampra/cmm074 .

46. McGovern MP, Boroujerdi MA, Taylor MW, Williams DJ, Hannaford PC, Lefevre KE, Simpson CR. The effect of the UK incentive-based contract on the management of patients with coronary heart disease in primary care. Fam Pract. 2008;25:33–9. https://doi.org/10.1093/fampra/cmm073.

47. Kojima G, Iliffe S, Jivraj S, Walters K. Association between frailty and quality of life among community-dwelling older people: a systematic review and meta-analysis. J Epidemiol Community Health. 2016;70:716–21. https://doi.org/10.1136/jech-2015-206717 .

48. Frailty, polypharmacy and deprescribing. Drug Ther Bull 2016;54:69–72. doi: https://doi.org/10.1136/dtb.2016.6.0408 .

49. Eisele M, Kaduszkiewicz H, König H-H, Lange C, Wiese B, Prokein J, et al. Determinants of health-related quality of life in older primary care patients: results of the longitudinal observational AgeCoDe study. Br J Gen Pract. 2015;65:e716–23. https://doi.org/10.3399/bjgp15X687337 .

50. Puth M-T, Weckbecker K, Schmid M, Münster E. Prevalence of multimorbidity in Germany: impact of age and educational level in a cross-sectional study on 19,294 adults. BMC Public Health. 2017;17:826. https://doi.org/10.1186/s12889-017-4833-3 .

51. Montiel-Luque A, Núñez-Montenegro AJ, Martín-Aurioles E, Canca-Sánchez JC, Toro-Toro MC, González-Correa JA. Medication-related factors associated with health-related quality of life in patients older than 65 years with polypharmacy. PLoS One. 2017; https://doi.org/10.1371/journal.pone.0171320 .

16

Views of family physicians on heterosexual sexual function in older adults

Inbar Levkovich[1]*[ID], Ateret Gewirtz-Meydan[2], Khaled Karkabi[3] and Liat Ayalon[2]

Abstract

Background: Sexual functioning among older adults has received little attention in research and clinical practice, although it is an integral part of old age. As older adults tend to consume health services and to visit family physicians more frequently, these care-providers serve as gatekeepers in the case of sexual concerns. The present study evaluated the perceptions of family physicians regarding sexuality in older adults.

Method: Qualitative interviews with 16 family physicians were conducted. We used in-depth, semi-structured interviews.

Results: Three main themes emerged: 1. Family physicians described having difficulty in raising questions about sexuality to older patients. 2. Family physicians tended towards the biological side of the spectrum, focusing on the patient's medical problem and asking physiological questions. 3. Family physicians mainly related to medication administered to their male patients, whereas a minority also described the guidance they provided to older individuals and couples.

Conclusions: The study shows that family physicians tend not to initiate discourse with older patients on sexuality, but rather discuss sexuality mostly in conjunction with other medical conditions. Implications for research and practice are discussed.

Keywords: Sexuality, Primary care, Psychogeriatrics, Health aging, Aging

Background

Sexuality is an important part of human health and well-being over the life cycle and in old age [1–3]. Sexuality represents people's sexual interest in and attraction to others as well as their capacity to have erotic experiences [4]. An individual's sexuality includes his or her attitudes, values, knowledge and behaviors [5]. Sexuality is different from sex. Sexuality is a much broader term, has many components, and includes much more than sexual intercourse [4, 6]. Sex, on the other hand, is a biological construct that encapsulates the anatomical, physiological, genetic, and hormonal variations that exist in species [6]. "Older adults" are traditionally defined as being over the age of 65 [7, 8]. The classified respondents between the aged 65–74 as "young old", aged 75–84 as "old old", and those aged 85 and older as "oldest old" [7, 8].

Sexual function and sexual satisfaction among the older adult population have received little attention in

research and clinical practice, although they are an integral part of old age and despite the fact that this age group may be characterized by sexual changes [9, 10]. Studies have shown that many older adults are interested in engaging in sex and are sexually active in their later years [11]. Surveys conducted in several countries have found that older adults attest to the importance of sexual activity in their lives and the sense of security it provides [12–14]. A study in which 3000 older adults were interviewed found that although the level of interest in sexuality was lower among older adults, 59% of participants aged 75–85 reported the importance of sexuality to their lives [11].

Studies indicate that the prevalence of symptoms and complaints increases with age - as much as double in comparison to young people [15]. It was also found that as age advances, there is a diminished interest in sexuality, and sexual activity is less frequent in comparison with younger ages [11, 16]. In interviews with 44 people aged 50–92, it was found that adults over 70 were less interested in sexuality in comparison with younger adults in this age range [16]. In a cohort study spanning

* Correspondence: inbar.lev2@gmail.com; inbar.lev@gmail.com
[1]The Division of Family Medicine, Department of Family Medicine, The Ruth & Bruce Rappaport Faculty of Medicine, Technion-Israel Institute of Technology, 6 Hashachaf St., Bat-Galim, 35013 Haifa, Israel
Full list of author information is available at the end of the article

10 years, data from 3032 respondents aged 25–74 were analyzed; the results showed that, among men, sexual interest remained stable across age groups whereas women's interest declined. Thus, the literature suggests that desire does not always decline as men and women age [17]. It is, rather, a complex component which is influenced by many variables [13].

One such variable concerns physiological and biological changes that occur with age.

It has been suggested that it is not age that causes the decline in sexual activity, but rather the natural physiological changes and common health problems that accompany older adults [16]. Hormonal changes associated with older adults are mainly reflected in the slowing down of sexual response and a decrease in the intensity of sexual arousal and pleasure. Among women, a decline in estrogen levels, which is characteristic of the post-menopausal period, causes atrophy (e.g, dryness, burning, dyspareunia) of the external female organs and a decrease in orgasm intensity [9]. As a result, women experience post-menopausal emotional changes [18]. The most prevalent sexual problems among women were low desire (43%), difficulties related to vaginal lubrication (39%), and inability to climax (34%) [17]. Women expressed less interest in non-sexual activities such as holding hands, kissing, hugging, and in masturbating or sexual activity [19]. After the age of 50, more women (56.6%) reported a cessation in sexual activity at some time, due to various reasons compared to men (16.6%), who remained sexually active (83.4%) [19].

In men, free testosterone decline causes a slowdown in response to sexual arousal, which consequently leads to a need for stronger, longer-lasting physical stimulation in order to achieve an erection. Penile erection is not as firm as in younger age groups, the amount of sperm lessens and there is a decrease in the intensity of ejaculation. In addition, there may be a decrease in sex drive [20] and endocrinal changes ('male menopause') [21]. There are many biomedical reasons for erectile dysfunction (ED), such as medication [22], diseases and surgeries [23], diabetes [24], and cardiovascular problems [25]. However, contrary to general opinion, Mazur and others [26] were unable to find a direct link between sexual desire and low free testosterone levels or depression in older men.

Although these changes are valid and likely affect the sexual function of older men and women, other factors are also important. The biopsychosocial model [17, 18] supports the approach that biological, psychological (including thoughts, emotions, and behaviors) and social factors affect one's health condition. The model promotes the perception of the human being as a whole, whereby the body and mind are interconnected and are in constant interaction with the social environment [27, 28]. Hence, in addition to medical conditions and health problems, emotional factors, such as depression and anxiety, affect sexual

activity at any age, but increase in frequency as aging progresses [22]. Meaningful life events such as retirement, death of a loved one, absence of a spouse and loss of privacy following relocation to an institutionalized setting are some of the causes of sexual disorders among older adults [2, 21].

Healthcare providers, including physicians, nurses, social workers, and psychologists, are required to understand the complexity of the psychological and biological factors that affect sexual function in old age, in order to help older adults cope with issues concerning sexuality [21]. Because older adults tend to consume health services and to visit family physicians more frequently [29, 30], these care-providers serve as gatekeepers in the case of sexual concerns [29, 30]. Little research has been conducted about older people's experiences of talking to family physicians about sexual function. Most participants said they did not discuss sexual issues with their healthcare providers, and the physician did not raise the issue [3]. For those individuals who did discuss sexual with their healthcare providers, negative and stigmatizing responses were common [31]. Barriers to discussing sexual issues with one's physician include personal embarrassment, lack of knowledge and awareness, and fear of wasting the doctor's time [16, 32]. Others said they did not consider sexual dysfunction to be a medical problem or a problem that could be treated by a doctor [32].

Other barriers to discussing sexual issues with older adults concern the physicians. Studies reporting family physicians' knowledge of sexuality in old age were inconsistent. Whereas some studies indicate appropriate or adequate knowledge, others show limited knowledge among family physicians in this field [33–35]. Moreover, the average medical staff's personal sense of comfort and confidence to discuss old-age sexuality with patients is low [36]. Additional barriers to discussing sexual concerns are lack of time, lack of communication skills and a general desire to avoid the subject [33, 37]. Health care professionals often assume that sexual function in older adults is beyond the scope of their expertise [4]. For instance, family physicians discuss sexual issues more often with young people than with older adults, and may regard sexuality as an intimate, private subject that should not be discussed in old age [38–40], thereby expressing ageist attitudes towards older adults.

An understanding of the impact of sexual orientation on older adults' life experiences may assist healthcare professionals in their efforts to determine appropriate interventions. Until recently, the literature has tended to disregard the sexual orientation of older adults. For example, many studies were framed from a heteronormative perspective, while very few studies have explored older lesbian, gay, bisexual, transgender, queer and intersex individuals (LGBTQ&I) [41]. Many LGBTQ&I older adults have built vibrant communities and a sensibility that they can count on each other [41]. Many LGBTQ&I older adults have also created close, intimate families of choice, comprised of loved ones, including current and former partners and friends [42]. In the Gay and Gray Project [43], over three-quarters of the respondents reported having active sexual lives and over half felt their sexuality had an important positive impact on their lives. Yet, population estimates suggest that one-third to one-half of older gay and bisexual men live alone, without adequate services or support [44, 45]. In the CAP project, 61% of the gay and 53% of the bisexual male participants reported experiencing loneliness [44]. Older LGBTQ&I adults face unique issues that can impede their well-being [44]. In a mixed methods study, participants identified that both ageism and heterosexism presented challenges when attempting to secure adequate housing and receive emotional support. Legal issues were another identified source of primary concern for the elderly with regard to a lack of legal protection for "married" same sex couples compared to opposite sex couples [46]. Family physicians may ignore LGBTQ&I needs and preferences due to discomfort, uncertainty or lack of LGBTQ&I -specific health knowledge [47–51]. This might reinforce heteronormative status quo and stereotypes [52].

Because family physicians are the main *gatekeepers* for a variety of medical and psychosocial issues concerning older adults [53] and in light of the lack of empirical knowledge concerning the way physicians perceive sexuality in older adults, the goal of this qualitative study was to investigate the perceptions of family physicians regarding sexuality in older adults.

Method

The study used a qualitative-phenomenological approach [54]. This approach attempts to obtain an in-depth understanding of the phenomenon by entering the world and experiences of the participants. The qualitative-phenomenological research approach was chosen to enable family physicians to tell their stories and give meaning to their experiences. The descriptive power of this approach allows for an in-depth understanding of the family physicians' perceptions of sexuality in older adults. Such research is based on small samples composed of a limited number of 'information-rich' informants, where depth is exchanged for representativeness [55, 56].

Sample and population

This study was supported by a grant from the Israel National Institute for Health Policy Research No. 16/2016/א. The present study focused on a sample of family physicians. Recruitment occurred via emails sent to family

physicians displayed in a variety of health clinics. Physicians were offered to participate in the study after receiving a comprehensive explanation of the study's purpose. Participants were 16 family physicians, aged 36–64. The majority were born in Israel; 13 worked in 'Clalit Health Services' and three worked in 'Maccabi Healthcare Services', the largest and second-largest health funds in Israel, respectively. Half of the participants were women. Seven physicians worked in urban clinics; the other nine worked in rural clinics.

Instrument

The data were collected using in-depth, semi-structured interviews. We designed the interview guide with questions to allow the participants to share their stories openly. The interview guide included several questions: "Tell me about sexual function in older adults;" "What are your reactions (thoughts, feelings, behaviors) when patients consult you about sexual function in older adults?"; "How do you handle sexual dysfunction in older adults?"; "What are the advantages and disadvantages of the treatment given to alleviate sexual dysfunction?"; "How do sexual difficulties among older adults differ from those of younger adults?" The interviewer encouraged physicians to narrate their experiences in their own words [57] Table 1.

Procedure

The Meir Medical Center Hospital Ethics Committee approved study No. 0262–16-MMC. The researchers identified the participants and requested their written consent to participate in the study. Prior to conducting the interviews, interviewers were required to undergo a reflection process [58], including the ability to reflect on the identities, social locations, assumptions, and life experiences they bring to the research endeavor, along with their interactions with interviewees. For example, the interviewers were asked how they identify themselves in relation to the subject - sexuality in older adults – and were requested to express their emotions, attitudes and opinions. Strong relational skills and competence in self-reflexivity helped to ensure that interviewers were authentic, attentive, able to critically examine their own reactions and responses, and address any awkward moments that might arise in the interview interaction.

The researchers identified the participants and requested their written consent to participate in the study. The participants then underwent an in-depth interview in their clinics or homes. Interviews were conducted in Hebrew, and lasted approximately 1 hour. Each interview was tape-recorded and later transcribed verbatim. At the end of the all the interviews, we performed the data analysis.

Table 1 Interview questions posed to family physicians for the qualitative analysis

1	How do you define sexuality?
2	Tell me about sexual function in older adults.
3	Do the reasons for engaging in intimate relations differ between young adults and older adults?
4	In your opinion, what reasons might elderly individuals have for refraining from engaging in intimate relations?
5	In your opinion, which factors might influence the levels of sexual function and sexual satisfaction in older adults?
6	How do you think society/the media perceives sexuality among the elderly?
7	How does treatment of sexual function differ between younger adults and older adults?
8	Tell me about contacting/referring patients to different specialists in relation to sexual function difficulties among the elderly.
9	What are the advantages/disadvantages of contacting different specialists in relation to sexual dysfunction in older adults?
10	In your opinion, how is it possible to create open lines of communication about sexual function between elderly patients and their physicians?

Data analysis

We used content analysis in this study. Where appropriate, we paraphrased and generalized respondents' statements. We organized similar passages by topic in order to identify individual influential factors, and then combined similar factors into major categories, to identify the main themes. Content analysis is used to unobtrusively explore large amounts of textual information, so as to determine trends and patterns of words used their frequency, and their relationships. Data analysis consisted of the following stages: 1. We first read all the data several times, to achieve immersion and obtain a sense of the text as a whole. 2. Open coding: The researcher (I.L.) first read each interview transcript line-by-line, jotting down notes to capture and identify initial units of meaning emerging from the data, and to allow the subthemes and their names to flow from the data [55]. 4. The researcher (L.A.) then reviewed the larger themes and discussed them with I.L. 4. Axial coding: The researchers gradually detected context and content-related associations between themes and sub-themes. Then, they compared all of the interviews to consolidate meaning and named the themes. Next, the researchers examined the interrelationships among the initial codes and sorted them into higher-order theoretical codes [55]. 5. Integration: The core themes that emerged from the data were reordered conceptually and placed back into context, enabling the analysis and integration of large amounts of data and the generation of abstractions and interpretations [59].

Reflecting on our experiences, we established biases, and prejudices regarding sexuality, older adults and family physicians [60, 61] during all the study's stages. The researcher (I.L.) interviewed the family physicians, sharing her thoughts and feelings which arose during the interviews and data analysis. For example: initiated by some family physicians' attitudes about sexuality in old age, she expressed a feeling of unfairness concerning the way women are treated by family physicians with regard to sexuality.

Results

Analysis of the qualitative interviews identified three main themes. The themes can be placed on a continuum of psychosocial factors at one end vs. biological factors at the opposite end, with most physicians leaning towards the biological end of the continuum as they initiate conversations with patients, perform diagnoses or recommend treatment for sexual dysfunction in older adults.

The first theme addressed the difficulty of asking questions related to sexuality: **"I hear nothing because I ask nothing"; family physicians refrain from initiating a conversation about sexuality with older adults** - Family physicians described having difficulty in raising questions about sexuality with their older patients, due to work overload and the lack of time; they also felt that this issue was not their top priority when talking with these patients and that questions concerning such intimate issues might harm their relationship with the patient. In those cases where they felt at ease asking questions about sexuality, it was done when sexuality was seen as being part of a variety of medical conditions, so that the biological-medical model guided them. **The second theme dealt with the challenge involved in the diagnosis: "Trying to understand where the difficulty lies"** - Family physicians described that most sexuality-related visits were made by males and the main complaint was erectile dysfunction. A variety of diagnostic questions focusing on the physiological aspects were described, including a physical examination. Only a small number of women turned to their family physicians; some came to receive medication for their husband or described gynaecological problems, from which a discourse on sexual function ensued. The third theme that emerged was: **"There are medications that can be offered";** treatment of sexual function in older adults - Family physicians mainly described medication administered to men, and a minority also described counselling, which included individual or couple's guidance to coordinate mutual expectations, encourage intimacy and referral for further treatment. However, the predominant view was that the main treatment which can be offered to patients is pharmacological.

Theme 1: "I hear nothing because I ask nothing"; family physicians refrain from initiating a conversation about sexuality with older adults.

Most of the family physicians who were interviewed said they do not ask older patients about sexual functioning and sexual difficulties on a regular basis. Many family physicians explained that the focus of the doctor-patient encounter is medical and other topics receive a lower priority. Much of the physician's attention is focused on illnesses, medication and diagnosis; therefore, the subject of sexual problems is often perceived as being less significant. Some family physicians emphasized the importance of the subject, but noted that in regard to older adults, a range of higher-priority medical issues require attention and should be examined. These physicians expressed a preference for the biological approach within the model, which attributes a rather limited importance to the psychosocial parts:

"I feel that it (sexual dysfunction) is very important, but it always gets lost among all the other issues and diseases and things that need to be done... the mammography and the other tests, and the drugs... it is very often neglected". (Family physician 5)

Family physicians have reported certain limitations that prevent them from asking about sexual function: workload, time constraints, and fear of offending patients were mentioned as the main factors. The physicians described the health system as demanding and the available resources as significantly inadequate. Anger, frustration, and even despair were expressed regarding the limited time available for the physician-patient interaction. In addition, physicians wondered whether questions about sexuality would not be perceived as an insensitive violation of the physician-patient relationship, with little time dedicated to each session, and the physician's sense of inability to create the necessary intimacy and closeness needed to facilitate a discourse on these personal issues:

"If someone makes an appointment, waits for 2 weeks and has a list of four or five medical problems, while other people are waiting outside, and we barely have 10 minutes, then how can I casually ask: How is your sexual function?" (Family physician 2)

Most family physicians explained that discourse with older patients on sexual function and satisfaction usually takes place with those patients who suffer from chronic disorders. The catalyst for the conversation is the patient's state of health, the common illnesses for which

the patient came in or the medication he or she takes or is expected to take. Because of the barriers to discussing the subject described by the physicians, a sense of relief and confidence was described when the conversation revolved around the physician's areas of strength, i.e., illnesses and medications, and those which he or she felt were within his or her field of expertise. These physicians tended towards the biological side of the model:

"Yesterday, I saw an older patient, who came in only because he wanted to stop taking his diabetes medication because his diabetes had stabilized, and he had been diabetic for a very long time. Incidentally, he also mentioned a prostate problem...he wanted to undergo a protein test, and this opened up a conversation on sexual function". (Family physician 6)

A minority of family physicians described the catalyst for sexual questions in older age not as the medical condition, but as the patient's emotional state. These physicians said that once they identify emotional distress or somatisation among patients, they ask them about sexual function. In their view, sexual dysfunction is not purely organic; it has emotional implications or may be caused by the patient's emotional distress. Emotional distress may contribute to sexual-function difficulties; therefore, questions and clarifications should be initiated on this issue as well. While these physicians emphasized the model's psychosocial aspects in the context of sexuality, they also described barriers which prevented them from asking directly and openly about sexual function, because they felt that such a conversation was less appropriate within the physician-patient encounter:

"A 70-year-old woman with a lot of somatization...and I could understand that much of it was related to the tension at home. But when I delicately tried to ask her whether anything might be bothering or troubling her daily, it [sexual functioning] didn't come up. I imagine it's a very difficult thing to talk about...so I didn't ask her directly about her sex life... I felt it would be too intrusive, invasive and painful". (Family physician 1)

Theme 2: "Trying to understand where the difficulty lies"; diagnosis of sexuality in older adults Diagnosis, which constitutes an essential component in patients' assessment, helps physicians focus on relevant clarification of the illness, e.g., the reason for referral to treatment, current symptoms, past illnesses, etc. Within the present research, family physicians described collecting diverse patients' diagnoses, along a biological-psychosocial continuum.

Most family physicians tended towards the biological end, preferring to focus on medical problems, and ask physiological questions, sometimes including a physical examination. The physicians described the manner in which they ask the patient which symptoms he or she is experiencing and for how long: Is it a libido problem or erectile dysfunction? Does he have a morning erection? Which medication(s) is he/she taking? What are his or her illnesses and risk factors? It seems physicians felt more at ease diagnosing on the basis of a variety of questions, similar to the way they diagnose any other illness, thoroughly and in a way which avoids dealing emotionally with sexual dysfunction:

> "So, I ask them what we're dealing with, how long...or what problems they have... If there are also urination problems, since that's more prostate-related, a clarification can be made in this direction...However, many times it's just the erection [problem]...either they don't have a morning erection, or the erection is too short". (Family physician 4)

Although most interviewees were more inclined towards the biological aspect, some showed a tendency towards the psychosocial aspect, examining the patient and his or her world as a whole, including family, marital and personal issues, which the patient brings from his or her world and may affect his or her condition.

A minority of the physicians focused on the patient's intimacy issues and checked whether the patient was in a relationship, having sex, whether any changes had occurred in the relationship, and which spouse complained about a difficulty. Their questions made room for exploring the medical and physiological aspects, although this was considered a secondary priority and came after a variety of generic questions. These physicians perceived the comprehensive clarification as being deep and thorough; some described a number of sessions in which they conducted a preliminary diagnosis and later invited the couple in order to ascertain a more complete idea of the situation, thereby eventually reaching the root of the problem. These physicians described the diagnosis as starting with questions on intimacy, rather than the patient's physiological state, and only afterwards asking about the patient's health condition, as needed:

> "I always start out by asking about the couple's intimacy, how they are together. Do they still sleep in the same bed? Are they still having sex? I do this gradually, in order to get an idea about their current status". (Family physician 6)

Theme 3: "There are medications that can be offered", treatment of sexual function in older adults.
Most family physicians reported perceiving treatment of sexual function in older adults as a pharmacological

treatment administered to men suffering from impotence. The physicians described a typical encounter in which the patient asks for medication on his or her own initiative or describes a related difficulty, followed by a short diagnosis, after which treatment is offered. The physicians discuss the treatment's advantages and disadvantages with the patient and make adjustments in case the patient is taking additional medication. With the exception of patients with complex problems, whose treatments include implants and injections, the physicians described the treatment as a one-time session, followed by the automatic prescription of medication:

> "Viagra and Cialis. ...Viagra isn't really a regular treatment. You can take it whenever you feel like it... but you have to know that you are about to have sex, so you need to take it ahead of time. You have to prepare. And even if a man doesn't have the desire, he'll still get an erection; and if he doesn't have sex it [the erection] will be maintained...Some other medications should be avoided, especially by coronary heart disease patients. You have to be a bit careful...". (Family physician 4)

Some family physicians stated that women seek treatment for sexual dysfunction in old age significantly less frequently than men. The treatment of women also focused on the biological aspect, including the prescription of medication and locally-applied ointments:

> "For women, local vaginal estrogen therapy is very effective. In cases of vaginal dryness and other complaints, I would suggest this treatment around menopause and up to a very old age – even to patients who haven't received it previously (why is this mentioned?). I also prescribe this treatment for patients aged 70 and up. This usually helps significantly. In many cases, once the physical complaints and symptoms improve, desire also increases". (Family physician 5)

A minority of the interviewed family physicians described care of patients with sexual dysfunction as a legitimate part of their role, advising couples to prolong foreplay and be more receptive to each other's needs, in an attempt to reduce the tension associated with penetration and reinforce intimacy. Some of the physicians described the difficulty of conducting these types of counseling sessions, claiming they are not qualified psychologists, and mentioning the short meeting time available in light of the patients' great needs. The physicians also said they usually postpone visits with patients with whom they would like to discuss the issue of sexual function to the end of the day, or ask them to schedule a double appointment, which will allow time for a more in-depth discussion:

"I talk about prolonging the foreplay, being more receptive to each other's needs... reducing the stress surrounding sexual function...placing more emphasis on intimacy, the needs of the other partner...and reducing the focus on penetration. Sex is not only penetration, there's a lot more between foreplay and penetration". (Family physician 12)

Referral to sexual therapy occurred in rare cases; physicians argued that most patients either are not interested or the physicians themselves do not suggest it. In more complex patients, such as those with implants and injections, physicians prescribed longer sessions, consultation with other specialists and referral to sexual therapy. Many physicians described the limitations of sexual therapy, in terms of the mobility of older adults: the distance between home and clinic and the high costs. Hence, most of the treatment options remain in the realm of the family physician.

Discussion

The study's objective was to expand the understanding of family physicians' perceptions regarding sexuality among older adults.

The current study shows that most family physicians do not initiate discourse on this subject and discuss sexuality mostly in relation to common illnesses. Most physicians tended to perform a diagnosis that focused on the physiological aspects, discussing the symptoms, prevalence of the disorder, medication, other illnesses, etc. A minority of physicians examined intimacy and marital relations as an integral part of the diagnosis. The proposed treatment entailed mostly drug therapy for men, while a small number of family physicians said they discussed the couple's sexual expectations and their difficulties, and attempted to reduce the stress associated with penetration.

The family physicians who participated in this study tended not to initiate a discussion on sexual matters with their older patients. This finding supports previous research that indicated medical staffs' low levels of self-confidence and personal comfort to discuss these issues [36]. The physicians described a large number of discourse barriers including lack of time, workload, and a feeling that this subject was beyond the scope of their expertise and was too intimate [37, 38]. Family physicians expressed frustration at the system's demand to meet various health measures; therefore, the issue of sexual function was pushed down to the bottom of the list. Family physicians are pressured to deliver an increasing number of preventive services, follow guidelines, engage in evidence-based practice, and deliver patient-centered care; they struggle with how much control they have over their time. Many older adults have more than one chronic disease and one of the greatest challenges for family physicians is the provision of optimal care for older adults with multiple chronic conditions.

When physicians initiated discourse with patients, it mainly revolved around common illnesses. Our study is supported by similar studies in which physicians preferred to discuss sexual dysfunction mainly in combination with old-age risk factors, e.g., hypertension and diabetes, in comparison with patients without risk factors [62]. Coronary heart disease, psychiatric disorders and psychological disorders were found to be disorders in which physicians turn to patients for evaluation of sexual function [63, 64]. It is possible that when the discourse takes place around the focal point of the physician's expertise, i.e., the physiological field, the family physician feels more confident in making a diagnosis and providing a satisfactory solution. Despite changes in the way older people view sexuality, when they face sexual problems significant barriers to seeking physicians' help have been identified [65]: some of which relate to the patient (e.g., embarrassment), some to the physician (e.g., ageist attitudes), and others to the geographical or cultural location of the individual (e.g., difficulty in accessing services). Some older people feel more comfortable talking about illness or medication than about their sexual dysfunction [20].

Most sexual complaints brought up in physician-patient discourse - whether through the initiative of the physician or the patient - are related to impotence in men. Consistently, according to the physicians, most patients with sexual dysfunction are men. Studies show that the impotence rate varies according to age, beginning at 2% for men under 40 and going up to 71% for men over the age of 70 [64, 66]. The diagnostic process, which is biological, examines the patient's symptoms, prevalence of the disorder, background illnesses, medication taken by the patient, and sometimes a physiological evaluation. There are also non-physiological reasons for these difficulties. Psychological problems, such as depression and its related medication, have been associated with sexual dysfunction in older age [20]. However, sexual dysfunctions in older age, due to emotional distress, were less frequently diagnosed and treated compared to young adults [20].

In this study, the treatment administered to male patients was most often identified as PDE5 inhibitor therapy (such as Viagra, Levitra ™ or Cialis ™). This treatment has been described by physicians as first-line, safe and highly effective for sexual dysfunction [67, 68], for use upon demand or on a daily basis [69]. According to an international survey of 12,563 people, only 7% of those who reported ED actually used medication, but

74% claimed they would like to receive medical treatment [70]. In other words, there is a considerable public preference for medical treatment.

Family physicians, in our study, claimed that sexual function has greater significance for men than for women, as the latter have a higher need for intimacy and communication and are more willing to accept a decrease in libido. This is despite studies which indicate a rate of 25–63% of sexual dysfunction among older women, pointing to a lack of estrogen as the main cause [71, 72]. In the English Longitudinal Study of Ageing (ELSA), among 6201 participants (56% women) aged 50 to > 90 [73], compared to men, women of all ages reported lower levels of concern about their sexual activities and functioning, together with lower levels of dissatisfaction with their overall sex lives [74–76]. However, it has been found that physicians treating women with gynecological symptoms recognize a difficulty in sexual functioning, but only very few opt to discuss the matter with them [77]. These findings suggest that family physicians tend not to initiate discourse about sexual functioning with older adults, due to their high workload, time constraints, and fear of offending their patients. Most physicians tended to focus on the physiological aspects of the patient and less on psychological aspects such as intimacy and relationships.

The present study can contribute to the improvement of the family physician's approach to the subject of sexual functioning in old age. The study emphasizes the numerous barriers which may prevent family physicians from addressing sexual functioning among the population of older adults when it comes to discussing the matter: increased workload, lack of time, fear of offending patients and harming the physician-patient relationship, and the many demands made by the health system, thereby pushing the issue of sexuality down to the bottom of the list of priorities. Although specialization in family medicine is based on the biopsychosocial model, it appears that in the area of sexual functioning and sexual satisfaction in older adults, the social aspect is still somewhat lacking. Based on previous studies, this is a significant issue in the lives of older people, who would like their family physicians to initiate discussions about this subject [3, 78]. The present study indicates that both diagnosis and treatment lean towards the biological end of the biopsychosocial model, and that the focus of communication on the subject is with male patients and on the administration of drug treatment. The research offers practical recommendations for training physicians, including guidance on the importance of sexuality in older age and improving communication with older patients [20, 38], so that family physicians may feel more comfortable about inquiring into the psychosocial aspects, in addition to the biological factors.

It is recommended to ask the patient's permission to talk about a personal issue [79], for example: "Are you experiencing any difficulty with sexual functioning?", "What is your sexual orientation?" or "People taking this medication sometimes report problems with sexual function; is that something you are familiar with?" [20]. Another important consideration concerns the use of medication such as Viagra, for instance. Viagra affects more than a man's erection. It also influences the nature of the sexual relationship that he and his partner share; therefore, we recommended that family physicians include women in the discussion about Viagra and give them an opportunity to be part of the medical consultations and decision-making process regarding a partner's treatment of erectile difficulties [80].

As the study has demonstrated, a significant barrier is physicians' heavy workload and busy schedule. Unfortunately, this cannot be easily overcome. Because sexual issues are an important part of general health and are often connected to other medical issues, health policy should advocate educating physicians on how to make time to address and give priority to sexuality. One possible proposal is to create an intervention program to increase physicians' awareness, so as to be able to identify when they may be sidestepping discussion of a sensitive topic because they are pressed for time or even personally fatigued and overloaded. The program should also legitimize this, and address any guilt, shame or uncomfortable feelings the physician might be feeling or suppressing because he did not give the patient enough time. When the physician is able to recognize this, he can then express to the patient that he realizes he has introduced an important topic. He and the patient can then discuss how they would like to discuss matters further, and encourage him to make an additional appointment in order to give the subject its due attention.In addition, as older people frequently visit their physician accompanied by a family member, physicians should be sensitive in ascertaining whether the patient feels comfortable discussing these issues in their presence [20]. In addition, as older people frequently visit their physician accompanied by a family member, physicians should be sensitive in ascertaining whether the patient feels comfortable discussing these issues in their presence [20].

When most communication concerning sexual difficulties is focused on biological aspects, the message conveyed to patients is that their difficulty is medical, although often this issue, in fact, represents a biopsychosocial problem [40]. Training family physicians in these matters can help them to deal with these barriers and gain a deeper understanding of the topic, thereby increasing their confidence in communicating the issue to their patients. Finally, it is important to acknowledge some of the limitations of the present study. The main limitation of this study is that generalization to broader populations ought to be done with caution. As a qualitative study, we were concerned with generating an in-depth exploration of participants' understandings and practices, and therefore, the findings presented here are not generalizable. Another limitation is that the research was carried out with a relatively small number of participants - family physicians from Israel. Cultural issues as well as sexual orientation were not directly examined in the present study. An understanding of the impact of cultural and sexual orientation on older adults' life experiences may assist healthcare professionals in their efforts to determine appropriate interventions. However, this was not the focus of the present study and was not brought up by physicians. There is a need to design curricula to ensure that physicians develop the necessary skills needed to provide comprehensive sexual health care to LGBTQ&I patients. Such curricula include information about sexual orientation and gender identity and tools to address these issues [81].

Conclusions

Sexual function remains important to older adults and should be recognized as an integral part of their general wellbeing and health. The present study presents the views of 16 family physicians on sexuality in older adults. We found that family physicians have difficulty raising questions about sexuality with older patients, due to workload, time constraints, and fear of offending their patients. Most physicians tended to concentrate on the patient's medical history, focusing on the physiological aspects, while only a minority of the physicians examined intimacy and marital relations as an integral part of the routine check-up. Family physicians reported that most of the sexuality-related visits were made by men and the main complaint was erectile dysfunction; the treatment most often administered to male patients was PDE5 inhibitor therapy. The current study provides practical recommendations for training family physicians, including stressing the importance of sexuality among the older population, and improving physician-patient communication - conducted with discretion and in complete confidentiality. It is recommended to ask the patient's permission, at the beginning of the conversation, to discuss a personal issue. It would also be wise to advise patients to schedule a double appointment or an appointment at the end of the day, when the physician is more available.

Abbreviation
ED: Erectile dysfunction

Funding
This study was supported by a grant from the Israel National Institute for Health Policy. The funders had no role in study design, data collection and analysis, decision to publish, or preparation of the manuscript.

Authors' contributions
I.L. designed the study, collected the data and wrote the paper. A.G.M. designed the study and assisted in the writing of the article/the writing process. K.K. assisted in the writing process. L.A. designed the study, supervised the data collection, and assisted in the data analysis and the writing process. All authors read and approved the final version of the manuscript.

Competing interests
The authors declare that they have no competing interests.

Author details
[1]The Division of Family Medicine, Department of Family Medicine, The Ruth & Bruce Rappaport Faculty of Medicine, Technion-Israel Institute of Technology, 6 Hashachaf St., Bat-Galim, 35013 Haifa, Israel. [2]The Louis and Gaby Weisfeld School of Social Work, Bar-Ilan University, Ramat Gan, Israel. [3]Department of Family Medicine, The Ruth & Bruce Rappaport Faculty of Medicine, Technion-Israel Institute of Technology, Clalit Health Services, Western Galilee District, Haifa, Israel.

References
1. Fisher LL, Anderson G, Chapagain M, et al. Sex, romance and relationships: AARP survey of midlife and older adults. Washington, DC: American Association of Retired Persons; 2010.
2. DeLamater J. Sexual expression in later life: a review and synthesis. J Sex Res. 2012;49(2–3):125–41.
3. Kasif T, Band-Winterstein T. Older widows' perspectives on sexuality: a life course perspective. J Aging Stud. 2017;41:1–9.
4. Haesler E, Bauer M, Fetherstonhaugh D. Sexuality, sexual health and older people: a systematic review of research on the knowledge and attitudes of health professionals. Nurse Educ Today. 2016;40:57–71.
5. Anderson R. Positive sexuality and its impact on overall well-being. Bundesgesundheitsblatt Gesundheitsforschung Gesundheitsschutz. 2013; 56(2):208–14.
6. Johnson JL, Repta R. Sex and gender. In: Oliffe JL, Greaves L, editors. Designing and conducting gender, sex, and health research. Los Angeles: SAGE; 2012. p. 17–37.
7. Terner M, Reason B, McKeag AM, Tipper B, Webster G. Chronic conditions more than age drive health system use in Canadian seniors. Healthc Q. 2011;14(3):19–22.
8. Liu R, Wu S, Hao Y, Gu J, Fang J, Cai N, Zhang J. The Chinese version of the world health organization quality of life instrument-older adults module (WHOQOL-OLD): psychometric evaluation. Health Qual Life Outcomes. 2013;11(1):156.
9. Latif EZ, Diamond MP. Arriving at the diagnosis of female sexual dysfunction. Fertil Steril. 2013;100(4):898–904.
10. Shifren JL, Monz BU, Russo PA, Segreti A, Johannes CB. Sexual problems and distress in United States women: prevalence and correlates. Obstet Gynecol. 2008;112(5):970–8.
11. Lindau ST, Schumm LP, Laumann EO, Levinson W, O'muircheartaigh CA, Waite LJ. A study of sexuality and health among older adults in the United States. New Engl J Med. 2007;357(8):762–74.
12. Beutel ME, Stöbel-Richter Y, Brähler E. Sexual desire and sexual activity of men and women across their lifespans: results from a representative German community survey. BJU Int. 2008;101(1):76–82.
13. Kontula O, Haavio-Mannila E. The impact of aging on human sexual activity and sexual desire. J Sex Res. 2009;46(1):46–56.
14. Mercer CH, Tanton C, Prah P, et al. Changes in sexual attitudes and lifestyles in Britain through the life course and over time: findings from the National Surveys of sexual attitudes and lifestyles (Natsal). Lancet. 2013;382(9907):1781–94.
15. Laux G, Kuehlein T, Rosemann T, Szecsenyi J. Co-and multimorbidity patterns in primary care based on episodes of care: results from the German CONTENT project. BMC Health Serv Res. 2008;8(1):8–14.
16. Gott M, Hinchliff S. How important is sex in later life? The views of older people. Soc Sci Med. 2003;56(8):1617–28.

17. Lindau ST, Gavrilova N. Sex, health, and years of sexually active life gained due to good health: evidence from two US population based cross sectional surveys of ageing. BMJ. 2010;340:c810.

18. Makara-Studzinska MT, Krys-Noszczyk KM, Jakiel G. Epidemiology of the symptoms of menopause - an intercontinental review. Menopause Rev. 2014;13(3):203–11.

19. Kalra G, Subramanyam A, Pinto C. Sexuality: desire, activity and intimacy in the elderly. Indian J Psychiatry. 2011;53(4):300–6.

20. Taylor A, Gosney MA. Sexuality in older age: essential considerations for healthcare professionals. Age Ageing. 2011;40(5):538–43.

21. Hillman J. Sexual issues and aging within the context of work with older adult patients. Prof Psychol Res Pr. 2008;39(3):290–7.

22. Gregorian Jr RS, Golden KA, Bahce A, Goodman C, Kwong WJ, Khan ZM. Antidepressant-induced sexual dysfunction. Ann Pharmacother. 2002;36(10): 1577–89.

23. Mehraban D, Naderi GH, Yahyazadeh SR, Amirchaghmaghi M. Sexual dysfunction in aging men with lower urinary tract symptoms. Urol J. 2008; 5(5):260–4.

24. Giugliano F, Maiorino M, Bellastella G, Gicchino M, Giugliano D, Esposito K. Determinants of erectile dysfunction in type 2 diabetes. Int J Impot Res. 2010;22(3):204–9.

25. Morgentaler A. A 66-year-old man with sexual dysfunction. JAMA. 2004; 291(24):2994–3003.

26. Mazur A, Mueller U, Krause W, Booth A. Causes of sexual decline in aging married men: Germany and America. Int J Impot Res. 2002;14(2):101–6.

27. Engel GL. The need for a new medical model: a challenge for biomedicine. Science. 1977;196(4286):129–36.

28. Engel GL. The clinical application of the biopsychosocial model. Am J Psychiatry. 1980;137:535–44.

29. Botica M, Zelić I, Pavlić Renar I, Bergman Marković B, Stojadinović Grgurević S, Botica I. Structure of visits persons with diabetes in croatian family practice–analysis of reasons for encounter and treatment procedures using the ICPC-2. Coll Antropol. 2006;30(3):495–9.

30. Månsson J, Nilsson G, Strender L, Björkelund C. Reasons for encounters, investigations, referrals, diagnoses and treatments in general practice in Sweden—a multicentre pilot study using electronic patient records. Eur J Gen Pract. 2011;17(2):87–94.

31. Fileborn B, Lyons A, Heywood W, et al. Talking to healthcare providers about sex in later life: findings from a qualitative study with older Australian men and women. Australas J Ageing. 2017; https://doi.org/10.1111/ajag.12450.

32. Moreira ED, Glasser DB, Nicolosi A, Duarte FG, Gingell C. Sexual problems and help-seeking behaviour in adults in the United Kingdom and continental Europe. BJU Int. 2008;101(8):1005–11.

33. Dogan S, Demir B, Eker E, Karim S. Knowledge and Attitudes of doctors toward the sexuality of older people in Turkey. Int Psychogeriatr. 2008; 20(5):1019–27.

34. Mahieu L, Van Elssen K, Gastmans C. Nurses' perceptions of sexuality in institutionalized elderly: a literature review. Int J Nurs Stud. 2011;48(9):1140–54.

35. Snyder RJ, Zweig RA. Medical and psychology students' knowledge and attitudes regarding aging and sexuality. Gerontol Geriatr Educ. 2010; 31(3):235–55.

36. Gilmer MJ, Meyer A, Davidson J, Koziol-McLain J. Staff beliefs about sexuality in aged residential care. Nurs Prax N Z. 2010;26(3):17–25.

37. Bouman WP, Arcelus J, Benbow SM. Nottingham study of sexuality and ageing (NoSSA II). Attitudes of care staff regarding sexuality and residents: a study in residential and nursing homes. Sex Relation Ther. 2007;22(1):45–61.

38. Gott M, Galena E, Hinchliff S, Elford H. "Opening a can of worms": GP and practice nurse barriers to talking about sexual health in primary care. Fam Pract. 2004;21(5):528–36.

39. Langer-Most O, Langer N. Aging and sexuality: how much do gynecologists know and care? J Women Aging. 2010;22(4):283–9.

40. Gewirtz-Meydan A, Ayalon L. Physicians' response to sexual dysfunction presented by a younger vs. an older adult. Int J Geriatr Psychiatry. 2016; https://doi.org/10.1002/gps.4638.

41. Brown MT, Grossman BR. Same-sex sexual relationships in the national social life, health and aging project: making a case for data collection. J Gerontol Soc Work. 2014;57(2–4):108–29.

42. Heaphy B. Choice and its limits in older lesbian and gay narratives of relational life. J GLBT Fam Stud. 2009;5(1 2):119 38.

43. Gay and Gray Project. Lifting the lid on sexuality and ageing: report of a research project into the needs, wants, fears and aspirations of older lesbians and gay men. Bournemouth: Help and Care; 2006.

44. Fredriksen-Goldsen KI, Kim HJ, Hoy-Ellis CP, et al. Addressing the needs of LGBT older adults in San Francisco. Seattle: University of Washington; 2013.

45. Wallace SP, Cochran SD, Durazo EM, Ford CL. The health of aging lesbian, gay and bisexual adults in California. Policy Brief UCLA Cent Health Policy Res. 2011;PB2011–2:1–8.

46. Orel NA. Investigating the needs and concerns of lesbian, gay, bisexual, and transgender older adults: the use of qualitative and quantitative methodology. J Homosex. 2014;61(1):53–78.

47. Stott DB. The training needs of general practitioners in the exploration of sexual health matters and providing sexual healthcare to lesbian, gay and bisexual patients. Med Teach. 2013;35(9):752–9.

48. Colledge L, Hickson F, Reid D, Weatherburn P. Poorer mental health in UK bisexual women than lesbians: evidence from the UK 2007 stonewall Women's health survey. J Public Health. 2015;37(3):427–37.

49. Carabez R, Pellegrini M, Mankovitz A, Eliason M, Ciano M, Scott M. "Never in all my years…": nurses' education about LGBT health. J Prof Nurs. 2015; 31(4):323–9.

50. Martos AJ, Wilson PA, Meyer IH. Lesbian, gay, bisexual, and transgender (LGBT) health services in the United States: origins, evolution, and contemporary landscape. PLoS One. 2017;12(7):e0180544.

51. Parameshwaran V, Cockbain BC, Hillyard M, Price JR. Is the lack of specific lesbian, gay, bisexual, transgender and queer/questioning (LGBTQ) health care education in medical school a cause for concern? Evidence from a survey of knowledge and practice among UK medical students. J Homosex. 2017;64(3):367–81.

52. Robertson WJ. 'Believe it or not': the medical framing of rectal foreign bodies. Cult Health Sex. 2017;19(8):815–28.

53. Hughes AK, Wittmann D. Aging sexuality: knowledge and perceptions of preparation among US primary care providers. J Sex Marital Ther. 2015;41(3):304–13.

54. Patton MQ. Two decades of developments in qualitative inquiry a personal, experiential perspective. Qual Soc Work. 2002;1(3):261–83.

55. Strauss AL. Qualitative analysis for social scientists. Cambridge: Cambridge University Press; 1987.

56. Creswell JW, Poth CN. Qualitative inquiry research methods: Choosing among five approaches. 4th ed. Los Angeles, London, New Delhi: Sage; 2018.

57. Clandinin DJ, Connelly FM. Narrative inquiry: experience and story in qualitative research. Educ Res. 2000;6:94–118.

58. Finlay L, Gough B. Reflexivity: A practical guide for researchers in health and social sciences. Malden: Blackwell Science; 2003.

59. Shkedi A. Words that try to touch: Qual Res-theory and implementation. Tel Aviv: Ramot; 2003.

60. Tufford L, Newman P. Bracketing in qualitative research. Qual Soc Work. 2010;11:80–96.

61. Finlay L. Phenomenology for therapists: Researching the lived world. Chichester: Wiley-Blackwell; 2011.

62. Perttula E. Physician attitudes and behaviour regarding erectile dysfunction in at-risk patients from a rural community. Postgrad Med J. 1999;75(880):83–5.

63. Gandaglia G, Briganti A, Jackson G, et al. A systematic review of the association between erectile dysfunction and cardiovascular disease. Eur Urol. 2014;65(5):968–78.

64. Campbell MM, Stein DJ. Sexual dysfunction: a systematic review of south african research. S Afr Med J. 2014;104(6):439–40.

65. Hinchliff S, Gott M. Seeking medical help for sexual concerns in mid-and later life: a review of the literature. J Sex Res. 2011;48(2–3):106–17.

66. Rosen RC, Fisher WA, Eardley I, Niederberger C, Nadel A, Sand M. The multinational Men's attitudes to life events and sexuality (MALES) study: I. Prevalence of erectile dysfunction and related health concerns in the general population. Cur Med Res Opin. 2004;20(5):607–17.

67. Buvat J, Montorsi F, Maggi M, et al. Hypogonadal men nonresponders to the PDE5 inhibitor tadalafil benefit from normalization of testosterone levels with a 1% hydroalcoholic testosterone gel in the treatment of erectile dysfunction (TADTEST study). J Sex Med. 2011;8:284 93.

68. Morelli A, Filippi S, Mancina R, et al. Androgens regulate phosphodiesterase type 5 expression and functional activity in corpora cavernosa. Endocrinology. 2004;145(5):2253 63.

69. Smith WB, McCaslin IR, Gokce A, Mandava SH, Trost L, Hellstrom WJ. PDE5 inhibitors: considerations for preference and long-term adherence. Int J Clin Pract. 2013;67(8):768–80.   –
70. Mulhall J, King R, Glina S, Hvidsten K. Importance of and satisfaction with sex among men and women worldwide: results of the global better sex survey. J Sex Med. 2008;5(4):788–95.
71. Addis IB, Van Den Eeden SK, Wassel-Fyr CL, Vittinghoff E, Brown JS, Thom DH. Reproductive risk factors for incontinence study at Kaiser study group. Sexual activity and function in middle-aged and older women. Obstet Gynecol. 2016;107(4):755–64.
72. Ambler DR, Bieber EJ, Diamond MP. Sexual function in elderly women: a review of current literature. Rev Obstet Gynecol. 2012;5(1):16–27.
73. Lee DM, Nazroo J, O'Connor DB, Blake M, Pendleton N. Sexual health and well-being among older men and women in England: findings from the English longitudinal study of ageing. Arch Sex Behav. 2016;45(1):133–44.
74. Hendrickx L, Gijs L, Enzlin P. Age-related prevalence rates of sexual difficulties, sexual dysfunctions, and sexual distress in heterosexual women: results from an online survey in Flanders. J Sex Med. 2015;12(2):424–35.
75. Rosen RC, Shifren JL, Monz BU, Odom DM, Russo PA, Johannes CB. Correlates of sexually related personal distress in women with low sexual desire. J Sex Med. 2009;6(6):1549–60.
76. Stephenson KR, Meston CM. Why is impaired sexual function distressing to women? The primacy of pleasure in female sexual dysfunction. J Sex Med. 2015;12(3):728–37.
77. Stead M, Brown J, Fallowfield L, Selby P. Lack of communication between healthcare professionals and women with ovarian cancer about sexual issues. Br J Cancer. 2003;88(5):666–71.
78. Bauer M, Haesler E, Fetherstonhaugh D. Let's talk about sex: older people's views on the recognition of sexuality and sexual health in the health-care setting. Health Expect. 2015;19:1237–50.
79. Hillman JL. Clinical perspectives on elderly sexuality. New York: Springer science & business media; 2000.
80. Potts A, Gavey N, Grace VM, Vares T. The downside of Viagra: women's experiences and concerns. Sociol Health Illn. 2003;25(7):697–719.
81. McNair RP, Hegarty K. Guidelines for the primary care of lesbian, gay, and bisexual people: a systematic review. Ann Fam Med. 2010;8(6):533–41.

17

Validity and reliability of the patient assessment on chronic illness care (PACIC) questionnaire: the Malay version

Suraya Abdul-Razak[1,2]*[iD], Anis Safura Ramli[1,2], Siti Fatimah Badlishah-Sham[1], Jamaiyah Haniff[3] and for the EMPOWER-PAR Investigators

Abstract

Background: Majority of patients with chronic illnesses such as diabetes, receive care at primary care setting. Efforts have been made to restructure diabetes care in the Malaysian primary care setting in accordance with the Chronic Care Model (CCM). The Patient Assessment on Chronic Illness Care (PACIC) is a validated self-report tool to measure the extent to which patients with chronic illness receive care that aligns with the CCM. To date, no validated tool is available to evaluate healthcare delivery based on the CCM in the Malay language. Thus, the study aimed to translate the PACIC into the Malay language and validate the questionnaire among patients with diabetes in the Malaysian public primary care setting.

Methods: The English version of the PACIC questionnaire is a 20-item scale measuring five key components, which are patient activation, decision support, goal setting, problem solving and follow-up care. The PACIC underwent forward - backward translation and cross cultural adaptation process to produce the PACIC-Malay version (PACIC-M). Reliability was tested using internal consistencies and test-retest reliability analyses, while construct validity was tested using the exploratory factor analysis (EFA).

Results: The content of PACIC-M and the original version were conceptually equivalent. Overall, the internal consistency by Cronbach's α was .94 and the intra-class correlation coefficient was .93. One item was deleted (item 1) when the factor loading was < 0.4. The factor analyses using promax identified three components ('Goal Setting/Tailoring and Problem solving/Contextual', 'follow-up/coordination' and 'patient activation and delivery system design/ decision support'); explaining 61.2% of the variation. The Kaiser-Meyer-Olkin (KMO) was 0.93 and Bartlett's test of sphericity was $p = .000$. Therefore, the final version of the PACIC-M consisted of 19 items, framed within three components.

Conclusion: The findings demonstrated that the PACIC-M measured different dimensions from the English version of PACIC. It is however; highly reliable and valid to be used in assessing three CCM model subscales. Further confirmatory factor analysis of PACIC-M should be conducted to confirm this new model.

Keywords: Validation, Reliability, PACIC, Cultural adaption, Malaysia

* Correspondence: drsuraya.abdulrazak@gmail.com;
suraya617@salam.uitm.edu.my
[1]Primary Care Medicine Discipline, Faculty of Medicine, Universiti Teknologi MARA, Selayang Campus, Jalan Prima Selayang 7, 68100 Batu Caves, Selangor, Malaysia
[2]Institute of Pathology, Laboratory and Forensic Medicine (I-PPerForM), Universiti Teknologi MARA, Sungai Buloh Campus, Jalan Hospital, 47000 Sungai Buloh, Selangor, Malaysia
Full list of author information is available at the end of the article

Background

The Chronic Care Model (CCM) is being widely used to assess and improve chronic illness care in the primary care setting [1, 2]. This model represents a conceptual framework based on well documented gaps between clinical research findings and real practice [2, 3]. It recommends a proactive and planned care approach than of reactive and unplanned care, in order to deliver high quality and patient-centred chronic disease care to the population [2]. The six dimensions of CCM include healthcare organisation, delivery system design, clinical information system, patient self-management support, decision support and use of community resource [2].

The evidence on effectiveness of one or more of CCM key elements in improving Type 2 Diabetes Mellitus (T2DM) outcomes, congestive heart failure, asthma and depression are well established in developed countries [4–6]. Although the evidence of its effectiveness in developing countries are scarce, emerging evidence from Malaysia and the Philippines shows reductions of Haemoglobin A1c (HbA1C) and improvement in the proportion of patients achieving good glycaemic controls following implementation of the CCM, support restructuring of care in limited resource settings [7, 8]. With the increasing burden of chronic diseases in developing countries, measures to restructure chronic illness care using multifaceted interventions based on the CCM are required to improve delivery and quality of chronic care over time.

In Malaysia, the implementation of essential components of the CCM in the public primary care setting has been shown to be feasible [9]. The EMPOWER Participatory Action Research (EMPOWER-PAR) Study has pragmatically implemented at least three components of the CCM framework at selected public primary care clinics which include creating or strengthening the diabetes care team (delivery system design), utilizing the clinical practice guideline (CPG) by the care team (decision support) and empowering patients with self-management skills through utilization of the Global Cardiovascular Risks Self-Management Booklet© (patient self-management support) [7]. In addition, various programs by the Ministry of Health to transform the non-communicable disease care has introduced positive changes at the ground level to improve chronic care delivery including dedicated clinic specifically for T2DM [10]. There were good provisions for CPG training in most clinics, with a comprehensive national data registry for T2DM and adequacy of staff willing to be trained, providing a good opportunity for CCM implementation. With the increasing effort to restructure chronic illness care in accordance with the CCM particularly for T2DM in the Malaysian primary care setting, assessment of healthcare delivery, not only from the healthcare providers' perspectives, but also from the patients' perspectives are pivotal to improve chronic care quality.

The Patient Assessment Chronic Illness Care (PACIC) questionnaire is a patient reported instrument to assess quality of patient-centred care for chronic illness consistent with the CCM [11]. The PACIC is the the most appropriate instrument to measure the experience of people receiving integrated chronic care due to its psychometric characteristics, perceived applicability and relevance [12]. It was developed by Glasgow et al. in the English language and consisted of 20 items (Q1-Q20) with each item scored on a 5-point likert scale with 1 being "Almost Never" and 5 being "Almost Always". The items were aggregated to five scale constructs that is congruent to components of the CCM but these constructs do not map perfectly onto the CCM components [11]. The five scale constructs in PACIC are patient activation; delivery system design/decision support; goal setting/tailoring; problem solving/contextual and follow-up/coordination. Each scale construct is scored by averaging the score of items answered within each scale and the overall PACIC is scored by averaging across all 20-items.

The PACIC helps healthcare providers to better understand the integration of CCM in their practices and to empower patients to be the evaluator of care they receive and avoid physicians over-reporting the CCM elements of chronic care delivered [13]. Thus, health care delivery as advocated by the CCM in the Malaysian primary care setting particularly for T2DM needs evaluation. Therefore, the objectives of this study were to translate the PACIC into the Malay language and to validate the tool among patients with T2DM receiving care at public primary care clinics.

Methods
Study design and participants
This cross sectional study involved three phases i) adaptation and translation ii) face validation and iii) field testing and psychometric evaluation of the PACIC-Malay (PACIC-M) version. It was conducted between March 2013 and March 2014. Figure 1 outlines the three phases of the translation and validation processes.

Phase 1: Adaptation and translation process
The PACIC English version underwent adaptation process including content validation by a group of five family physicians. The expert panel rated the relevance of each item to the conceptual framework. Table 1 describes the rating criteria used by expert panels to assess the content validity. The rating template measures relevance, clarity, simplicity and ambiguity of PACIC-M in a scale of 1 to 4. Then, adaptations to the original questionnaire were made to suit the objectives of the study, local language and culture. The translation process into the Malay language was carried out via two forward translations. The first forward translation was done by a family physician who

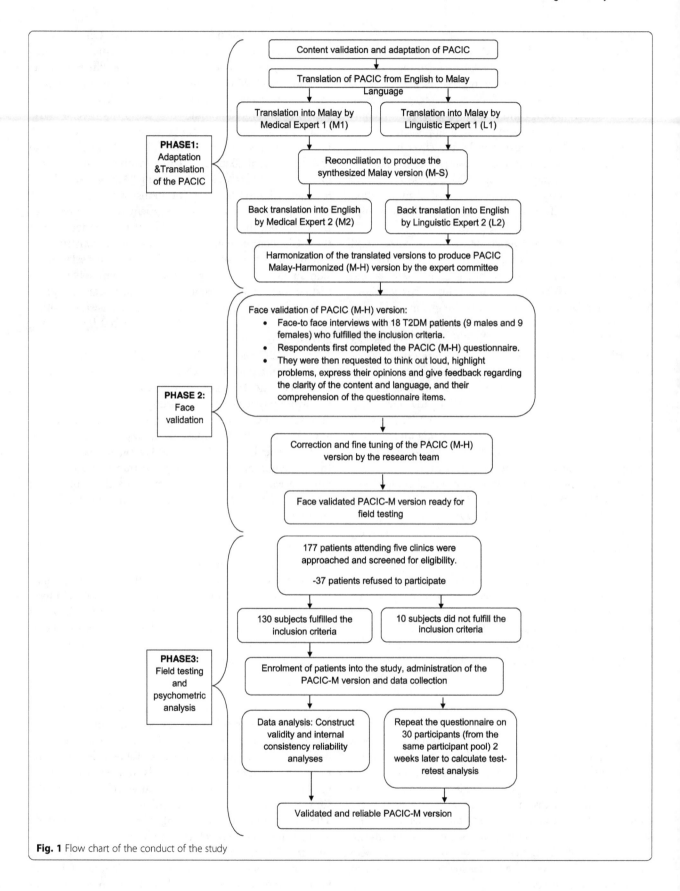

Fig. 1 Flow chart of the conduct of the study

Table 1 Rating criteria for measuring content validity of PACIC-M

Relevance

1 = not relevant

2 = item need some revision

3 = relevant but need minor revision

4 = very relevant

Clarity

1 = not clear

2 = item need some revision

3 = clear but need minor revision

4 = very clear

Simplicity

1 = not simple

2 = item need some revision

3 = simple but need some minor revision

4 = very simple

Ambiguity

1 = doubtful

2 = item need some revision

3 = no doubt

4 = meaning is clear

had direct involvement in diabetes care at public primary care clinic, and was not blinded to the study objectives. The second translator was a certified translator who was blinded to the study objectives. Each translator produced the M1 and L1 versions, which were later back translated into English independently by another certified translator and a family physician producing M2 and L2 versions, respectively. The forward and backward translations were conducted in accordance with the guidelines for cross-cultural adaptation and translation studies [14, 15]. An expert panel consisting of researchers and translators, reviewed the translated Malay versions to produce a synthesized Malay version prior to the back translation into the English language. This harmonization process ensured inter-translation validity between these versions to produce the PACIC M-harmonised version which was ready for face validation among the target population i.e. T2DM patients.

Phase 2: Face validation
The main objective of the face validation was to identify and solve any potential problems related to comprehension among the target population. The face validity testing was conducted with 18 T2DM patients (9 males and 9 females) who fulfilled the inclusion criteria. The inclusion criteria included T2DM patients aged ≥18 years who have received care at least once in the last 1 year at the public primary care clinics and were able to read

and write in the Malay language. Foreigners, pregnant women and patients with Type 1 Diabetes Mellitus, mental disorders, visual impairment and those who did not give informed consent were excluded from the study. Respondents completed the PACIC M-harmonised version and they were later requested to think out loud, highlight problems, express their opinions and give feedback regarding the clarity of the content and language, and their comprehension of the questionnaire items. Following their feedback, the questionnaire was further refined to produce the final version of PACIC-M, which was ready for the psychometric evaluations.

Phase 3: Field testing and psychometric evaluation
The final version of the PACIC-M was field tested amongst patients who fulfilled the same inclusion criteria as in Phase 2. However, patients who participated in Phase 2 and 3 were mutually exclusive, as those who participated in Phase 2 were not re-selected for Phase 3. The sampling frame for Phase 3 was T2DM patients from the five public primary care clinics participated in the EMPOWER-PAR study [7]. A detailed EMPOWER-PAR study protocol was described elsewhere [16].

Test-retest
Thirty participants who were recruited in Phase 3 participated in the test-retest of the PACIC-M, in which they were given a date to return to the clinic after two to 4 weeks. Upon their return, they were given the same questionnaire to complete for the test-retest reliability analysis.

Sample size
The sample size for Phase 3 was calculated using the subject to item ratio. A minimum of 100 participants were needed (20 items × 5 = 100) based on Gorsuch's for which a subject to item ratio 5:1 was used [17]. By taking into account of a 30% non-responder rate, the sample size was increased to 130 participants.

Sampling method
Consecutive sampling was adopted to recruit T2DM patients from the five clinics over a 2-week recruitment period i.e. 26 patients from each clinic, giving a total of 130 participants. Patients with T2DM who attended the clinic on the day of the data collection were consecutively approached and invited to participate in the study. This sampling method was chosen as there was difficulty to conduct probability sampling as the clinics only had paper based registry for their T2DM patients. A briefing to explain the purpose of the study was held to the respondents who were interested to participate and information sheets about the study were also distributed. Those who agreed to participate were then screened for

eligibility according to the inclusion and exclusion criteria. Those who were eligible were recruited into the study and written informed consent was obtained.

Data collection

Demographic data was collected and participants were given the self-administered PACIC-M questionnaire. Instructions were given on how to fill up the questionnaire and they were reminded to answer the questions themselves rather than getting their family members to complete it. Upon completion, the questionnaires were returned to the investigators who then checked for completeness.

Statistical analysis

Data entry and statistical analysis were performed using IBM SPSS Statistics Version 21 (IBM Corp., Armonk, NY, USA). Psychometric elements of PACIC-M were then examined in three parts:

First, data was assessed for quality and data suitability for factor analysis. Data quality was assessed with mean, standard deviation, and the extent of floor and ceiling effects for all items. Floor and ceiling effects between 1 and 15% were considered as optimal [18]. Sampling adequacy was assessed using the Kaiser-Meyer-Olkin (KMO) measure value and appropriateness of data was conducted using the Bartlett's test of sphericity. The KMO value of > 0.50 [19] with a significant Bartlett's test of sphericity with a p-value of < 0.05 [20] were considered suitable for factor analysis.

Secondly, exploratory factor analysis (EFA) using principal component analysis (PCA) with promax rotation (Eigenvalue > 1) was conducted to examine the PACIC-M dimensionality and construct validity i.e. the number and type of subscales in the instrument. Only factors with values of ≥0.40 were considered. Significance of a factor loading will depend on the sample size. Typically, researchers take a loading of an absolute value > 0.3 to be important but only appropriate if the sample size is 300 [21]. With a sample size of 130, a higher loading is chosen to be considered significant. Items were excluded if they met one of the following criteria; i) weak loadings (failing to load above 0.39 on any component), ii) general loadings of 0.40 on more than one component, iii) 30% of the responses were missing or iv) 80% of item responses were the same (floor/ceiling effect).

Thirdly, reliability of the PACIC-M was assessed using internal inconsistency and test retest reliability analyses. To represent high internal consistencies, Cronbach alpha of 0.5–0.7 for groups' comparisons [22] and average item-total correlation in a moderate range between > 0.3 and > 0.9 were considered as reliable. Cronbach alpha value of > 0.9 was considered as redundant, while correlation near 0 indicated no meaningful construct [23]. The test-retest reliability was assessed using the intra-class

correlation coefficient (ICC) [24]. ICC values of > 0.7 indicated that PACIC-M was stable over time, values between 0.4–0.7 indicated fair reliability while values of < 0.4 indicated poor reliability [25]. The inter-item correlations between domains (item discriminant validity) and the overall PACIC-M (internal item convergence) was assessed using Spearman correlation due to non-normal distributions of the variables. Correlation value of ≥0.4 was considered adequate to support the internal consistency of the instrument [26].

Results

The content validation, translation, adaptation and face validation of PACIC-M

A group of five family physicians found that the content of all 20 items of the PACIC English version were relevant to the conceptual framework. The two forward translators from English to the Malay language agreed on most items. However, several items in the original questionnaire were adapted to suit the local language and Malaysian culture e.g. 'healthcare team' as used in the introductory wording is not a well-known term in the primary healthcare setting in Malaysia and among our patients. The patients might be in contact with a diabetes healthcare team but many may not be aware of this term as the team members may change regularly due to constraints in staffing faced by the public primary care clinics. The closest concept to healthcare team is healthcare providers i.e. the health clinic as a whole. Another word with ambiguous meaning was 'treatment' in items 1, 2, 9 and 13 in which treatment may mean medication in the day to day Malay language. The word 'treatment' was initially translated to 'rawatan', however, after the face validation process, examples of 'treatment' (i.e. medications, exercise, diet) were added to these items to increase the clarity. During the face validation process, all of the respondents found all of the 20 items were relevant to their chronic care. However, to improve clarity of the questionnaire, several respondents suggested that the items be changed from statements regarding their care to questions such as 'I was asked' to 'Were you asked' for all items. Following their feedback, the questionnaire was further refined and proof-read for spelling and grammar to produce the final version of PACIC-M.

Field testing and psychometric evaluation

A total of 177 patients were approached, 37 refused to participate and 10 did not fulfil the inclusion and exclusion criteria. In total, 130 questionnaires were administered and all were returned. Table 2 shows the demographic characteristics of the respondents. The mean age was 48.5 ± 7.3 years. More than half were females (56.9%), attained secondary education (51.2%) and there were more Malays (45.7%) than other races (see Table 2).

Table 2 Demographic characteristics of the respondents (N = 130)

Characteristics	
Age in years	
Mean ± SD	48.5 ± 7.3
Median (min, max)	49.0 (32, 64)
Gender[a] n, (%)	
Male	55 (42.6)
Female	74 (56.9)
Race[a] n, (%)	
Malay	59 (45.7)
Chinese	21 (16.3)
Indian	47 (36.2)
Others	2 (1.6)
Educational level n, (%)	
Primary School	44 (34.1)
Secondary School	66 (51.2)
College/University	20 (14.7)
Number of co-morbid n, (%)	
0	9 (6.9)
1	46 (35.4)
2	14 (10.8)
≥ 3	61 (46.9)

[a]one missing data

Table 3 shows the descriptive statistics of the 20 item PACIC-M: mean, standard deviation (SD), percentage of respondents achieving the lowest score (indicating no satisfaction) and percentage of respondents achieving the highest score (indicating full satisfaction).

There was no missing data for individual items for PACIC-M. The floor effect (percent of patients answering "None of the time" to any given item) exceeded 15% in item 16 and the ceiling effect (percent of patient answering "All of the time" to any given item) was not prominent, with none of the item exceeded 15%.

Overall, PACIC-M score was 2.53 (±0.48) out of possible score of 5, ranging between 2.45 (±0.60) for item 4: "Given a written list of things I should do to improve my health" and 2.64 (±0.57) for item 6 "Shown how what I did to take care of myself influenced my condition". When grouped together as five predetermined subscales, the subscale score ranged between 2.49 (±0.60) for subscale 5: "follow-up/coordination" and 2.54 (±0.49) for subscale 1: "patient activation". Floor and ceiling effect for the entire PACIC-M was 0% respectively.

The KMO revealed an excellent value of 0.93 and the Bartlett's test of sphericity value was significant (1565.7, p = .000). Both of these values indicated that the data set was suitable for further factor analysis. Using the PCA with promax rotation, we identified three components explaining 61.2% of the total variance. The first component with Eigenvalue of 9.853 explained 49.3% of the total variance, while the second component with an Eigenvalue of 1.379 explained 6.9% of the total variance. The third component with Eigenvalue of 1.012 explained 5.1% of the total variance. Table 4 shows the results of factor loadings of the PACIC-M 3-component structure. Factor loading for item 1 was below 0.4 for all components identified de-novo. Component one which consisted of items 6,7,8,9,10,11,12,13,14 and 15 was labelled as 'goal setting/tailoring and problem solving/contextual'. Component two which consisted of items 16, 17, 18, 19 and 20 was labelled as 'follow-up/coordination'. The third component which consisted of items 2, 3, 4 and 5 was labelled as 'patient activation and delivery system design/ decision support'.

Table 5 shows the score distributions and reliability of PACIC-M. The Cronbach alpha value for the overall PACIC-M was 0.94 and ICC was 0.93. The Cronbach alpha values for two subscales 'goal setting/tailoring and problem solving/contextual' and 'follow-up/coordination' was greater than 0.9, respectively which is high for a brief scale [22]. One subscale i.e. 'patient activation and delivery system design/decision support' had a Cronbach alpha value of 0.77.

Table 6 shows the Spearman correlations between the original PACIC subscales and the overall score. The correlations between the overall and PACIC subscales were found to be generally higher than correlations between subscales. Correlations between subscales were positive but lower, ranging between 0.41 for 'patient activation' and 'problem solving/contextual', and 0.80 for 'goal setting/tailoring' and 'problem solving/contextual'.

Meanwhile, Fig. 2 shows the summary of the matrix scatter plot of mean score for PACIC subscales.

Discussion

The implementation of CCM to guide chronic disease management system change for T2DM in the Malaysian primary care setting highlights a pressing need for a practical and validated tool to evaluate the quality of patient-centred care which is consistent with the CCM. This was the first study to translate, adapt and validate the PACIC questionnaire into the Malay language among patients with T2DM whom received care at the public primary care clinics in Malaysia. The PACIC-M had undergone rigorous process according to established guidelines for translating, adapting and validating a questionnaire [14, 15].

Our study shows that the overall and individual subscales PACIC-M scores were comparable to other studies [11, 27]. The floor and ceiling effect in this study was better than studies conducted in the Danish populations [28, 29], and similar to a Spanish validation of PACIC delivered in ambulatory clinic where the staff received

Table 3 Descriptive statistics of 20-item PACIC-M questionnaire, grouped into 5 subscales ($N = 130$)

Items	Mean Score	(SD)	Z-Skew	Floor N (%)	Ceiling N (%)
Overall PACIC-M score	2.53	0.48	−2.3	0 (0)	0 (0)
Patient activation	2.54	0.49	−6.4	4 (3.1)	0 (0)
Q1	2.53	0.64	−4.0	9 (6.9)	0 (0)
Q2	2.52	0.65	−4.9	11 (8.5)	0 (0)
Q3	2.55	0.62	−5.1	9 (6.9)	0 (0)
Delivery system design/decision support	2.53	0.48	−5.7	2 (1.5)	0 (0)
Q4	2.45	0.60	−2.8	7 (5.4)	0 (0)
Q5	2.48	0.64	−4.0	10 (7.7)	0 (0)
Q6	2.64	0.57	−6.2	6 (4.6)	0 (0)
Goal setting/tailoring	2.53	0.46	−4.6	0 (0)	0 (0)
Q7	2.52	0.60	−4.0	7 (5.4)	0 (0)
Q8	2.56	0.60	−4.8	7 (5.4)	0 (0)
Q9	2.46	0.66	−4.0	12 (9.2)	0 (0)
Q10	2.55	0.61	−4.7	8 (6.2)	0 (0)
Q11	2.55	0.61	−4.7	8 (6.2)	0 (0)
Problem solving/contextual	2.52	0.51	−4.3	0 (0)	0 (0)
Q12	2.48	0.61	−3.4	8 (6.2)	0 (0)
Q13	2.52	0.60	−3.9	7 (5.4)	0 (0)
Q14	2.54	0.64	−5.0	10 (7.7)	0 (0)
Q15	2.54	0.68	−2.8	11 (8.5)	1 (0.8)
Follow-up/coordination	2.49	0.60	−5.2	6 (4.6)	0 (0)
Q16	2.40	0.75	−3.8	21 (16.2)	0 (0)
Q17	2.51	0.67	−4.9	13 (10.0)	0 (0)
Q18	2.58	0.71	−6.0	16 (12.3)	0 (0)
Q19	2.48	0.70	−3.9	14 (10.8)	0 (0)
Q20	2.46	0.71	−4.4	16 (12.3)	0 (0)

intensive training in CCM [30]. Our findings have also shown that the internal consistency for overall PACIC-M is very high and comparable to the original PACIC instrument and to most of the other validated PACIC done in various European countries [11, 27, 29]. The instrument is stable over time which is similar with Glasgow et al. [11] and Rosemann et al. [27] The inter-item correlations among the subscales were found to be high and this is comparable to other studies [11, 27].

The final validated PACIC-M consisted of 19 items framed within the following three components i) goal setting/tailoring and problem solving/contextual, ii) follow-up/coordination, and iii) patient activation and delivery system design/ decision support. Item 1 was removed as it did not load onto any of the three components. Like others who translated the PACIC into different languages [31–33], we were unable to confirm the 5-component structure model in the factorial examination in patient responses to PACIC-M instrument. PACIC-M was unable to identify all components of the

CCM, in which it was inadequate to provide information about individual construct of CCM as expected. Our findings suggest almost half of the PACIC-M variability was explained by component 1 (item 6 to15), which is a combination of 'goal setting/tailoring and problem solving/contextual'. This component is positively correlated to component 2 (follow-up/coordination) and component 3 (patient activation and delivery system design/ decision support). Our findings of the 3-component structure of the PACIC-M is a reflection of the EMPOWER-PAR intervention which reinforced the national clinical guideline recommendations for diabetes care through individualized goal setting of treatment targets, problem solving skills, follow-up and coordination of care by the healthcare team [7, 16]. It also reflects the use of Global Cardiovascular Risks Self-Management Booklet which supports goal setting and problem solving skills through effective communication and patient empowerment [7, 16]. These three components were found to be positively correlated

Table 4 Factor loadings of the PACIC-M reveals 3-component structure

| | Component | | |
	1	2	3
Q1	0.307	0.218	0.215
Q2	−0.255	0.063	**0.915**
Q3	0.138	−0.101	**0.783**
Q4	0.055	0.009	**0.659**
Q5	0.329	0.006	**0.546**
Q6	**0.410**	0.336	0.198
Q7	**0.606**	0.001	0.069
Q8	**0.546**	0.328	−0.147
Q9	**0.901**	−0.225	0.053
Q10	**0.576**	0.210	−0.006
Q11	**0.573**	0.202	−0.014
Q12	**0.745**	0.071	−0.071
Q13	**0.722**	0.108	−0.073
Q14	**0.515**	0.295	0.030
Q15	**0.870**	−0.110	−0.006
Q16	0.295	**0.465**	0.015
Q17	−0.161	**0.906**	0.150
Q18	−0.023	**0.833**	0.109
Q19	0.037	**0.938**	−0.155
Q20	0.041	**0.908**	−0.062

Extraction Method: Principal Component Analysis
Rotation Method: Promax with Kaiser Normalization
Note: Factor loadings > 0.40 appear in bold

which signifies prominence of these three subscales in the selected clinics.

In the development of PACIC, Glasgow et al. conducted confirmatory factor analysis (CFA) and concluded that the five scales identified were moderately fit [11]. It was further highlighted that the correlation and reliability coefficients reported by Glasgow et al. underestimated the true parameters when Cronbach's alpha and Pearson's correlation was used when a normal data from ordinal scale was assumed [34]. It was argued that the 5-point likert score used to measure the score was

Table 5 Reliability of PACIC-M

	Cronbach alpha	Intra-class correlation
Overall PACIC-M	0.94	0.93
PACIC-M Scales		
Goal setting/tailoring and problem solving/contextual	0.91	
Follow-up/coordination	0.90	
Patient activation and delivery system design/ decision support	0.77	

ordinal but was used in the manner appropriate for interval measurement, in which interpretation of mean score used by Glasgow et al. should be based upon equidistance between two points [34, 35]. Subsequently, published factor analyses found conflicting results, in which only two out of seven studies reported unequivocal results to support the 5-factor structure while others suggested a variety of techniques for further validation [35]. It was subsequently translated and validated in the primary care setting among Danish populations [28, 29, 31] and German populations [27]. These studies have shown mixed results and further validation study was suggested.

Our study highlights an interesting finding when patients' responses may not conform to the expectations of the design of the questionnaire, such that analyses of the responses can reveal aspects of care delivery deemed important for the patients. Patients may be conscious of clinical targets and self-care as dominated by the two subscales following utilization of the self-management booklet but may be unaware of system delivery re-design which is important to healthcare providers. The 20-items of PACIC was designed to assess patients' perspectives, of which patient's experiences of chronic illness care and their understanding of CCM concept is substantial in order to match the person interpreting the results. This finding affirms that patients understanding and interpretation may vary and may be influenced by individual patient's factor and care delivery already implemented in the chronic disease management system. However, confirmatory factor analysis of the PACIC-M is recommended to confirm the 3-component model found in this study.

Study limitations

This study has several limitations. The final PACIC-M consisted of 19 items, with Item 1 was deleted when the factor loading was < 0.4. We consider the deletion is appropriate when significance of a factor loading will depend on the sample size, in which a higher loading is needed if the sample size is small [21]. Typically, researchers take a loading of an absolute value > 0.3 to be important, and only appropriate if the sample size is 300 [21]. With a sample size of 130, a higher loading was chosen to be significant for our study. Secondly, the PACIC-M was administered to T2DM patients who were able to read and understand the Malay language. Therefore, the findings of this study could only be generalised and the usability of PACIC-M could only be extended to individuals with T2DM who could read and understand the Malay language. There is a need to translate and validate this questionnaire into other languages such as Mandarin and Tamil to give better utilisation in a multi ethnic Malaysian population. For item discriminant

Table 6 Spearman correlations between the original PACIC subscales and the overall score

	Patient activation	Delivery system design/decision support	Goal setting/ tailoring	Problem solving/ contextual	Follow-up/ coordination
Patient activation	1	.623[a]	.455[a]	.408[a]	.523[a]
Delivery system design/decision support		1	.587[a]	.582[a]	.589[a]
Goal setting/tailoring			1	.807[a]	.689[a]
Problem solving/Contextual				1	.692[a]
Follow-up/coordination					1
Overall score	.671[a]	.748[a]	.877[a]	.858[a]	.872[a]

[a]Correlation is significant at the 0.01 level (2-tailed)

validity, we were not able to test the hypothesized scales with other measurement tool as none were available in the Malay language. Other limitation includes the consecutive sampling method used in this study which may be vulnerable to sampling bias. However, measures were taken to ensure that all T2DM patients who attended the clinics on the data collection days were approached and invited to participate.

Implications for clinical practice and future research
The validated PACIC-M serves as an important patient reported instrument to measure the quality of patient-centred care for T2DM which is consistent with the CCM in the Malaysian primary care setting. This information would be pivotal in guiding the healthcare professionals and policy makers to make the necessary changes to the chronic disease delivery system, to ensure that patients are satisfied with the

care that they receive. However, to strengthen the validity of the PACIC-M, further validation study which includes confirmatory factor analysis is recommended. Future research may also include utilisation of the PACIC-M to evaluate the impact of a CCM-based intervention on the perceived quality of care as received by the patients.

Conclusions
The PACIC-M contains 19 items which are framed within 3-component model. It is a valid and reliable tool which can be used to measure the perception of T2DM patients towards the care that they receive and whether the care is congruent with the CCM elements. However, further validation study which includes confirmatory factor analysis is recommended to strengthen the validity of the PACIC-M.

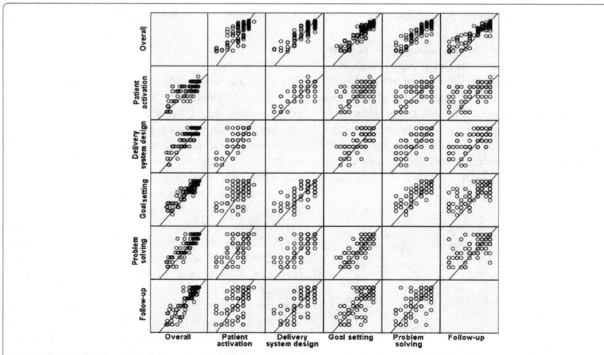

Fig. 2 Matrix plot of mean score for overall, patient activation, decision support, goal setting and follow up

Abbreviations

CCM: Chronic care model; CFA: Confirmatory factor analysis; CPG: Clinical practice guideline; EFA: Exploratory factor analysis; EMPOWER-PAR: EMPOWER participatory action research; HbA1C: Haemoglobin A1c; ICC: Intra-class correlation coefficient; KMO: Kaiser-Meyer-Olkin; MOH: Ministry of Health; PACIC: Patient assessment on chronic illness care; PACIC-M: PACIC-Malay version; PCA: Principal component analysis; Q1-Q20: Item 1-item 20; SD: Standard deviation; T2DM: Type 2 diabetes mellitus; UiTM: Universiti Teknologi MARA

Acknowledgements

We would like to thank the EMPOWER-PAR Investigators: Professor Dr. Ng Chirk Jenn, Dr. Inderjit Singh Ludher, Dr. Suhazeli Abdullah, Professor Dr. Teng Cheong Lieng, Dr. Verna K. M. Lee, Dr. Ng Kien Keat, Dr. Farnaza Ariffin, Dr. Hasidah Abdul-Hamid, Dr. Mazapuspavina Md Yasin, Dr. Nafiza Mat-Nasir, Dr. Maizatullifah Miskan, Dr. Yong-Rafidah Abdul Rahman, Dr. Mastura Ismail, Mr. Wilson H. H. Low and Staff Nurse Sarimah Mahmood for their contributions towards the EMPOWER-PAR Study. We also wish to thank Dr. Maryam Hannah Daud, Dr. Khamsiah Abdul Shukor and Dr. Syarifah Azimah Wan Ali for their assistance in data collection at the study sites.

Funding

This work was supported by the Ministry of Higher Education (MOHE) Malaysia:
Exploratory Research Grant Scheme (ERGS) no: ERGS/PHASE 1–2011/(Health and Clinical Sciences)/ (Universiti Teknologi MARA)/(JPT.S (BPKI) 2000/09/01/ 018 959) or 600-RMI/ERGS 5/3 (28/2011) and by the Ministry of Health (MOH).
Malaysia: Major Research Grant Scheme (NMRR ID -11-250-8769). The funding bodies did not play any role in the design of the study, or in data collection, analysis or interpretation, or in writing the manuscript.

Authors' contributions

SAR drafted the manuscript. ASR and JH conceptualized, designed and acquired the funding for the study. SAR and SFB analysed and interpreted the data. ASR, JH and SFB revised it critically for important intellectual content. All authors have read and given approval of the final manuscript. Each author has participated sufficiently in the work to take public responsibility for appropriate portions of the content as described above. All authors agreed to be accountable for all aspects of the work to ensure that questions related to the accuracy or integrity of any part of the work would be appropriately investigated and resolved.

Ethics approval and consent to participate

We had obtained written permission from Professor Russell E. Glasgow to adapt, translate and validate the PACIC questionnaire. This validation study was approved by the institutional Ethics Committee of Universiti Teknologi MARA (UiTM) and the Medical Research Ethics Committee of the Ministry of Health (MOH), Malaysia. Patient information sheets were distributed in two languages i.e. Malay and English. Written informed consent was obtained from all participants prior to their study enrolment. Confidentiality of personal information was ensured at all times. Enrolment was done by the investigators and not the participants' attending doctors to reduce participants' perceived coercion to participate in the study.

Competing interests

The authors declare that they have no competing interests.

Author details

[1]Primary Care Medicine Discipline, Faculty of Medicine, Universiti Teknologi MARA, Selayang Campus, Jalan Prima Selayang 7, 68100 Batu Caves, Selangor, Malaysia. [2]Institute of Pathology, Laboratory and Forensic Medicine (I-PPerForM), Universiti Teknologi MARA, Sungai Buloh Campus, Jalan Hospital, 47000 Sungai Buloh, Selangor, Malaysia.[3]National Clinical Research Centre, Ministry of Health, Kuala Lumpur, Malaysia.

References

1. Bodenheimer T, Wagner E, Grumbach K. Improving primary care for patients. JAMA. 2002;288(15):1990–14.
2. Rothman AA, Wagner EH. Future of primary care chronic illness management : what is the role of primary care ? Ann Intern Med. 2003;138:256–61.
3. Bensing J. Bridging the gap. The separate worlds of evidence-based medicine and patient-centered medicine. Patient Educ Couns. 2000;39(1):17–25.
4. Glasgow RE, Whitesides H, Nelson CC, King DK. Use of the patient assessment of chronic illness care (PACIC) with diabetic patients: relationship to patient characteristics, receipt of care, and self-management. Diabetes Care. 2005;28(11):2655–61.
5. Tsai AC, Morton SC, Mangione CM, Keeler EB. A meta-analysis of interventions to improve care for chronic illnesses. Am J Manag Care. 2005;11(8):478–88.
6. Drewes HW, Steuten LMG, Lemmens LC, Baan CA, Boshuizen HC, Elissen AMJ, et al. The effectiveness of chronic care management for heart failure: meta-regression analyses to explain the heterogeneity in outcomes. Health Serv Res. 2012;47(5):1926–59.
7. Ramli AS, Selvarajah S, Daud MH, Haniff J, Abdul-Razak S, TMI T-A-B-S, et al. Effectiveness of the EMPOWER-PAR intervention in improving clinical outcomes of type 2 diabetes mellitus in primary care: a pragmatic cluster randomised controlled trial. BMC Fam Pract. 2016;17(1):157.
8. Ku G, Kegels G. Implementing elements of a context-adapted chronic care model to improve first-line diabetes care: effects on assessment of chronic illness care and glycaemic control among people with diabetes enrolled to the first-line diabetes care (FiLDCare) project in the Northern Philippines. Prim Heal Care Res Dev. 2015;16(5):481–91.
9. Ariffin F, Ramli AS, Daud MH, Haniff J, Abdul-Razak S, Selvarajah S, et al. Feasibility of implementing chronic care model in the Malaysian public primary care setting. Med J Malaysia. 2017;72(2):106–12.
10. Mustapha FI, Omar ZA, Mihat O, Noh K, Hassan N, Bakar RA, et al. Addressing non-communicable diseases in Malaysia : an integrative process of systems and community. BMC Public Health. 2014;14(Suppl 2):S4.
11. Glasgow RE, Wagner EH, Schaefer J, Mahoney LD, Reid RJ, Greene SM. Development and validation of the patient assessment of chronic illness care (PACIC). Med Care. 2005;43(5):436–44.
12. Vrijhoef HJM, Berbee R, Wagner EH, Steuten LMG. Quality of integrated chronic care measured by patient survey: identification, selection and application of most appropriate instruments. Health Expect. 2009;12(4):417–29.
13. Hibbard JH. Engaging health care consumers to improve the quality of care. Med Care. 2003;41(1 Suppl):I61–70.
14. Wild D, Grove A, Martin M, Eremenco S, McElroy S, Verjee-Lorenz A, et al. Principles of good practice for the translation and vultural adaptation process for patient-reported outcomes (PRO) measures: report of the ISPOR task force for translating adaptation. Value Heal. 2005;8(2):94–104.
15. Gjersing L, Caplehorn JRM, Clausen T. Cross-cultural adaptation of research instruments: language, setting, time and statistical considerations. BMC Med Res Methodol. 2010;10:13.
16. Ramli AS, Lakshmanan S, Haniff J, Selvarajah S, Tong SF, Bujang M-A, et al. Study protocol of EMPOWER participatory action research (EMPOWER-PAR): a pragmatic cluster randomised controlled trial of multifaceted chronic disease management strategies to improve diabetes and hypertension outcomes in primary care. BMC Fam Pract. 2014;15(1):151.
17. Gorsuch RL. Factor analysis. 2nd ed. Hillsdale: Lawrence Erlbaum Associates; 1983.
18. McHorney CA, Tarlov A. Individual-patient monitoring in clinical practice: are available health status surveys adequate? Qual Life Res. 1995;4(4):293–307.
19. K A B. A new incremental fit index for general structural equation models. Sociol Methods Res. 1989;17(3):303–16.

20. Bentler P. Comparative fit indexes in structural models. Psycho Bull. 1990;
     107:238–46.
21. Stevens J. Applied multivariate statistics for the social sciences. 4th ed.
     Hillsdale: Mahwah: Erlbaum, L; 2002.
22. Sitzia J. How valid and reliable are patient satisfaction data? An analysis of
     195 studies. Int J Qual Heal Care. 1999;11(4):319–28.
23. Streiner DL, Norman GR. Health measurement scales: a practical guide to
     their development and use. Oxford: Oxford University Press; 2008.
24. Shrout PE, Fleiss JL. Intraclass correlations: uses in assessing rater reliability.
     Psychol Bull. 1979;86(2):420–8.
25. Cicchetti DV. Guidelines, criteria, and rules of thumb for evaluating normed
     and standardized assessment instruments in psychology. Psychol Assess.
     1994;6(4):284–90.
26. Maccallum RC, Browne MW, Sugawara HM. Power analysis and determination
     of sample size for covariance structure modeling of fit involving a particular
     measure of model. Psychol Methods. 1996;13(2):130–49.
27. Rosemann T, Laux G, Droesemeyer S, Gensichen J, Szecsenyi J. Evaluation of
     a culturally adapted German version of the patient assessment of chronic
     illness care (PACIC 5A) questionnaire in a sample of osteoarthritis patients. J
     Eval Clin Pract. 2007;13(5):806–13.
28. Maindal HT, Sokolowski I, Vedsted P. Adaptation, data quality and
     confirmatory factor analysis of the Danish version of the PACIC
     questionnaire. Eur J Pub Health. 2012;22(1):31–6.
29. Wensing M, van Lieshout J, Jung HP, Hermsen J, Rosemann T. The patients
     assessment chronic illness care (PACIC) questionnaire in the Netherlands: a
     validation study in rural general practice. BMC Health Serv Res. 2008;8:182.
30. Aragones A, Schaefer EW, Stevens D, Gourevitch MN, Glasgow RE, Shah NR,
     et al. Validation of the Spanish translation of the patient assessment of
     chronic illness care (PACIC) survey. Prev Chronic Dis. 2008;5(4):A113.
31. Fan J, McCoy RG, Ziegenfuss JY, Smith SA, Borah BJ, Deming JR, et al. Evaluating
     the structure of the patient assessment of chronic illness care (PACIC) survey
     from the Patient's perspective. Ann Behav Med. 2015;49(1):104–11.
32. Tusek-Bunc K, Petek-Ster M, Ster B, Petek D, Kersnik J. Validation of the
     Slovenian version of patient assessment of chronic illness care (PACIC) in
     patients with coronary heart disease. Coll Antropol. 2014;38(2):437–44.
33. Taggart J, Chan B, Jayasinghe UW, Christl B, Proudfoot J, Crookes P, et al.
     Patients assessment of chronic illness care (PACIC) in two Australian studies:
     structure and utility. J Eval Clin Pract. 2011;17(2):215–21.
34. Gugiu C, Coryn CLS, Applegate B. Structure and measurement properties of
     the patient assessment of chronic illness care instrument. J Eval Clin Pract.
     2010;16(3):509–16.
35. Spicer J, Budge C, Carryer J. Taking the PACIC back to basics: the structure
     of the patient assessment of chronic illness care. J Eval Clin Pract. 2012;
     18(2):307–12.

GP/GPN partner* perspectives on clinical placements for student nurses in general practice: can a community of practice help to change the prevailing culture within general practice?

Robin Lewis[1]* and Shona Kelly[2]

Abstract

Background: The UK Government document *5 year forward view* describes the need to move chronic disease management from secondary to primary care, which will require a significant increase in the numbers of General Practice Nurses (GPNs). Until recently, there has been no specific recruitment strategy to address this increased need. In recent times, a number of solutions have been suggested to address this impending GPN recruitment crisis. For example, Health Education England (HEE) commission General Practitioners (GPs), who are members of the Advanced Training Practice Scheme (ATPS), to provide placements for student nurses within general practice.

Methods: A descriptive qualitative study was undertaken, in which data were collected using semi-structured interviews with 16 GPs and 2 GPN partners*. Qualitative analysis used a framework approach and themes were cross-checked within the team and member checking was undertaken with a convenience sample of GPs. The research had ethical approval and anonymity and confidentiality were maintained.

Results: From the GP perspective, there were two key themes that emerged from the data. The first theme of *'fishing in the same small pond'* included succession planning for the general practice workforce, the 'merry go round' of poaching staff from other practices, and the myths and misunderstandings that have grown up around general practice nursing. The second theme, *'growing your own,'* looked at the impact of the student nurse placements as a means to address the crisis in GPN recruitment. There was recognition of the need for cultural change in the way that GPNs are recruited, and that the ATPS was one way of helping to achieve that change. There were however a number of challenges to sustaining this cultural shift, such as the financial constrains placed upon the GP practice, and the need to function as a 'small business'.

Conclusions: Despite all the challenges, the evidence is that, through the Community of Practice (CoP), the ATPS scheme is beginning to 'bear fruit', and there is a subtle but discernible move by GPs from a 'why *would* we?' to 'why *wouldn't* we?' invest in education and training for nurses in general practice.
N.B. The term GPN partner* denotes a GPN who is a 'full partner' in the practice business, holding the same NHS contracts and the same status as a GP. For the purposes of the paper itself, the term GP will be used to denote both types of partner.

Keywords: General practice, Workforce, Placements, Nurse education, Organisational culture, Community of practice

* Correspondence: r.p.lewis@shu.ac.uk
[1]Department of Nursing and Midwifery, Sheffield Hallam University, Sheffield
S10 2BP, England
Full list of author information is available at the end of the article

Background

There is constant reference in the UK media to an 'impending workforce crisis' in UK general practice, set against the backdrop of the Health Education England (HEE) report into primary care [1] and the Royal College of General Practitioners (RCGP) Practice Forum Report [2]. Both of these reports concluded that General Practitioner (GP) partners are finding it harder to recruit GP trainees and to replace those GPs who are increasingly opting to retire. This occurs at the same time as the current 'direction of travel' within NHS England is to move more and more services from secondary care into primary care; in particular chronic disease management. NHS England's 5 Year Forward View [3] outlined plans to move more services into the community however it is acknowledged that if general practice is to be able to meet this future demand, the necessary human resources must be put in place to support that transition.

General practitioners (GPs) are doctors that work in primary care. They treat common medical conditions and refer patients to hospital and other services for urgent and specialist treatment. In some parts of the UK there is a significant shortfall in the number of General Practitioners (GPs), and the age profiles of GPs are such that there is significant concern over the supply of appropriately trained GPs to fill future vacancies. Despite initiatives to increase the numbers of GP training opportunities available, applications to GP training nationally continue to fall. Some parts of the UK particularly in the north of England, significantly struggle to recruit sufficient numbers of GP trainees [4]. This chronic shortage of GPs has had a number of consequences for general practice, specifically the enhanced profile of the General Practice Nurse (GPN) [5]. Central to this study, the GPN role has evolved and developed to address some of these workforce issues. In particular, chronic disease management and surveillance now comes under the aegis of the GPN [7].

This has resulted in GPNs taking on more responsibility for running long term conditions clinics such as those for chronic asthma and diabetes [6, 7]. This 'extended' clinical responsibility requires specialist education and training, including training to 'independently prescribe' medications [6, 7]. However, the age profile of GPNs is not dissimilar to those of GPs, with a recent Queen's Nursing Institute (QNI) report [8] identifying that approximately 33% of GPNs are due to retire within the next 5 years. If there is no clear recruitment and retention strategy in place to increase the numbers of GPNs to both replace those GPNs due to retire and to address the increasing workload being transferred to general practice, then there is a 'perfect storm' brewing in which there will be an acute shortage of both GPs

and GPNs at a time when the workload in primary care will be at its greatest [5].

It has been argued [9–13] that at least part of the forthcoming GPN recruitment crisis relates to the dearth of general practice placements available for student nurses in the UK. Unlike medicine, there is no established culture of student nurses spending time on placement in general practice. This means that many student nurses do not know what general practice nursing is or what it has to offer, and conversely many GPs are unaware of the current situation in nurse education [9]. This clearly needs to be addressed, and one practical way to do this is to increase the number of clinical placements for student nurses within general practice. However, the QNI survey [8] also found that only 27% of GPs offered placements for undergraduate nursing students, compared to 61.5% offering placements to undergraduate medical students.

It is clear that these matters are not unique to the UK. The Australian government has similarly invested in providing incentives for general practices to employ more GPNs, however the same issues remain as in the UK [14]. The move to treat an ageing population with increasingly complex healthcare needs in primary care, allied to challenges in addressing shortages in the primary care workforce mean that Australia is facing many of the issues being addressed here. In New Zealand, the picture is slightly different. The development of a Primary Health Care Strategy [15] in 2001 highlighted the need to invest in the development of Practice Nursing as a career, with an associated national career pathway for GPNs. This means that in New Zealand, significant advances have been made in recent times to both recruit and retain GPNs.

In recent times, there have been a number of proposed solutions to the shortage of student nurse placements in general practice, and to positively influence the developing GPN recruitment crisis in the UK [9–13]. In a number of areas within the UK, GPs have been specifically commissioned by HEE to provide placements for student nurses. These schemes are part of the wider National Training Hubs Initiative (NTHI). This is a targeted response to two key government documents: The GP Forward View [16] and The 5 Year Forward View [3]. It brings together primary care and higher education institutions such as Sheffield Hallam University in the UK, enabling the development of the networks required to support future workforce planning. As part of the NTHI, this Advanced Training Practice Scheme (ATPS) within the north of the UK provides General Practice (GP) placements for undergraduate student nurses that offer opportunities for students to gain experience in a general practice setting. In addition, further workforce transformation initiatives such as the 'GPN Ready' scheme (to support the recruitment of new graduate nurses) have also been developed under the ATPS banner. This particular ATPS covers a large geographical area in the North of the UK, which is predominantly urban in nature, with a population with higher than average indices of deprivation [15]. It is a partnership between the participating GP practices and SHU, and is specifically designed to provide opportunities for student nurses at all levels of training to gain an in-depth and sustained exposure to, and experience of, general practice nursing [13]. The idea is that this dedicated exposure to general practice will encourage the students to consider applying for a GPN post on graduation.

Students' career intentions upon graduation are influenced by their perceptions of the different clinical areas in which they work [17]. Popular clinical environments such as those in acute care are viewed as being dynamic, exciting and challenging places in which to work, and much of this information appears to come from students' working knowledge of the area and from positive placement experiences. Consequently, there has been no real opportunity for students to positively experience general practice, and all the evidence points to a lack of knowledge and understanding of the role of the GPN and all that it has to offer.

This is borne out by the findings from a study carried out by Bloomfield et al. [18] which looked at students' career intentions in relation to primary care in Australia. The study compared tertiary care, secondary care and primary care as potential career options. The authors found that primary care was not regarded seriously as a viable career option by the majority of the students that were surveyed. In addition, there have been a number of studies from Australia that have looked specifically at students' experiences of general practice placements [19, 20]. The findings from these studies reported a generally positive student experience, and although the placements did provide some impetus for consideration of a career in general practice, little is currently known regarding the true impact of primary care placements upon students' career intentions or on the GPs themselves.

Communities of practice (CoP)

The theoretical approach used in this study is based upon Lave & Wenger's idea of a 'community of practice' (CoP) [21]. According to Lave & Wenger, a community of practice (CoP) is a *socially situated, practice-based* approach to learning, in which the learning that takes place is viewed in terms of a series of collective, relational and social processes (as opposed to an individual, solitary process of knowledge acquisition). It involves a complex relationship between novice(s) and expert(s), being socialised into the practice and developing an identity within that practice community.

As a theoretical lens through which to view the general practice placements, CoP are clearly attractive because they use a *socially constructed* approach to learning, in that learning is seen as much more than simply the individual acquisition of knowledge [21]. It is argued that the CoP as a community of learning enables the development of positive personal relationships and ways of interacting, together with a mutually constructed sense of identity. As Ranmuthugala et al. note [22], a strong learning community promotes healthy interactions and work-based relationships based upon mutual trust and respect. The successful CoP may be characterised in terms of a shared *domain* of interest, a *community* that pursues that shared interest and the open and unbiased *sharing* of knowledge, information and resources. The development of a work-based identity is key, in that it enables the GPs to visualise how the neophyte GPN might 'fit in' and positively influence the general practice team [23].

By adopting a socially constructed approach to learning, learning is seen as much more than simply the acquisition of knowledge. Therefore, by using the CoP we may gain a better understanding of the processes by which the GPs' views and perceptions are formed. This will enable us to address the key aims of the study, which are outlined below:

Aims and objectives

The overarching aim of the study was to explore GP perceptions of the student nurse placement in general practice. There were a number of specific objectives relating to the examination of:

1) GPN recruitment: culture and practice
2) The effectiveness of the ATPS 'model' of student nurse placements
3) General Practice as a career for new graduate nurses

Methods
Context for the study

The ATPS being studied was one of the first of the Practice placement networks to be formed, and has been in existence since 2009 [1]. The overarching philosophy of the scheme is to promote sustainable cultural change in general practice, by widening student nurse access to general practice placements. Through the ATPS, GPs are also supported to 'grown their own' GPNs by recruiting new graduate nurses. As the ATPS becomes fully embedded, the idea of 'growing your own' is beginning to change the prevailing culture within general practice. Partner HEIs such as SHU work closely with the GPs to provide support for the students (proto-GPNs) through the ATPS placements and the recruitment of new graduates into a GPN post (neophyte GPN) and afterwards (emergent GPN).

Study design

A descriptive, qualitative approach was used for the study. This involved the use of semi-structured, one to one interviews with 16 GPs and 2 GPN partners. Although it may be seen as a 'low inference' approach to interpretation of the data, the descriptive qualitative study design is a pragmatic way for the researcher to gain an authentic and in-depth insight into the perceptions, thoughts and experiences of the participants. This type of study design may be regarded as a useful means for addressing many research questions in health care, since it is an effective way in which to look at the experiences of health professionals and their views on the way that health care systems are organised.

Cohort and sample

A purposive, cross-sectional sample of GPs was drawn from the population of 37 practices currently participating in the ATPS programme. The GPs in these practices were approached by letter and a follow up phone call. The sample was based upon data relating to the number of GPs and GPNs within the practice and the length of time the practice has participated in the ATPS programme.

Data collection

Data collection was carried out using semi-structured interviews with an interview schedule (please refer to Additional file 1 for details) based upon the findings from a rapid review of the existing literature. There were seven questions in the interview schedule, and these related to the views of the GP on general practice as a placement for student nurses. The questions were used as prompts for the interviewer and as a framework to guide the dialogue. The interviews were conducted by a member of the study team and took place at a date and time of the participants' choosing. With the participant's consent the interviews were digitally recorded, with each interview lasting approximately 15–20 min. Data collection continued until saturation was reached.

Research governance

Following an agreement in principle to take part, formal written consent was obtained from all interview participants prior to the interviews taking place. Ethical approval for the study was obtained from the SHU Faculty Research Ethics Committee (Ref: H447). SHU Research governance protocols were adhered to throughout the study. All data was anonymised to maintain confidentiality and to ensure that no individual could be recognised in any subsequent report. Paper based data is kept securely in a locked drawer and electronic data and information relating to this research is kept on a password-protected computer on a network storage system that adheres to Home Office Standards of Data Security. This data will be kept for a minimum of 7 years in accordance with SHU guidelines.

Data analysis

The interview transcripts were anonymised and each transcript was allocated a unique code. They were entered into Quirkos© software for analysis and cross-checked for accuracy by the team. Once it had been cross-checked, the data was analysed following the National Centre for Social Research 'Framework' guidelines [24]. This approach has emerged from applied health and social policy research and analysis. It involves a systematic processing, sifting, charting and sorting of material into key issues and themes. It also permits both within- and across-case comparisons and allows the integration of existing knowledge from previous research and policy into the emerging analysis. All transcripts were analysed independently by all four members of the research team and the interpretation of data was also cross-checked within the team. Member checking was also used, as were direct quotes from the participants. The use of these techniques both enriches and enhances the link between the respondents' experiences and the analysis of the data (25).

Results

There were two key themes that emerged from the data. The first theme (Table 1) looked back at what had gone before, with the recognition that things needed to change. This included issues such as the culture of general practice, the need for succession planning and the poaching of experienced staff from other practices. The second theme (Table 2) looked at the impact of the student nurse placements. This included the need to address the longstanding cultural issues and the need to invest in the GPN workforce.

Fishing in the same small pond

The first theme of 'fishing in the same small pond' included the lack of infrastructure and succession planning for the general practice workforce, the 'merry go round' of poaching staff from other practices and the various misunderstandings that have grown up around general

Table 1 Themes and sub-themes

Theme One:	Sub-themes:
"Fishing in the same small pond"	• Succession planning
	• The recruitment 'merry go round'
	• Cultural antecedents
	• Adapt to survive

Table 2 Themes and sub-themes

Theme Two:	Sub-themes:
"Growing your own staff"	• The need for 'new blood'
	• The need for some fine tuning
	• Investing in the future workforce
	• Green shoots of cultural change

practice nursing (see Table 1). The care delivery 'model' for general practice has remained largely unchanged since the inception of the NHS and general practice continues to be run by small, independently-run businesses, contracted to provide a portfolio of defined health services to a registered list of patients. These businesses are owned and run by one or more GP/GPN 'partners' who hold the various NHS patient care contract(s).

Succession planning

For the most part the culture and practice of GPN recruitment had also not fundamentally changed in decades. The age profile of both GPs and GPNs within the UK meant that a significant proportion of the GP and GPN population were nearing retirement age. From a practical point of view, this GP commented on the 'perfect storm' that was brewing within general practice:

> "... there are lots of GPs round here who are coming up to retirement, and they have all got practice nurses that are coming up to retirement too ..."

This GP was also pragmatic in the approach to GPN recruitment. The difficulties in recruitment were clear, and the GP acknowledged the need for a fresh look at the subject:

> "We had some real difficulty filling that last vacancy ... we've got a number of people [GPNs] approaching retirement and that gives us an opportunity to perhaps do things a bit differently next time ..."

When a GPN leaves a practice there is a hiatus caused by the recruitment processes. The economies of scale in general practice (i.e. small to medium businesses working in small, socially isolated teams) mean that when they do recruit a GPN, the practice will attempt to recruit an experienced, competent nurse who won't need much training and can therefore 'hit the ground running'. Inevitably this desire simply reinforces the idea that newly qualified nurses and general practice are not suited to each other. Older, more experienced nurses were often recruited from secondary care settings. There were however, a number of reservations voiced regarding the motives of these nurses. For example, this GP commented:

> "I think [the] hospital nurses want to come into primary care because it's a Monday to Friday nine-to-five job ... they've done a few years in hospital with shifts and nights and everything else, seven days a week and then they start thinking, actually, I quite fancy a job that's a bit more family-friendly. It's not always ... 'I really want to work in primary care'..."

The recruitment 'merry go round'

In spite of the numbers of nurses recruited from secondary care, experienced GPNs remained at a premium. The dwindling numbers of GPNs and the increasing need for skilled, experienced nurses to take on chronic disease management to meet UK Government monitoring (QOF: Quality Outcomes Framework) targets meant that they were (and still are) much in demand. This situation has led to a GPN recruitment 'merry go round'. In an assessment of the current situation, this GP remarked:

> "There's going to be a much greater demand for practice nurses and particularly the more highly skilled ones that can manage their own caseload ..."

It is not difficult to see how and why the 'merry go round' has existed to date, but there was a realisation that it was becoming unsustainable:

> "I do understand that we are poaching them [GPNs] from each other ... You know, obviously, there's not enough nurses around (sic) and it does seem to me they just swap from one practice to another ... "

This GP also reflected upon the futile nature of 'poaching' of GPNs from other practices. There was also recognition of the increasing difficulties in recruiting experienced GPNs.

> "They just poach from other practices, but [even] that's dried up now ... they've been taking from secondary care too ... So we're all just fishing in the same small pond, aren't we?"

Cultural antecedents

The current situation clearly has a number of historical and cultural antecedents. There has been an historic lack of communication between general practice and nurse education, and this has led to a number of misunderstandings. For example, this GP expressed frustration over the current situation:

> "We've had to work hard to get an understanding from some of the GPs and from quite a lot of university

*teachers and from quite a lot of student nurses too that they [nurses] **do not*** need secondary care experience before they go into primary care ... and that's the problem"*

* Denotes heavy emphasis placed on these words by respondent

There was also a widespread frustration amongst the GPs that most of the nursing students' placement time was still spent on hospital wards. Although the balance between the number of primary and secondary placements is slowly changing, the comment of this GP was typical:

"I don't know how many of the students will actually try and get into general practice... most of them go into the hospitals [when they qualify] as that's where they have all their training..."

Working in acute care was also perceived as being much more much more attractive to the students than working in primary care. This GP noted ruefully:

" ... They all seem to think that working in a hospital is sexier (sic) than working in a GP surgery ..."

This then became a self-fulfilling prophesy in which GPs did not actively seek to recruit new graduate nurses, and new graduate nurses did not apply for GPN posts. However, the findings from another component of this evaluation [20] indicated that the students with general practice placements were beginning to appreciate the role of the GPN and the opportunities that it provided. The prospect of working in general practice upon graduation was now seen as attractive to many of them.

Adapt to survive

There did seem to be an acknowledgement of the need to change the culture of GPN recruitment and retention. The demands for new ways of working proposed in the *5 Year Forward View*, together with the longstanding difficulties in GP recruitment meant that the skill mix within general practice that had existed for years needed to be updated to meet the requirements of the twenty-first century patient. The GPs were candid in their assessment of the need to 'adapt to survive':

"I mean ... 'traditional' general practice needs to adapt ... previously you had say five or six GPs, a couple of nurses and one HCA [in a practice] but the skill mix is not needed like that anymore ... "

This GP went on to say that:

"... there are some practices who are already beginning to change, so they'll have three GPs, four or five nurses, of which three will prescribe and one's an ACP [Advanced Clinical Practitioner], and five or six HCAs"

The development of non-medical staff within general practice has been ad hoc and informal, and this has meant that the infrastructure required for sustainable workforce change has not been a priority. The accelerated expansion of non-medical roles in more recent times has resulted in a 'patchwork' of different roles and different titles. The introduction of the ACP role is a good example of this. The title of ACP is not regulated in the same way as the title of GP, but an ACP is generally considered to be a fully autonomous practitioner, educated to Masters Level, managing their own caseload in the same way as the GP.

However a number of experienced GPNs had already developed a high level of autonomy through for example the ability to independently prescribe medication. There was however the realisation that this cohort of GPNs was dwindling due to retirement and that the traditional recruitment methods were becoming obsolete. Although experienced GPNs were highly sought after, they were seen to have their drawbacks. This GPN partner commented:

"What you don't want is loads of other people's 'baggage', which you generally get with somebody who's come from somewhere else ... 'we don't do it that way; I do it this way'... far better then, to recruit newly qualifieds (sic) and 'grow your own'?"

Growing your own staff

The second theme *'growing your own,'* looked at the impact of the student nurse placements upon the looming workforce crisis. As we can see from the first theme, there was already acknowledgement of the need for cultural change, and in this second theme, recognition that the ATPS was one way to achieve that change. There were however a number of challenges to this, including the often competing demands of the GPNs for education and the practice as a 'small business'.

The findings here (see Table 2) show that the philosophical approach of 'growing your own' GPNs had begun to gain some traction, albeit on a small scale, within general practice. This GP in particular could see the benefits of 'growing your own' GPNs, and was also clear that the current situation was becoming untenable. There was a need for 'new blood'.

" ... GPs need to understand that if they want a new nurse, they can either try and poach one off [the] 'roundabout', which just recycles what's there, does

nothing for the gene pool or they can take somebody straight from training ... and train them up themselves ..."

Through the CoP, the student nurses were beginning to have a small but discernible impact on general practice. One GP summarised the benefits of the ATPS scheme. From a partner's point of view, the new graduate nurses would be free of any 'bad habits', unlike some of the GPNs they had previously employed.

"I suppose they'll not come with any of the preconceived ideas of, you know, 'this happens in the practice that I used to work in before'... from the beginning you're teaching them how you want it to work here from the very start. I think that's got to be a good thing..."

Again, there was recognition that 'new blood' was needed. This GP was clear that there was a need to re-invigorate the GPN role, and to attract new, dynamic graduate nurses:

"We've got to encourage the younger generation... I think we've got this fixed idea of what practice nurses are, and we think of the 'old school' nurses and so many things have changed now... So I think we would encourage new young nurses to come in..."

There were a number of other benefits highlighted by the respondents. For example, the influence of the CoP was such that the student nurses kept the other staff 'on their toes'. As this GP astutely noted:

"I think there are several advantages [to the ATPS] having somebody helps you keep up to date [...] that also helps the practice [...] It gives a different perspective because the nurses that are training are doing other things [...] so they've got a slightly different angle on things..."

There was also recognition of the need for change, and the benefits that younger, newly graduated staff would bring to the practices. Commenting upon the presence of the student nurses in her practice, this GP was enthusiastic about the possibilities:

"I think they [the student nurses] bring a fresh and different outlook, different skills too... I would hope that we'd be able to develop them and they'd stay... like I say it's growing your own isn't it..?"

This quotation seemed to encapsulate the developing influence of the ATPS and the new CoP. Finally, the

parallels with medical training placements were becoming clear. As this GP noted:

It's a win-win situation [the ATPS]. If they like the practice and you like them, then you know they're coming up... that's what we do with the [GP] trainees. I mean most of the partners here have been ex-trainees in this practice because it's much better to recruit someone you know who's worked here. And they know what you're like so it's about getting the right fit, isn't it?"

The need for some 'fine tuning'

Although the CoP generated by the ATPS placements was generally seen as 'a good thing' by the majority of the respondents, there were still a number of issues to be addressed. Initially, the students undertook 6 week placements which were deemed to be the minimum length of time for the students to gain sufficient exposure to general practice to make an informed decision about the placement. This GP argued for longer placements to be the norm:

"We are trying to address it [the shortage of GPNs]. We're taking student nurses now and that's great. But they only came for like a six week block in a three-year training programme. It's not enough. We need them for longer but I don't know how we would get around that [...] I think they do need more exposure to primary care..."

Despite the progress being made through the CoP, there was still some evidence of a residual lack of understanding between general practice and nurse education. Having experienced the ATPS, a number of the GPs wanted the students to return each year for a placement. This GP was clear what was needed for the practice to grow its own GPNs.

"Realistically, if you really wanted grow your own, you would have them in the first year, then the second year and then you would have them back in the third year, back to you at your practice, and then you'd offer them a job at the end of it. That's where this [ATPS] would come in..."

This GP was clear that the partnership between general practice and the HEIs providing nurse education are vital to the long term sustainability of the ATPS. The GP identified that there was still some 'room for improvement'.

"It needs to be a proper partnership between you [the HEIs] and us then we all benefit don't we? I don't

think we understand enough [about each other] *but having them* [the students] *helps..."*

Investing in the future workforce

In the UK, the education and training for GPNs is funded primarily by the business. There is some limited access to government funding; however this tends to be regional and ad hoc. The issues over the funding of education meant that there were still some challenges to the recruitment of new graduate nurses. For example, this GP was worried that a newly qualified nurse would not stay in post. Having been used to longevity in their practice staff (one of the GPNs had been with their practice for over 20 years), this was clearly a concern.

"... I think there's perhaps a worry that somebody at that [early] *stage of their career is more likely to be looking for the next job..."*

Another concern was the disparity between what hours the newly qualified nurses would expect and what hours would be available. Given that the GPN role has historically not been the domain of newly-qualified RNs, this is not surprising. Stereotypically, older nurses with children will generally prefer part time, child-friendly working patterns. This very subtly feeds into the idea that general practice is no place for young, new graduate nurses. As this GP noted:

"The younger ones... they'll all want full time hours... you are going to get [some] *smaller practices who don't always need full-time nurses... then what?"*

From a strategic workforce perspective, the ATPS placements may be seen as the first phase of a much wider, long term project to address the recruitment and retention of GPNs in general practice. Once recruited, the need for a more formalised framework of education and training for new graduate GPNs was also becoming clear, albeit rather slowly. Inevitably, this raised the issue of the financial investment required for nurse education and training. The fact that general practices are medically-dominated small businesses means that the provision of education for non-medical staff has not always been a high priority and the needs of the practice were always seen as taking precedence. As this GP noted when asked about financial support for neophyte GPN education and training:

"We'd have to think... 'what would that enable them to do and does it fit with what we want them to do?'..."

There was a clear tension between the needs of the practice and the needs of the staff. This was made clear by one of the GPs who said:

"We're a business in the same way everyone else is (sic) *and therefore it's not like a hospital... you're not going to train someone at your own cost are you?"*

This was a recurrent theme, linked to the GPN recruitment 'merry go round' already described. Clearly this had happened before. Although expressed in a rather convoluted manner, this GP did make the point that:

"... it would be a disincentive to encourage increasing training (sic) *if you think that somebody who's better trained might get poached by another practice in order to get a pay rise..."*

This seems to relate to a largely unfounded perception that, once trained, the GPNs would simply 'follow the money'. Whilst some of the GPNs were clearly 'economically mobile', the vast majority of the GPNs were viewed as being driven by the perceived quality of their terms and conditions rather than purely by financial concerns.

Green shoots of cultural change

The effective provision of GPN education and training for the neophyte GPNs clearly required a good 'fit' between the perceived needs of the practice and the GP partners and the developmental needs of the GPNs involved. The most interesting aspect of the study was that in spite of all their reservations, a number of the GPs interviewed did appear to be moving from a "why *should* we invest in our practice nursing workforce?" perspective to a "why *shouldn't* we invest in our practice nursing workforce?" perspective.

From a workforce perspective, this subtle but crucial change in emphasis may be seen as vindication of the success of the ATPS and the CoP that developed as a result. Some of the more forward thinking GPs had realised the benefit to them of a well-educated and well-supported GPN workforce. As this GP noted, when asked about the ATPS:

"...This [ATPS] *has been a massive but necessary change when you think that general practices are still, the majority, are very much 'corner shops' all doing their own thing..."*

When asked to look into the future:

"... I think in the future you're going to get practices working together to employ nurses to meet the

demand. It will have to happen ... but they may have to work across practices..."

As a final thought, some of the respondents were already thinking about the longer term impact of the ATPS:

"What's next then? Well, in my mind the [long term] *plan would be to make the ATPS, now they're well-established, to make them proper educational hubs for doctors and nurses alike ..."*

Discussion

The well-documented and widely reported fall in the number of GP trainees has meant that the GPN role has assumed a much greater significance within the provision of general practice services. The realisation that a substantial number of existing GPNs are nearing retirement age at a time when more and more services are being moved into primary care has raised the prospect of a 'perfect storm' within the general practice workforce. There are a number of issues that affect the ability of general practice as a whole to address this impending 'storm'. Primarily, these relate to the prevailing culture within general practice. This is complex and socially constructed, with a medical *hegemony* that is both extremely powerful and firmly embedded [25, 26]. There is a widespread agreement that the number of GPNs needs to be increased if primary care is to meet future demand; however the culture of general practice makes this difficult to achieve [27].

The RCGP *Roadmap to Excellence* report [2] clearly articulated the need to attract more new graduate nurses into general practice if the predicted increases in workload and complexity of care are to be satisfactorily addressed in the future. In order to address this predicted shortfall in GPN numbers, there has been a move to increase the numbers of new graduate nurses entering general practice. This has met with some resistance, and to better understand the situation, we need to look at the historical and cultural antecedents [1, 9–13]. Traditionally there has been little or no incentive for GPs to consider employing new graduate nurses. GPNs are employed by the partners and not the NHS, and are therefore seen as a 'cost' to the business [4]. However, GPNs contribute a significant amount of income to general practice through meeting UK Quality Outcomes Framework (QOF) monitoring targets for long term conditions [6, 7]. Consequently, GPs prefer to recruit experienced nurses, rather than invest in new graduate nurses and absorb the costs involved in providing them with the education and training required for the role. When a GPN post becomes vacant, there is evidence of a GPN recruitment 'merry go round' in which new

GPNs are often appointed by being 'poached' from other GP practices [13].

The findings from a companion paper [27], which looked at student nurse perceptions of general practice placements, found that graduating student nurses are often under the (mis)impression that they 'need' to have secondary care experience before applying for a GPN post [10]. These myths have had the effect of both dissuading new graduates from applying for GPN posts, and continuing to 'excuse' GPs from considering them. As with most myths, they have assumed a certain degree of truth. Historically, this has resulted in a situation in which new graduate nurses do not feature in general practice. The overarching philosophy of the ATPS is therefore to promote lasting cultural change within general practice. Through the ATPS, GPs are fully supported to 'grown their own' GPNs by recruiting new graduate nurses. As the ATPS becomes fully embedded, the idea of 'growing your own' is beginning to change the prevailing culture within general practice [9, 10]. In order to better appreciate the theoretical context in which this cultural shift is currently taking place, the ATPS may be considered in terms of an embryonic CoP [22]. From a pedagogical perspective, the GPs learn about student nurses through their participation in the shared social practices of the general practice team [23]. It may be argued that the GPs' learning is therefore seen in terms of a process in which they learn to view the students as 'proto-GPNs', through the students' adoption of a new, albeit temporary identity. The CoP also provided the students with the opportunity to positively influence the social context in which the learning takes place [22]. From a cultural perspective, this social and contextual learning is clearly vital in positively influencing the GPs perceptions of 'new' nurses. According to Lave and Wenger, the students' emerging identity will enable the GPs to modify their perceptions of, and attitudes towards the student nurses and their role in general practice. The regular interaction with the student nurses through the CoP will, it is argued; positively influence the GPs' perceptions over the benefits of recruiting new graduate nurses. The successful facilitation of a Community of Practice (CoP) for placements within general practice is used to provide GPs with the knowledge and understanding needed to gain a much more useful and authentic insight into the benefits of 'modern' nurse education [13].

Conclusions

There is some, albeit fragile, evidence within this study of a cultural shift in general practice towards the proactive recruitment of new graduate nurses. This has been predicated upon the development of a CoP, which has enabled the GPs to develop a better understanding of the benefits to their practice of employing new graduate nurses. This understanding has emerged through socially-situated interaction mediated by the CoP [21]. This degree of culture change has taken time, patience and a great deal of persistence. Despite the challenges, the evidence is that the ATPS scheme is beginning to 'bear fruit', and there is a subtle but discernible move by GPs from a 'why *would* we?' to 'why *wouldn't* we?' recruit new graduate nurses into general practice and invest in their education and training.

Abbreviations

ACP: Advanced Clinical Practitioner; ATPS: Advanced Training Practice Scheme; CoP: Community of practice; GP: General Practitioner; GPN: General Practice Nurse; HCA: Health care assistant; HEE: Health Education England; HEI: Higher Education Institution; NHS: National Health Service (UK); NTHI: National Training Hubs Initiative; QNI: Queen's Nursing Institute; QOF: Quality Outcomes Framework; RCGP: Royal College of General Practitioners; UK: United Kingdom

Acknowledgements

Many thanks to Dr. Peter Lane and to Mrs. Louise Berwick for their unstinting help and support throughout the study. Thanks also to the GPs who gave their valuable time to be interviewed.

Funding

Funding for this research was provided under a 'small grants' contract from Health Education England (Yorkshire & Humber Region) UK. HEYH (the funding body) had no role whatsoever in the design of the study or the writing of the manuscript.

Authors' contributions

RL conceived of the project, conducted and analysed the interviews. SK independently reviewed the transcripts and confirmed the themes. Both authors contributed to the writing of the paper, and approved the final manuscript.

Authors' information

RL is a Senior Lecturer in the Department of Nursing and Midwifery. His research focuses on the impact of workforce re-organisation and the effect of new roles in healthcare.
SK is Professor of Interdisciplinary Health in the Faculty of Health & Wellbeing. She has worked on healthcare provision in Canada, Australia and the UK.

Competing interests

The authors declare that they have no competing interests.

Author details

[1]Department of Nursing and Midwifery, Sheffield Hallam University, Sheffield S10 2BP, England. [2]Department of Social Work, Social Care and Community Services, Sheffield Hallam University, Collegiate Crescent, Sheffield S10 2BP, England.

References

1. Health Education England: Yorkshire & the Humber. A Future Workforce Strategy for General Practice. Leeds: Health Education England; 2014.
2. Royal College of General Practitioners. Nursing in Primary Care - 'a roadmap to excellence' (report of an event). Royal College of General Practitioners; 2014. http://www.rcgp.org.uk/policy/rcgp-policy-areas/primary-care-development.aspx. Accessed 27 Mar 2018.
3. NHS England. Five-year forward view. NHS England; 2014. https://www.england.nhs.uk/wp-content/uploads/2014/10/5yfv-web.pdf. Accessed 27 Mar 2018.
4. British Medical Association. General practice in the UK. BMA: London; 2014.
5. Royal College of General Practitioners. The 2022 GP: a vision for general practice in the future NHS. London: Royal College of General Practitioners; 2013.
6. Ball J, Maben J, Griffiths P. Practice nursing: what do we know? Br J Gen Pract. 2015;65(630):10–1.
7. Griffiths P, Maben J, Murrells T. Organisational quality, nurse staffing and the quality of chronic disease management in primary care: observational study using routinely collected data. Int J Nurs Studies. 2011;48(10):1199–210.
8. Queen's Nursing Institute. General practice nursing in the 21st century: a time of opportunity. London: Queen's Nursing Institute; 2015.
9. Lane P, Peake C. A scheme to increase practice nurse numbers. Nurs Times. 2015;111(13):22–57.
10. Lewis R, Kelly S. Would growing our own practice nurses solve the workforce crisis? Pract Nurs. 2017;28(4):2–4.
11. McLaren WK, Quinlivan L. Developing student nurse placements in general practice. General Pract Nurs. 2016;2(1):54–9.
12. Gale J, Ooms A, Sharples K, Marks-Maran D. The experiences of student nurses on placements with practice nurses: a pilot study. Nurse Educ Pract. 2015;16:225–34.
13. Lewis R, Kelly S, Berwick L. An Evaluation of the Health Educ England working across Yorkshire & the Humber Advanced Training Practice Scheme (ATPS). Sheffield Hallam University; 2017. https://www.hee.nhs.uk/news-blogs-events/news/independent-evaluation-advanced-practices-scheme-atps-across-yorkshire-humber.
14. Parker R, Keleher H, Francis K, Abdulwadud O. Practice nursing in Australia: a review of education and career pathways. BMC Nurs. 2009;8:5.
15. NZ Ministry of Health. Evaluation of the eleven primary health care nursing innovation projects: a report. NZ: Ministry of Health Wellington; 2007.
16. NHS England. General practice: forward view. London: NHS England; 2016.
17. McKenna L, Brooks I. Graduate entry students' early perceptions of their future nursing careers. Nurse Educ Pract. 2018;28:292–5.
18. Bloomfield J, Gordon C, Williams A, Aggar C. Nursing students' intentions to enter primary care as a career option: findings from a national survey. Collegian. 2015;22:161–7.
19. McInness S, Peters K, Hardy J, Halcomb E. Clinical placements in Australian general practice: the experience of pre-registration nursing students. Nurse Educ Pract. 2015a;15:437–42.
20. McInness S, Peters K, Hardy J, Halcomb E. Clinical placements in Australian general practice: the views of registered nurse mentors and pre-registration nursing students. Nurse Educ Pract. 2015b;15:443–9.
21. Lave J, Wenger E. Situated learning: legitimate peripheral participation. New York: Cambridge University Press; 1991.
22. Ranmuthugala G, et al. How and why are communities of practice established in the healthcare sector? A systematic review of the literature. BMC Health Serv Res. 2011;11:273.
23. Chandler L, Fry A. Can communities of practice make a meaningful contribution to sustainable service improvement in health and social care? J Integrated Care. 2009;17:41–8.
24. Ritchie J, Lewis J. Qualitative research practice: a guide for social science students and researchers. London: Sage; 2003.
25. Boyce R. Emerging from the shadow of medicine: allied health as a 'professional community' subculture. Health Sociol Rev. 2006;15(5):520–34.

19

Perceptions of shared care among survivors of colorectal cancer from non-English-speaking and English-speaking backgrounds

Lawrence Tan[1]*[iD], Gisselle Gallego[2], Thi Thao Cam Nguyen[3], Les Bokey[4] and Jennifer Reath[1]

Abstract

Background: Colorectal cancer (CRC) survivors experience difficulty navigating complex care pathways. Sharing care between GPs and specialist services has been proposed to improve health outcomes in cancer survivors following hospital discharge. Culturally and Linguistically Diverse (CALD) groups are known to have poorer outcomes following cancer treatment but little is known about their perceptions of shared care following surgery for CRC. This study aimed to explore how non-English-speaking and English-speaking patients perceive care to be coordinated amongst various health practitioners.

Methods: This was a qualitative study using data from face to face semi-structured interviews and one focus group in a culturally diverse area of Sydney with non-English-speaking and English-speaking CRC survivors. Participants were recruited in community settings and were interviewed in English, Spanish or Vietnamese. Interviews were recorded, transcribed, and analysed by researchers fluent in those languages. Data were coded and analysed thematically.

Results: Twenty-two CRC survivors participated in the study. Participants from non-English-speaking and English-speaking groups described similar barriers to care, but non-English-speaking participants described additional communication difficulties and perceived discrimination. Non-English-speaking participants relied on family members and bilingual GPs for assistance with communication and care coordination. Factors that influenced the care pathways used by participants and how care was shared between the specialist and GP included patient and practitioner preference, accessibility, complexity of care needs, and requirements for assistance with understanding information and navigating the health system, that were particularly difficult for non-English-speaking CRC survivors.

Conclusions: Both non-English-speaking and English-speaking CRC survivors described a blend of specialist-led or GP-led care depending on the complexity of care required, informational needs, and how engaged and accessible they perceived the specialist or GP to be. Findings from this study highlight the role of the bilingual GP in assisting CALD participants to understand information and to navigate their care pathways following CRC surgery.

Keywords: Colorectal cancer, Survivorship, Care coordination, Cultural and linguistic diversity, General practice

* Correspondence: lawrence.tan@westernsydney.edu.au
[1]Department of General Practice, School of Medicine, Western Sydney University, Locked Bag 1797, Penrith, NSW 2751, Australia
Full list of author information is available at the end of the article

Background

Colorectal cancer (CRC) is the second-largest cause of cancer death in Australia. The five-year survival rate has risen from 48% in 1983–1987, to 64% in 2008–2012 [1]. Proposals have been made for the care of cancer survivors to be shared with general practitioners (GPs) rather than being exclusively specialist-centred. Hospital-based care tends to focus on detecting disease recurrence, while care shared with primary care services could potentially improve psychosocial support, care for other comorbidities, and preventive care [2, 3].

Cancer survivors have described multiple care needs following surgery, [4–6] and poor coordination of health care is a recurrent theme in cancer survivorship research [7]. A randomised controlled trial conducted in Australia comparing CRC follow up in general practice with surgical based follow-up showed no difference in patient satisfaction, detection of recurrence or mortality [8]. However cancer survivors, GPs and specialists have mixed feelings about shared care [9]. Some studies show patients are more satisfied with specialist care [10] even though shared care was found to be more cost-effective [11]. Elsewhere, patients were satisfied overall with follow-up in primary care unless they had more challenges in recovery, when the organisation of care became "complex and variable" [12]. They valued support from an "active" GP, and also reassurance from their specialists [13]. Concerns mentioned by GPs regarding participating in shared care for colorectal cancer survivors included time, cost, poor communication and inadequate transfer of information between specialist and GP settings [14–16].

Australia is a multicultural country with almost half of its population (49%) born overseas. According to the 2016 Census more than one-fifth (21%) of Australians spoke a language other than English at home [17]. This is important considering that people from minority culturally and linguistically diverse (CALD) backgrounds have lower screening rates, poorer cancer outcomes [18, 19] and greater informational needs [20]. For example, Caucasian cancer survivors in the United States of America (USA) were more likely to have follow-up screening, preventive care, access to mental health services and more frequent visits to their physician compared with patients from other ethnicities [21].

In Australia, patients can freely choose their GP. If required, the GP refers them to a private specialist, often taking into account the patient's preferences when selecting which specialist to refer to. Patients who go through the public hospital system have no choice of specialist. Public hospitals are free and visits to GPs (who provide community based primary health care) and community based specialists are cost-subsidised through a universal health insurance (Medicare). Private

insurance is also available for those who choose and can afford to purchase it, providing additional subsidies for private hospital access and choice of specialist. Cancer follow up is provided across all these settings, but no formal model of shared care for CRC survivors is currently in place. Little research has been undertaken on cancer survivorship in CALD communities in the Australian setting [22]. This study aimed to explore how CRC survivors from CALD backgrounds who speak languages other than English at home, as well as those from English-speaking backgrounds, perceive care to be coordinated amongst various health practitioners in an Australian setting.

Methods

Qualitative methodology was chosen to explore the experiences and perceptions of the participants [23] in order to help the researchers understand how they navigated the health system to overcome barriers to care, which relates to how they felt their care was being coordinated.

Setting

This qualitative study was undertaken between 2015 and 2016, mainly in South West Sydney. South West Sydney is known for its cultural diversity with 45% of the population speaking a language other than English at home. After Arabic, Vietnamese is the second-most common non-English language spoken at home. The next most frequently spoken languages are Mandarin, Cantonese and Hindi; Spanish being the tenth-most frequently spoken language [24].

Participants and recruitment

In order to represent a continuum of experiences, stratified purposive sampling [25] was used to recruit participants 6 weeks to 8 years following CRC surgery, who spoke either English, Spanish or Vietnamese at home. These three languages were spoken by members of the research team. We used the language spoken at home as a proxy for the cultural background participants identified with. Participants were recruited from community support groups, and GP and colorectal surgeon private rooms. None of the GPs treating the patients at the time of the CRC diagnosis and initial follow-up were involved in this research. Radio and newspaper announcements were made in the target languages. Potential participants were asked to contact the researchers. They were then informed verbally about the aim of the study and provided with a printed participant information statement that explained the aims of the research, and a consent form in their preferred language. These forms had been translated by translators from the

National Accreditation Authority for Translators and Interpreters. We set no formal exclusion criteria although one potential participant was excluded because he was still recovering in hospital, and another because she had a bowel resection during her breast cancer treatment, but did not actually have CRC. Participants were offered a small gift voucher as a token of appreciation for their time.

Data collection

Participants were given the option of a face-to-face or telephone interview, or participation in a focus group. All participants provided written informed consent except for two who were interviewed by phone, whose verbal consent to participate in the study was recorded after the consent form was read out to them as approved by the ethics committee. An interview guide with open-ended questions and prompts was prepared in English, Spanish and Vietnamese (Additional file 1). The interview guide was developed following a review of the literature and discussion within the research team. LT, a male GP researcher, is fluent in English and Spanish and conducted the Spanish interviews and some of the English interviews. TN, a female GP researcher, is a native speaker of Vietnamese and conducted some of the Vietnamese interviews. The remaining English and Vietnamese interviews were conducted by research assistants (a male and a female medical student trained in qualitative research interviewing, who are native speakers of both English and Vietnamese). In order to respect cultural preferences, Vietnamese interviews were conducted where possible by researchers of the same gender as the participants. Participants were asked to speak in their preferred language. Interviews were conducted in the patient's home, GP surgery, coffee shop or by telephone according to participant preference. Five participants were accompanied by a family member – one English-speaker, one Spanish-speaker and three Vietnamese-speakers. Interviews took between 30 to 45 min and concurrent field notes were taken. The focus group with three English-speaking participants was facilitated by LT together with a research assistant in a meeting room at a cancer survivor centre, that lasted for approximately 1 hour. Interviews and the focus group session were digitally recorded and transcribed in the original language. Participants were offered a copy of the transcripts to check. Transcriptions were performed by a professional transcription service in the original language and their integrity checked by the interviewer. Transcripts were analysed concurrently with the interviewing, which continued until no new themes emerged, suggesting data saturation [26] within the groups of participants studied.

Data analysis

Participants were de-identified and transcripts labelled with an individual number and letters denominating the gender and language(s) spoken. Vietnamese transcripts were translated by the bilingual interviewers. Spanish transcripts were analysed by LT and GG, who cross-checked their translations with each other and translated relevant excerpts into English for review by the research team. GG is a native speaker of Spanish who is fluent in English. A thematic analysis was conducted [26]. LT read and reread the transcripts and applied descriptive codes to the data. Initially, early transcripts were reviewed and coded independently by GG and JR and a tentative coding framework was agreed by all three researchers. This framework was applied to subsequent interview transcripts by LT and GG, and the framework reviewed and revised at regular team meetings including JR until all 22 interviews had been coded using the final agreed framework. At a later stage the codes were grouped into themes derived from the data. Illustrative quotes not in English were translated by the research assistants, TN and LT, then checked by a second native speaker of that language. Data were managed using Microsoft® Excel® 2016. Ethics approval was provided by the Western Sydney University Human Research Ethics Committee (approval number H9067).

Results

Twenty-two patients participated, of whom 10 spoke English at home, five spoke Spanish and four spoke Vietnamese. Two were bilingual Spanish-English, and one was bilingual Vietnamese-English. The three bilingual participants preferred to be interviewed in English. All the Vietnamese-speakers had been born in Vietnam and had migrated to Australia between 29 to 37 years ago. The Spanish-speakers came from Argentina, Chile, El Salvador and Uruguay. They had lived in Australia for 23 to 40 years. Three native English-speakers participated in a focus group and the remainder were interviewed individually. The English-speakers were all born in Australia or the United Kingdom, except for three who had been born in Croatia, Lebanon and the Netherlands. These three had come to Australia in childhood. In our study, most of the English-speaking participants had private insurance, while most of the Spanish-speaking ones did not have private insurance and used the public hospital service. Half of the Vietnamese-speakers had private health insurance. See Table 1 for other participant characteristics.

Participants described a complex blend of barriers to care, strategies used to meet their care needs and discussed how they perceived care to be coordinated between their care providers. Table 2 summarises the themes and subthemes identified.

Table 1 Participant characteristics (n = 22)

	Mean	Range
Age, years	65	38–88
Years since surgery	2.5	0.1–8
	N	%
Female	12	54.5
Relative present at interview	5	22.7
Private health insurance	14	63.6
Language spoken at home		
English	10	45
Spanish	5	23
Vietnamese	4	18
English-Spanish	2	9
English-Vietnamese	1	5
Cancer treatment		
Surgery only	7	32
Surgery plus chemotherapy	7	32
Surgery plus neoadjuvant therapy	4	18
Surgery plus radiotherapy	1	5
Surgery including colostomy	11	50

Barriers to care

Participants described numerous difficulties receiving the care they required, including getting appointments, navigating care pathways, understanding information, perceived discrimination, cost and logistical difficulties.

Both English-speaking and non-English-speaking participants found specialist and GP appointments could take a long time, but in general it was easier to get an appointment with a GP:

"It would always take a number of weeks to get to see [the specialist] because he was heavily booked" (Male English-speaker).

Table 2 Colorectal cancer survivorship themes

Barriers to Care	Cost
	Logistics
	Timeliness
	Language and communication
	Perceived discrimination
Strategies used to meet care needs	Family members
	Bilingual GP
	Private health insurance
Coordination of care	Variability in information flow
	Variability in GP and specialist involvement
	Role of the bilingual GP

Another barrier common to both groups was confusion about who to go to when care was required after hours:

"I ring up the hospital and ask them what I should do if I have this problem, they say, first of all you need to go to your GP doctor to let him have a look how serious is it. If that serious he would send - give you the letter referred you to hospital... at the time it's six o'clock, your GP doctor closed, what you going to do?" (Male bilingual Vietnamese-English speaker)

Communication was a particular barrier for non-English-speaking participants. They were sometimes unclear about what was being treated and what treatment had been given. For example, one of the Vietnamese-speaking participants described how she did not even know what surgery had been performed:

"[I] would look at the scar and try and guess what happened". (Female Vietnamese-speaker)

They were also unsure where or when to attend for follow-up, who to consult if problems arose, or what support services were available in the community. A bilingual English-Vietnamese speaker expressed both his difficulty understanding and his difficulty communicating in English, even though he chose to speak in that language:

"... but who will be the responsibility to help you, to understand what you do for first month, second month, third month, I don't know. For myself or for whoever Western, they can read it in English or they can understand thing would be good, but for traditional like, for my mum and if you don't have relationship with English I don't know what will be difficult for them" [sic].

Even though interpreters were available in hospital to assist with communication, some participants were reluctant to impose on interpreters' time.

"There were interpreters but I think that ...when you ask too many questions it feels like they don't like it" (Male Vietnamese-speaker)

Two of the five Vietnamese-speaking patients also described perceived discrimination, compounded by an inability to express themselves in English:

"The way she put the needle in was as if she thought of me like a dog or an animal! It was very painful but I couldn't say a word because no one understood my

language - Vietnamese. Therefore, I told her that I am in pain in Vietnamese 'dau' and I stared at her" (Female Vietnamese-speaker).

One described this as double-discrimination – because of his race, and also because of his inability to speak English:

"Asian people are already discriminated against and not being able to speak English; then those two factors combine" (Male Vietnamese-speaker).

He felt this contributed to a delay in diagnosis of a serious post-operative complication because it appeared to him that staff would not pay attention to his complaints of pain.

Many participants in both English-speaking and non-English-speaking groups described difficulty accessing their specialists because of cost. Other logistical issues included difficulty finding parking, and having to make sure they didn't eat or drink too much that day because of a lack of toilet facilities at the specialist's consulting rooms:

"You have one 15-minute session with your surgeon, and once that 15 minutes is up, there's the door for $100 and the next patient comes in" (Male English-speaker)

Strategies used to meet care needs

Non-English-speaking participants brought family members with them to specialist appointments, for emotional support as well as to interpret for them:

"Someone always goes with me, always" (Female Spanish-speaker).

Interestingly, an English-speaking participant who was hearing-impaired used the same strategy:

"... So I'm her second pair of ears" (sister of female English-speaker)

All non-English-speaking participants in our study had a bilingual GP whom they consulted. The bilingual GP assisted non-English-speaking participants by providing information and advice on how to navigate the health care system:

"Well if I didn't feel well in myself or something like that, then I would call my son to drive me to the [Vietnamese-speaking] family doctor. I could ask him this and that, and then he would direct me to who I

should call or where I should go" (Female Vietnamese-speaker).

One Spanish-speaking female participant described consulting a GP who only spoke English when her usual bilingual GP was unavailable. On this occasion she brought her daughter to the consultation to interpret for her.

Both non-English-speaking and English-speaking participants perceived private health insurance to facilitate in their cancer management by reducing the waiting time, providing additional private hospital benefits such as permission for family to stay over, and improved access to the specialist.

"I paid [for the colonoscopy in a private hospital], because the specialist said that if you wait [for a public hospital colonoscopy] it can take quite a while ... and I also bought medical insurance" (Female Vietnamese-speaker)

Coordination of care

Participants described a wide range of health professionals involved in their care, including stoma nurses, physiotherapists, psychologists and even a surgeon's receptionist who would assist by ringing up for appointments with other specialists. None of the participants described a formal shared care arrangement between specialist and primary care services, nor mentioned a written shared care plan. They described a variable information flow between their health providers, and tended to seek help from the health provider the participant felt was most involved or appropriate to meet their needs. Some participants assumed specialists and GPs were in communication, while others reported poor information flow:

"Yeah, and nothing's linked ... three different hospitals I've got to go to ... you've got to explain yourselves so many times, over and over again" (Female English-speaker)

Sometimes non-English-speaking and English-speaking participants or their relatives, would take the initiative to assist in the information flow:

"So I ended up trying to collect everything and I got something good off - the first person who had written up the story was the oncologist, I said 'Oh, can I have a copy of that, because that's got everything?' ... So it took me a while to get it all together and say 'OK, the person who has got to have this is my GP. And I've got to stick to this one GP" (Female English-speaker).

Both English-speaking and non-English-speaking background participants had a high degree of trust in their private specialist, particularly when there were complex care needs and they needed someone to coordinate everything:

"I wasn't really searching for too much information, I just basically left it in the hands of the Professor and his staff" (Male English speaker)

"Up front we asked [the private surgeon], we wanted somebody to be the manager of the whole thing and not have to talk to different doctors and wonder who is doing what." (Male English-speaker).

On the other hand, one participant felt devastated, starting to cry as she described how her oncologist seemed dismissive of her mental health concerns. Another felt rejected by the surgeon when seeking help for persistent diarrhoea following surgery:

"But afterwards I felt a lot of rejection; I went to complain, because I felt as if he didn't want to know anything more about it. He was washing his hands. That's how I felt." (Male Spanish-speaker)

Some English-speaking participants had little or no relationship with their GPs, with one not even recalling the GP's name. Following the initial diagnosis and referral, some English-speaking participants viewed GPs as irrelevant, only becoming involved in care after they had been discharged by the specialist:

"I don't know what I would expect from a GP afterwards, well, I haven't got a lot, so I don't, but I don't know what they can do. You've had the treatment, haven't you, and you're moving on, so there's not a lot they can do except keep an eye on you and I guess after I get cut adrift after these five years they'll take more of an active role" (Male English-speaker).

Other English-speaking patients only consulted GPs for non-cancer matters, although provision of preventive care was not mentioned:

"I've seen my GP for, I think I've just had to get a script for my blood pressure tablets and so on and so forth" (Male English-speaker)

For CRC-related issues they preferred to consult the surgeon, and sometimes the GP also appeared to defer to the surgeon:

"But anything more detailed, he would say 'of course, this is a matter be addressed by your surgeon,' which

is easier said than done when you've got to wait three and a half weeks to get an early appointment" (Male English-speaker)

Other participants described their GP as being engaged and pro-active in managing the cancer recovery process. One detected a post-operative wound infection when asked to make a house-call because of an unrelated issue. In this case the participant had not even been told to see the GP after the surgery:

"But that was for the ear he came, and that's when he says, 'I'll look at your wound while I'm here' [laughs]. So that's how. But they didn't say to me that I had to see my GP; they just said I had to see [the gastroenterologist] within 2-3 weeks" (Female English-speaker).

In another situation an involved GP was seen to provide good ongoing whole-person care when the participant felt specialist care was fragmented and did not address all her needs:

"You didn't realise how much you needed to rely on a GP for all the referrals and just to have somebody who collected all the information that came in, knew your history and could refer you to different people and if you came in and said 'look, I'm really low today and not doing well,' to know where you were at, to know where the medication was at and what to do and yeah, just to be that go-to person" (Female English-speaker).

In comparison with the English-speaking participants, bilingual GPs were perceived by many non-English-speaking participants to be key coordinators of care who could support the participant in their own language. These participants displayed a high level of trust in their bilingual GPs who could also explain what the follow-up arrangements were, and facilitate communication between the participant and the specialist or hospital without requiring assistance from family members or official interpreters:

"I would say [to the surgeon], 'Please, you have to write to my father's doctor, please you have to send him all the information because I don't go with him, because the [GP] speaks Spanish'" (daughter of male Spanish-speaker)

"Like, I felt that the [Vietnamese-speaking] GP was important because if anything happened, I would have to go get checked by the GP. I could talk to the GP, call

the GP, if I needed medication or had any troubles. I would have to tell the GP and the GP could contact the specialists. They all worked together." [Female Vietnamese-speaker]

Discussion

English-speaking and non-English-speaking CRC survivors had a similar range of barriers to care, but non-English-speaking patients faced additional difficulties due to communication issues and perceived discrimination. Participants in this study did not describe formal shared care arrangements, but described using GP-led, specialist-led or shared models of care depending on multiple factors such as ease of access, private insurance, presence of co-morbidities, complexity of care, and perceived interest or engagement by the GP or specialist. Bilingual GPs were described by participants as being key in coordinating care for participants who came from a non-English-speaking background.

The Primary Care Collaborative Cancer Clinical Trials Groups' principles statement on implementing shared care of cancer patients [27] emphasises that shared care should be acceptable and flexible; with clear expectations, communication pathways, implementation process, integration with existing processes and evaluation. Participants in this study did not always have expectations of shared care clarified, and mostly assumed the specialist and GP communicated with one another. Other studies have provided a different perspective from GPs who identified issues with information flow [28]. In our study, where communication was perceived to be deficient, participants or their carers often took steps to ensure their GP received the information, or took charge of the information themselves by asking for copies so they could show them to the next health professional consulted. Examples of deficiencies in care from our study included one participant developing a wound infection after the surgery, who had not been told to see her GP for post-operative review; another whose medication changes had not been communicated with the GP; and others who described hospital results not being available at the time of post-surgical consultation with the GP.

Specialist-led care rather than GP-led care was demonstrated in both non-English-speaking and English-speaking groups, particularly if they had more complicated cancer treatment, fewer co-morbidities, and easy access to specialist care. Participants who had private insurance in our study had a greater reliance on specialist-led care, similar to a previous study on patient experiences of the referral process for CRC [29]. Some participants considered GPs to be irrelevant in the care of cancer survivors until they had been discharged by the specialist. In other cases, GPs

themselves appeared to disengage from cancer survivor care, influencing the participant to seek specialist help.

On the other hand, GP-led care was perceived by participants in our study to be more important when participants had physical and emotional needs not addressed by specialists. Studies of Danish, US and Australian GPs similarly showed they were consulted by CRC patients with more complex comorbidities because they were more accessible and provided whole-person care [30–32].

In the absence of formal processes for sharing care, participants in this study described unclear expectations, communication pathways, implementation processes and integration of health care. They adopted a flexible approach using existing processes to seek help primarily from specialists, GPs or both, using informal shared care pathways. This appears to be a dynamic process depending on patient, GP and specialist preferences and taking into account particular health needs and difficulties with access and communication. This is summarised in Fig. 1, which describes care pathways used by CRC survivors according to their care needs, CALD status, and patient and health provider preferences. A recent study of care pathways used by Aboriginal and Torres Strait Islander cancer survivors also concluded that "one size does not fit all" [33].

Non-English-speaking participants had greater difficulty communicating with specialists, and understanding follow-up arrangements. They relied on bilingual GPs following CRC surgery to coordinate care, provide health information, follow-up results, assist with navigating the health care system, and provide emotional support. Bilingual GPs have been previously acknowledged to play a key role in promoting cancer screening [34], presumably because of shared language and cultural insights, but to our knowledge this is the first study describing the role of bilingual GPs in the care of CALD cancer survivors. Data on the number of bilingual GPs in Australia is limited, but one study showed 15.5% of 206 randomly-selected Australian GPs used a language other than English in their consultations [35]. Anecdotally, patients sometimes have long wait times or distances to travel to find a GP who speaks their language.

Findings from our study suggest the cultural and linguistic background of the CRC survivor can influence care pathways. Identifying non-English-speaking cancer survivors from a different cultural and linguistic background could be used to assist in determining the optimal shared care model, as well as factors such as cancer type, stage and comorbidities that are usually used for risk stratification of cancer survivors [36, 37]. Greater effort should be made by specialist services to share care with the bilingual GP consulted by the CALD CRC patient.

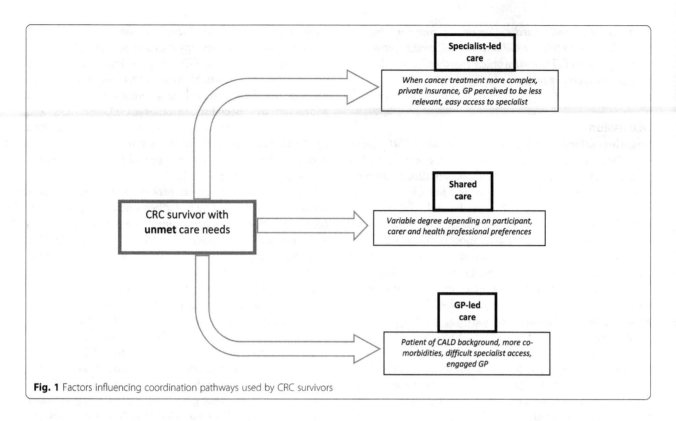

Fig. 1 Factors influencing coordination pathways used by CRC survivors

Implications for research and/or practice

Findings from this study reinforce recommendations to include GPs in the care of cancer patients and to support these GPs with the training, resources and pathways to access specialist advice when needed [34]. This study highlights the role of the bilingual GP in translating information and assisting CALD CRC survivors in navigating the health care system. Cancer services could take a more pro-active role to inform patients on the role of the GP in cancer care, including coordination of care, providing continuity, surveillance, cancer prevention, care for emotional needs and for other medical conditions (3). This would involve specific instructions to see the GP for follow-up [38] and clarification of care pathways [39] particularly when the patient comes from a CALD background and is more likely to experience barriers to care because of difficulties with communication and coordination of care. Online localised health pathways [40] are currently being developed which may help clarify expectations, communication and implementation of shared care for CRC survivors. These care pathways are primarily intended for GPs within each health district, but information for patients is being added, and in the future could include patient information in community languages. Proposed shared care plans [9, 41, 42] that include information for the patient, carers and GP would be particularly useful for patients with complex needs and those from CALD backgrounds. Multicultural state-wide health services could assist in connecting

cancer survivors with support groups and health services accessible for CALD groups. Further research is required concerning what support is required by bilingual GPs to assist them in caring for CALD cancer survivors.

Strengths and limitations

This study provides an important insight into the under-researched area of CALD cancer survivorship care. Strengths of the study included participant recruitment from community settings with a broad range of GP and specialist levels of engagement in their care. Interviews with non-English-speaking participants were conducted in their own language by researchers fluent in that language, thus respecting the voice of the informant. This study only included two CALD groups with small numbers in each group, hence the study findings may not be generalizable to other cultural groups. Nevertheless, similar experiences were described by both Spanish and Vietnamese groups. One of the participants had had his initial cancer treatment up to 8 years prior to the study, which may have affected his recollections of post-surgical care, however no substantial changes to the health system have been made since his treatment and his experiences were similar to that of other CRC survivors. Our methodology relied on patient perspectives that limited our ability to independently verify and evaluate the forms of shared care they described. Perspectives of cancer specialists, GPs and other health professionals caring for the participants were not obtained but may have provided additional insights. Further research seeking their perspectives is in progress. Our recruitment strategy may have sampled CRC survivors who were more engaged in follow-up care, reflecting the difficulty engaging more marginalised groups. Patient recruitment from hospital outpatient clinics may also have provided different perspectives on shared care for CRC. Care pathways for CRC survivors within the Australian health care system will differ from those in other countries, however with increasing globalisation and migration the specific care needs of patients from CALD groups and the role of the bilingual GP will be important to consider in future research.

Conclusions

Non-English-speaking CRC survivors report experiencing similar barriers to care as English-speaking CRC survivors, but experience greater informational and communication needs. Both non-English-speaking and English-speaking CRC survivors describe a blend of specialist-led, GP-led and informal shared care pathways, depending on the complexity of their care needs and perceived engagement and accessibility of the health professionals. Because of the additional challenges navigating care arrangements and the absence of more formal care coordination so far, non-English-speaking CRC survivors tend to rely on family members and bilingual GPs to coordinate their care following surgery. The development of formal shared care plans and localised health pathways should include communication of what CRC survivors can expect from the GP, specialists and other health professionals, particularly targeted at those with complex needs including those from CALD backgrounds.

Abbreviations

CALD: Culturally and linguistically diverse; CRC: Colorectal cancer; GP: General Practitioner; USA: United States of America

Acknowledgements
We would like to acknowledge the participants in this study, the Spanish Cancer Network, and our research assistants Danny Lam, Beatriz Martin and Lana Nguyen.

Funding
This study was funded by a grant from the Primary Collaborative Cancer Clinical Trials Group (PC4) and the Royal Australian College of General Practitioners. PC4 provided early advice on study design, but was not involved in data collection, analysis, interpretation or writing the manuscript.

Authors' contributions
LT, GG, LB and JR contributed to the conception and design of this study. LT and TN were involved in data collection. LT, GG, TN and JR analysed and interpreted the data. The manuscript was drafted by LT and GG and edited by JR. The final version was reviewed and approved by all authors.

Competing interests
The authors declare that they have no competing interests. One of the funding bodies, PC4, provided early advice on study design, but was not involved in data collection, analysis, interpretation or writing the manuscript. The other funding body, The Royal Australian College of General Practitioners, was not involved in the research process.

Author details
Department of General Practice, School of Medicine, Western Sydney University, Locked Bag 1797, Penrith, NSW 2751, Australia. [2]School of Medicine, University of Notre Dame, 140 Broadway, Sydney, NSW 2007, Australia. [3]Bonnyrigg Family Medical Centre, Bonnyrigg, NSW, Australia. [4]Department of Surgery, Western Sydney University, Locked Bag 1797, Penrith, NSW 2751, Australia.

References
1. Australian Institute of Health and Welfare. National Bowel Cancer Screening Program: monitoring report 2016. Canberra: AIHW; 2016.
2. Emery J. Cancer survivorship - the role of the GP. Aust Fam Physician. 2014;43(8): 521–5.
3. Hewitt M, Greenfield S, Stovall E. From cancer patient to cancer survivor: lost in transition. Washington: The National Academies Press; 2006.
4. Harrison JD, Young JM, Price MA, Butow P, Solomon MJ. What are the unmet supportive care needs of people with cancer? A systematic review. Support Care Cancer. 2009;17:1117–28.
5. Hoekstra RA, Heins MJ, Korevaar JC. Health care needs of cancer survivors in general practice: a systematic review. BMC Fam Pract. 2014;15:94.
6. Harrison JD, Young JM, Auld S, Masya L, Solomon MJ, Butow P. Quantifying postdischarge unmet supportive care needs of people with colorectal cancer: a clinical audit. Color Dis. 2011;13:1400–6.
7. Weller DP, Harris M. Cancer care: what role for the general practitioner? Med J Aust. 2008;189(2):59–60.
8. Wattchow D, Weller D, Esterman A, Pilotto L, McGorm K, Hammett Z, et al. General practice vs surgical-based follow-up for patients with colon cancer: randomised controlled trial. Br J Cancer. 2006;94:1116–21.
9. Emery JD, Shaw K, Williams B, Mazza D, Fallon-Ferguson J, Varlow M, et al. The role of primary care in early detection and follow-up of cancer. Nat Rev Clin Oncol. 2014;11:38–48.
10. Chubak J, Aiello Bowles EJ, Tuzzio L, Ludman E, Rutter CM, Reid RJ, et al. Perspectives of cancer survivors on the role of different healthcare providers in an integrated delivery system. J Cancer Surviv. 2014;8:229–2328.
11. Baena-Canada JM, Ramirez-Daffos P, Cortes-Carmona C, Rosado-Varela P, Nieto-Vera J, Benitez-Rodriguez E. Follow-up of long-term survivors of breast cancer in primary care versus specialist attention. Fam Pract. 2013;30:525–32.
12. Sisler JJ, Taylor-Brown J, Nugent Z, Bell D, Khawaja M, Czaykowski P, et al. Continuity of care of colorectal cancer survivors at the end of treatment: the oncology-primary care interface. J Cancer Surviv. 2012;6:468–75.
13. Urquhart R, Folkes A, Babineau J, Grunfeld E. Views of breast and colorectal cancer survivors on their routine follow-up care. Curr Oncol. 2012;19(6):294–301.
14. Johnson CE, Lizama N, Garg N, Ghish M, Emery J, Saunders C. Australian general practitioners' preferences for managing the care of people diagnosed with cancer. Asia Pac J Clin Oncol. 2014;10:e90–e8.
15. Mitchell G, Burridge LH, Colquist SP, Love A. General Practitioners' perceptions of their role in cancer care and factors which influence this role. Health Soc Care Commun. 2012;20(6):607–16.

16. Papagrigoriadis S, Koreli A. The needs of general practitioners in the follow-up of patients with colorectal cancer. Eur J Surg Oncol. 2001;27:541–4.

17. Australian Bureau of Statistics. 2016 Census: Multicultural 2017 [Available from: http://www.abs.gov.au/ausstats/abs@.nsf/lookup/Media%20Release3.]

18. Federation of Ethnic Communities' Council of Australia. Cancer and Culturally and Linguistically Diverse Communities. Deakin: ACT: Federation of Ethnic Communities' Council of Australia; 2010.

19. Dossett LA, Hudson JN, Morris AM, Lee MC, Roetzheim RG, Fetters MD, et al. The primary care provider (PCP)-cancer specialist relationship: a systematic analysis and mixed-methods review. CA Cancer J Clin. 2016;00(00):1–14.

20. Licqurish S, Phillipson L, Chiang P, Walker J, Walter F, Emery J. Cancer beliefs in ethnic minority populations:a review and meta-synthesis of qualitative studies. Euro J Cancer Care. 2016;26(e12556):1–13.

21. Treanor C, Donnelly M. An international review of the patterns and determinants of health service utilisation by adult cancer survivors. BMC Health Serv Res. 2012;12:316.

22. Jiwa M, Saunders C, Thompson SC, Rosenwax LK, Sargant S, Khong EL, et al. Timely cancer diagnosis and management as a chronic condition: opportunities for primary care. Med J Aust. 2008;189(2):78–82.

23. Ritchie J, Lewis J. Qualitative research practice. London: Sage; 2004.

24. WSROC. South West Subregion: languages spoken at home [cited 2016 November 9th, 2016]. Available from: http://profile.id.com.au/wsroc/language?WebID=220.

25. Patton MQ. Qualitative research & evaluation methods. 3rd ed. Thousand Oaks: Sage; 2000.

26. Miles M, Huberman M. Qualitative data analysis. 2nd ed. Beverley Hills: Sage; 1994.

27. The Primary Care Collaborative Cancer Clinical Trials Group. Implementing shared care of cancer patients in primary and specialist care setting. A Principles Statement 2014 [cited 2016 November 9th, 2016]. Available from: http://pc4tg.com.au/wp-content/uploads/2016/07/PC4-Principles-Statementshared-care-2016-1.pdf.

28. Walsh J, Harrison JD, Young JM, Butow PN, Solomon MJ, Masya L. What are the current barriers to effective cancer care coordination? A qualitative study. BMC Health Serv Res. 2010;10:132. https://doi.org/10.1186/1472-6963-10-132.

29. Pascoe S, Veitch C, Crossland LJ, Beilby JJ, Spigelman A, Stubbs J, et al. Patients' experiences of referral for colorectal cancer. BMC Fam Pract. 2013;14

30. Anvik T, Holtedahl KA, Mikalson H. "When patients have cancer, they stop seeing me" - the role of the general practitioner in early follow-up of patients with cancer - a qualitative study. BMC Fam Pract. 2006;7(19). https://doi.org/10.1186/1471-2296-7-19.

31. Haggstrom DA, Arora NK, Helft P, Clayman ML, Oakley-Girvan I. Follow-up care delivery among colorectal cancer survivors most often seen by primary and subspecialty care physicians. J Gen Intern Med. 2009;24(Suppl 2):472–9.

32. Goldsbury D, Harris M, Pascoe S, Barton M, Olver I, Spigelman A, et al. The varying role of the GP in the pathway between colonoscopy and surgery for colorectal cancer: a retrospective cohort study. BMJ Open. 2013;3(3): e002325.

33. Mieklejohn JA, Garvey G, Bailie R, Walpole E, Adams J, Williamson D, et al. Follow-up cancer care: perspectives of aboriginal and Torres Strait islander cancer survivors. Support Care Cancer. 2017;25(5):1597–605.

34. Phillipson L, Larsen-Truong K, Jones S, Pitts L. In: Sax Institute, editor. Improving cancer outcomes among culturally and linguistically diverse communities: an evidence check rapid review brokered by the sax institute. Cancer Institute NSW: Sydney; 2012.

35. Bayram C, Ryan R, Harrison C, Gardiner J, Bailes MJ, Obeyesekere N, et al. Consultations conducted in languages other than English in Australian general practice. Aust Fam Physician. 2016;45(1):9–13.

36. Nekhlyudov L, O'Malley D, Hudson SV. Integrating primary care providers in the care of cancer survivors: gaps in the evidence and future opportunities. Lancet Oncol. 2017;18:e30–8.

37. Jacobs LA, Shulman LN. Follow-up care of cancer survivors: challenges and solutions. Lancet Oncol. 2017;18:e19–29.

38. Adams E, Boulton M, Rose P, Lund S, Richardon A, Wilson S, et al. Views of cancer care: reviews in primary care. Br J Gen Pract. 2011;16(12):1231–72.

39. Rubin G, Berendson A, Crawford SM, Dommett R, Earle C, Emery J, et al. The expanding role of primary care in cancer control. Lancet Oncol. 2015; 16:1231–72.

40. McGeoch G, Anderson I, Gibson J, Gullery C, Kerr D, Shand B. Consensus pathways: evidence into practice. N Z Med J. 2015;128(1408):86–96.

41. Nielsen JD, Palshof T, Mainz J, Jensen AB, Olesen F. Randomised controlled trial of a shared care programme for newly referred cancer patients: bridging the gap between general practice and hospital. Qual Safety Health Care. 2003;12:263–72.

42. Walsh J, Young JM, Harrison JD, Butow P, Solomon MJ, Masya L, et al. What is important in cancer care coordination? A qualitative investigation. Euro J Cancer Care. 2011;20:220–7.

20

Factors related to intentional non-initiation of bisphosphonate treatment in patients with a high fracture risk in primary care

Karin M. A. Swart[1,2]* ⓘ, Myrthe van Vilsteren[1,2], Wesley van Hout[1], Esther Draak[1], Babette C. van der Zwaard[1], Henriette E. van der Horst[1], Jacqueline G. Hugtenburg[3] and Petra J. M. Elders[1]

Abstract

Background: Adherence to osteoporosis treatment is crucial for good treatment effects. However, adherence has been shown to be poor and a substantial part of the patients don't even initiate treatment. This study aimed to gain insight into the considerations of both osteoporosis patients and general practitioners (GP) concerning intentional non-initiation of bisphosphonate treatment.

Methods: Osteoporosis patients and GPs were recruited from the SALT Osteoporosis Study and a transmural fracture liaison service, both carried out in the Netherlands. Using questionnaires, we identified non-starters and starters of bisphosphonate treatment. Semi-structured interviews were conducted to gain a detailed overview of all considerations until saturation of the data was reached. Starters were asked to reflect on the considerations that were brought forward by the non-starters. Interviews were open coded and the codes were classified into main themes and subthemes using an inductive approach.

Results: 16 non-starters, 10 starters, and 13 GPs were interviewed. We identified three main themes: insufficient medical advice, attitudes towards medication use including concerns about side effects, and disease awareness. From patients' as well as GPs' perspective, insufficient or ambiguous information from the GP influenced the decision of the non-starters to not start bisphosphonates. In contrast, starters were either properly informed, or they collected information themselves. Patients' aversion towards medication, fear of side effects, and a low risk perception also contributed to not starting the medication, whereas starters were aware of their fracture risk and were confident of the outcome of the treatment. Concerns about osteoporosis treatment and its side effects were also expressed by several GPs. Some GPs appeared to have a limited understanding of the current osteoporosis guidelines and the indications for treatment.

Conclusions: Many reasons we found for not starting bisphosphonate treatment were related to the patients or the GPs themselves being insufficiently informed. Attitudes of the GPs were shown to play a role in the decision of patients not to start treatment. Interventions need to be developed that are aimed at GPs, and at education of patients.

Keywords: Bisphosphonates, Osteoporosis, Non-initiation, General practitioner

* Correspondence: k.swart@vumc.nl
[1]Department of General Practice and Elderly Care Medicine, Amsterdam Public Health research institute, Amsterdam UMC, Vrije Universiteit Amsterdam, De Boelelaan 1117, 1081 HV Amsterdam, Netherlands
[2]Stichting Artsen Laboratorium en Trombosedienst, Molenwerf 11, 1541 WR Koog aan de Zaan, Netherlands
Full list of author information is available at the end of the article

Background

Osteoporosis is a condition that affects 1.9 per 1000 men and 16.1 per 1000 women in the Netherlands [1]. The reduced density of the bone increases the risk of fractures [2]. Fractures are associated with increased morbidity and, especially hip fractures, are associated with increased mortality for many years after the fracture [3]. Fractures at an older age are a burden on the healthcare system. A study in the Netherlands estimated that the annual healthcare costs for osteoporosis-related fractures were almost 200 Million Euros per year in 2010 [4]. It is estimated that the costs for osteoporosis-related fractures will increase with 50% between 2010 and 2030, due to an ageing population [4].

Osteoporosis can be treated with bone-sparing drugs. Bisphosphonates inhibit bone resorption, thereby reducing the risk of future fractures [5, 6]. The authors of a Cochrane review concluded that the use of alendronate can lead to a relative risk reduction of 45% for vertebral fractures, 16% for non-vertebral fractures, and 39% for hip fractures [7]. However, the effectiveness of bisphosphonates is dependent on the adherence, i.e. the extent to which patients take their medication as prescribed [8]. A meta-analysis indicated that the fracture risk increases by approximately 30% in non-adherent patients compared to adherent patients [9]. It has been shown that adherence to bisphosphonates is poor, significantly threatening the anti-fracture efficacy as well as the cost-effectiveness [10].

The process of adherence involves initiation, implementation, and continuation of medication use. Non-adherence can be the result of late or non-starting of the treatment, sub-optimal implementation of the prescribed dosing scheme, and/or early discontinuation of the treatment [11]. The reasons that patients may have for being non-adherent may be intentional or non-intentional [12]. Unintentional non-adherence is related to forgetfulness and not knowing exactly how to use medicines. In contrast, intentional non-adherence has been described as an active process, in which patients beliefs and cognition may play an important role [12].

About 30% of osteoporosis patients do not start their prescribed medication [13]. Understanding of intentional non-initiation is essential to improve the overall adherence to bisphosphonate treatment. Few studies examined the reasons that patients have for not starting with their prescribed osteoporosis medication. Main reasons include limited knowledge of osteoporosis, fear of side effects, distrust in medication in general, and a lack of belief in medication effectiveness [14–17]. Although the importance of the role of health care providers in medication adherence in general has been recognized [18], considerations of general practitioners (GPs) regarding osteoporosis medication and their awareness of patients' intentional non-initiation have not been studied previously. Since bisphosphonates are effective in reducing fracture risk, thereby preventing serious consequences for the patients themselves and saving medical costs, it is important to thoroughly explore considerations of both patients and GPs about intentional non-initiation of bisphosphonates in patients at high fracture risk. In this study, we aimed to explore these considerations among non-starters, starters and GPs, with semi-structured interviews in order to provide a detailed overview of considerations that patients and GPs have.

Methods

We carried out a qualitative study in which we performed semi-structured interviews, based on thematic analysis with elements of grounded theory [19]. We interviewed patients who decided not to start taking bisphosphonates despite treatment advice (intentional non-initiation), to which we will refer as non-starters. Next, we interviewed patients who did start taking bisphosphonates and continued taking them for at least three months (adherent patients, to which we will refer as starters), and asked them to reflect on the reasons that we distilled from the non-starters for not initiating treatment. In addition, GPs of non-starters were interviewed.

Study population

Participants were recruited from a fracture prevention study and an ongoing fracture liaison service in the Netherlands. The common denominator of both is that the fracture risk assessment is centrally organised after which the GP receives the results of the evaluation and a treatment advice provided by an expert panel. From that point on, the GP is responsible for the initiation of treatment and for monitoring of the patient.

First, patients were recruited from the SALT Osteoporosis Study (SOS) [20]. The SOS is a pragmatic randomized controlled trial among women of 65 years and older in the Netherlands. It examines the effectiveness of a structured screening program and subsequent bisphosphonate treatment of patients with a high fractures risk, compared to usual care. Women with an absolute 10-years fracture risk according to the fracture risk assessment tool (FRAX) of main osteoporotic fractures including bone mineral density, and women with a prevalent vertebral fracture as determined with vertebral assessment, had an indication for bisphosphonate treatment. The treatment with bisphosphonates was initiated by the GP. By using the FRAX, the SOS protocol is less conservative than current practice in primary care in the Netherlands. Current practice according to Dutch guidelines for GPs consists of treating only patients with an increased fracture risk based on recent fracture, or several important risk factors for fractures and either low bone mineral density ($T < -2.5$) or prevalent vertebral fracture. Therefore, more patients have an indication for bisphosphonate treatment in the SOS than in usual care. Treatment initiation was documented as part of the study by the GP. Non-starters received a written request to participate in our qualitative interview via the GP and were approached for an interview if they indicated to be willing to participate.

Secondly, patients were recruited from a transmural fracture liaison service located in the Onze Lieve Vrouwe Gasthuis hospital in Amsterdam, the Netherlands. In this fracture liaison service, the GP has a central role in initiating osteoporosis screening and initiating and monitoring subsequent treatment. The service is offered to all patients aged 50 years or older who come to the emergency department of the Onze Lieve Vrouwe Gasthuis hospital with a fracture. In consultation with the GP, patients undergo an evaluation program, including dual x-ray absorptiometry and vertebral assessment. Evaluations and treatment advices are the responsibility of an expert team. Patients identified with a high fracture risk according to the Dutch guidelines for GPs have an indication for treatment with bisphosphonates. Accordingly, the GP initiates treatment. For this study, patients received a questionnaire several months after their visit to the fracture liaison service, in which we inquired whether treatment with bisphosphonates was initiated.

Non-starters were contacted with the request for an interview. We also contacted patients for an interview who indicated to have started and continued the treatment (starters). Furthermore, we contacted the GPs of the non-starters, and asked them for an interview. Not all GPs of the interviewed patients of this study were willing to participate in an interview. We therefore contacted additional GPs from the groups of GPs participating in the SOS study who had patients who had not started bisphosphonate treatment.

Interview procedure

The interviews with the patients were conducted face-to-face, at the patients' home. Prior to the interview, there was no relationship between the patient and the interviewer. Before the start of the actual interview, the purpose of the interview was explained, as well as the procedure (recording of the interview and confidentiality). Semi-structured interviews were performed using a topic list (see Additional file 1:Table S1 for the final version). The topic list was based on literature and expertise of the research team, and was completed during the study in an iterative process using the data from the interviews. The interviewer specifically asked whether the GP had advised to start bisphosphonate medication. The interviews with the GPs were performed at their practice or by phone.

The interviews with starters were performed after the interviews of the non-starters had been performed and analysed. The same topic list as the topic list for non-starters was used. In addition, the starters were asked to reflect on the main reasons of non-starters at the end of the interview. The interviewer started with open-ended questions and subsequently proceeded with more specific in-depth questions.

Seven interviewers of which one GP (female), three GPs in training (1 male and 2 female) and three medical students (3 female) carried out the interviews between March 2013 and September 2016. Training of the interviewers involved practice interviews plus evaluation with the principle investigator (PE). In order to ensure optimal quality of the interviews, all interviews were analysed on content as well as competence of the interviewing techniques and discussed with the interviewer before a new interview could be performed.

Analyses

The interviews were audio-recorded and transcribed verbatim. Transcripts were not returned to the participants for comments or corrections. The transcripts of the patient interviews were coded using the Atlas-ti qualitative data analysis software package, and the interviews with GPs were coded in Microsoft Excel 2007. Inductive analyses were performed. The interviews were analysed independently by two researchers (ED, WH, BZ, or MV). After individual coding of the interviews, the analyses were compared and discussed until consensus was reached. Disagreements were discussed with the principal investigator (PE), who also ensured the consistency of analysis method. The interviews were open-coded in the same order as the interviews were performed. The goal of open coding was to identify all aspects of the text that related to the research question. The labels of the open codes represented the text as closely as possible. In addition, these open codes were classified into main themes and subthemes. After each interview, the interview was analysed to find new themes. When there were no new themes after two subsequent interviews, we concluded that saturation was reached and ceased the interviews. The interviews of the starters were analysed to evaluated whether the reasons of non-starters were also expressed by starters, or whether they were refuted by starters.

Results

One patient was excluded because she was sure that her GP had advised her not to start treatment. We reached saturation of data after we interviewed 16 non-starters, 13 GPs, and 10 starters. Mean age of the patients was 76.3 years, 22 out of the 26 patients were female, and 10 out of 26 patients were recruited from the fracture liaison service. Of the non-starters, only 8 had had a previous fracture, whereas all starters had a previous fracture.

Among the patients without a previous fracture, one patient was identified with a vertebral fracture despite normal BMD. The mean duration of the interviews was 28:52 min for non-starters, 14:13 min for GPs and 11:12 min for starters. After analysis, we identified three main themes in the considerations patients and GPs had for not starting bisphosphonate treatment. These three themes, with subthemes, are described below.

Main theme I: Medical advise
Information to patients
Patients
Non-starters' knowledge on osteoporosis medication was limited: most of the non-starters did not know how bisphosphonates work. Many non-starters said that they had expected to have been given more information by the GP. Starters were either well informed and had been actively seeking information themselves, or they were rather passive and followed the instructions from their GP: "*I read about osteoporosis and its treatment before the consultation*" and "*a GP knows what he talks about. If he gives me advice, I follow it*".

Several non-starters reported that they had not fully understood the information: "*I would like to know to what extent I have it, whether it is really severe*". One non-starter mentioned that her impression was that the GP did not understand the explanation herself. Many non-starters felt their GP easily accepted their decision and thereby approved their decision. As one non-starter pointed out: "*And what did your GP tell you? Well, he said, if you do not want to take the medication, that's fine, it's up to you*". Furthermore, non-starters indicated that their GP gave mixed signals concerning whether or not to start with bisphosphonate treatment. Some non-starters said that some GPs in the end agreed with them to not start using bisphosphonates. As one non-starter explained: "*He (the GP) said, honestly, I don't think it's necessary for you to take the medication, I have forgotten why you should take the medication, because he said, you are a bit on the verge*". These issues were not recognized by the starters.

GPs
Some GPs acknowledged that risks and details were not fully discussed during the consultation and that in some cases, the patient made a decision based on too little information. Time constraints were mentioned as reason. Some GPs mentioned to have provided mixed signals concerning treatment: "*Uhm, I have talked about my doubts concerning this intervention towards my patient, yes*". The GPs sometimes did not question the decision of their patient not to start with the medication. The GPs gave the argument that they wish to respect the self-determination of the patient, and therefore, they would not go against the decision of their patient. Some GPs mentioned they felt unable to redirect the decision.

Assumptions about patients
GPs
GPs indicated that the decision of the patient fitted with the GPs' impression of the patients' beliefs concerning healthcare. One GP pointed out: "*This is what I expected, so I thought to myself, I'm not going to put too much energy in this*", or "*It makes no sense, she will stop anyway. I mean, whatever I prescribe her she will just quit*".

Main theme II: Medication
The theme medication concerns attitude towards preventive medication in general, attitude towards osteoporosis treatment, and side effects.

Attitude towards medication in general
Patients
Many non-starters indicated that they have an aversion against medication in general, and that they would rather not take any medicine: "*I just don't like pills, I think it's all poison*". Some non-starters only want to take medication that it is absolutely necessary: "*I think when you really need it, when something is life threatening, I would be okay with it*". The starters, in general, did not express an aversion against medication, although some starters were also critical about any medication they take. Some non-starters felt confident about their own health and had a preference for lifestyle interventions: "*I believe in my own healthy lifestyle*". Some of them also pointed out that they had a fear for side effects in general, or a distrust in the pharmaceutical industry: "*I am always afraid of side effects*", and "*There is a commercial aspect related to the pharmaceutical industry, I mean profit seeking*". Starters did not express a real aversion in the pharmaceutical industry. With respect to treatment duration one starter mentioned: "*I have a healthy distrust in the pharmaceutical industry. So I think that I would have checked this (the treatment duration) in due time*".

GPs
Some GPs mentioned that they have an aversion against preventive medicine in general: "*I doubt every form of preventive research or preventive treatment*".

Attitude towards osteoporosis treatment
Patients
Many non-starters were unsure about the effectiveness of osteoporosis medication: "*And my mom, who had terrible osteoporosis, she had to take a lot of stuff. She still had to get a new hip and new knee, despite all the*

medication". In contrast, starters generally trusted the treatment advice they received from their GP, and expressed no distrust in the effectiveness of osteoporosis medication: "*Before the GP called me, I was already convinced that I would start using the medication*", and: "*With this medication, you can really prevent something*". Furthermore, some starters expressed a positive attitude towards treatment: "*It is what it is. But luckily, there is treatment available*".

Many non-starters felt the intake instructions would result in practical problems, and they therefore preferred to take other medication such as calcium and vitamin D: "*Well, the period between taking the medication and eating is really too long for me*", and "*The only thing I did was starting to take calcium and those vitamins*". Some starters acknowledged that the intake of bisphosphonates is not very practical, but they got used to it, and did not see the intake instructions as a reason not to start with treatment: "*It took a lot of effort to get into the rhythm to start using the medication*".

GPs
Some GPs also doubted the effectiveness of osteoporosis treatment. One GP described: "*I think all that osteoporosis, it's very vague if I'm honest. What is meaningful, and what is not. The vitamin D, I also think that's a difficult subject*". Some GPs indicated that they were ambiguous about bisphosphonate treatment and its indication. "*If it's evident a patient has osteoporosis, then you can choose to protect them, but I think the indication to treat patients is more and more expanded*".

Side effects
Patients
Many non-starters expressed fear concerning the possible side effects of bisphosphonate treatment: "*I thought, I don't want those side effects, I already have fatigue, and I think I don't have a very strong stomach*", whereas starters had no fear for side effects before starting the medication: "*The information leaflet is miserable, but I just put it aside and just trust the medication*". Several non-starters indicated that side effects experienced by relatives or friends influenced their decision not to start bisphosphonate treatment. One non-starter explained: "*I know that my cousins, my sisters, all could not endure that stuff*". Another non-starter recalled: "*A friend of mine, she started a year ago. After the first box she said, I will stop with this mess, I'm not doing it any longer! She was done with it. She felt uncomfortable, so you have to take something that makes you feel bad, and you don't sense that your bones are weak. Why would you take it?*"

GPs
Some GPs agreed with the concern of possible side effects, and expected side effects to occur with specific patients: "*My idea was, those bisphosphonates are not going to work, she cannot handle that anyway. She always has complaints of her stomach and oesophagus*", and "*To give her bisphosphonates intravenously is also not going to work, because then she will feel sick for a year and I will be blamed for it*". Furthermore, some GPs thought that some patients are more prone to experience side effects: "*she asked me about the side effects of bisphosphonates. I told her. Then we both thought, this is going to be a mess, we should not do this*".

Main theme III: Disease awareness
This theme refers to the awareness of illness, prioritizing diseases, and risk acceptance.

Illness awareness
Patients
We observed a low risk perception in many non-starters. As one patient recalled: "*I thought about the facture risk in 5 or 10 years: there would be a risk, but in my opinion that was not enough to start taking medication*". The starters were more aware of the risks of osteoporosis than non-starters: "*It shocked me that I had osteoporosis, I realised that something was wrong*". Many non-starters indicated that they trusted their own health, and that they did not believe their diagnosis: "*I think I have pretty solid bones*", and "*I am not convinced that I am at a higher risk than anyone else*". Non-starters who had a fracture after a fall, did not link their fracture to osteoporosis: "*I broke my arm, my elbow, but then I had fallen from my bike. I think that even a 6-year old child with strong bones would have broken their elbow*". Several starters, however, acknowledged that fractures they had experienced could be the consequence of osteoporosis and not just from an accident: "*I suspected that something could be wrong. If you experience two fractures within 10 years, then something is probably wrong*". Some non-starters without fractures thought the absence of fractures was a proof of good bone health: "*I don't think I have it, well at least not very bad, because I have never had a fracture*".

GPs
GPs were not always aware of the guidelines, and therefore an increased fracture risk was not always recognized. As one GP recalled: "*The problem is not the treatment, but the diagnosis. She had a completely normal DXA result, and normal vitamin D levels. The only reason she got the diagnosis was that het risk for fractures was high was because she got a thoracic fracture due to a fall*". This GP apparently did not know that a

vertebral fracture is a very important risk factor for new fractures and an indication for bisphosphonates that is independent of bone mineral density results.

Prioritizing diseases
Patients
Some non-starters expressed that they prioritized other diseases they had, and that osteoporosis treatment therefore became less important: "*And then I got the diagnosis of breast cancer, so then the conversation about osteoporosis stopped*". The issue of prioritizing other diseases did not come up among the starters. They were more aware of their risk than non-starters and thought it was important to prevent subsequent fractures.

GPs
Some GPs prioritized other diseases as well: "*I thought it was much more important that she took her thyroid tablets, and she is not taking them. And that she took her acenocoumarol*".

Risk acceptance
Patients
Some non-starters indicated that they feel osteoporosis is related to aging: "*I don't think osteoporosis is a disease, it's just a part of getting older*". In contrast, starters did not accept osteoporosis as just a part of getting older: "*Do you think osteoporosis is a part of getting older? Well, yes it is. But to me that is not a reason to just accept it if there are good treatment options available for it*". Also, some non-starters rather accepted the risks and consequences of osteoporosis. As one non-starter described: "*I just take the risk to fall, then we will see what happens*". The starters were not willing to accept the risk of a fracture: "*I thought, I am not going to take the risk that I will get another fracture*". One starter also expressed: "*Being careful is always a good idea. But that does not mean you do not have to make sure your bones are as strong as possible. An accident can happen any time*" . A few non-starters indicated that they just felt too old to start osteoporosis treatment: "*I am 70 now, so how much longer do I have?*"

GPs
Also some GPs accepted the consequences of osteoporosis. One GP mentioned: "*So yes, the quality of life at this moment is more important than the probable prevention of fractures*".

Discussion
In this study, we analysed considerations of patients as well as GPs about not starting with osteoporosis treatment, despite an indication for treatment. Using semi-structured interviews, we found that these considerations focused on three main themes: medical advice, attitudes towards medication use, and disease awareness. For non-starters, insufficient information and the attitude of the GP, aversion of medication, fear of side effects, and a low risk perception contributed to non-starting their prescribed medication. Starters indicated to be properly informed, or they collected information themselves. They were aware of their fracture risk and were confident in the outcome of the treatment. For GPs, concerns about the effectiveness of osteoporosis treatment or its side effects were important considerations for not prescribing osteoporosis medication. Attitudes of the GPs were shown to play a role in the decision of patients not to start treatment.

To our knowledge, there are four studies available in which the reasons patients have for not starting bisphosphonate treatment were examined. Fear of side effects was reported as a primary reason for not starting with the medication in three of the studies [14, 15, 17]. Consistent with these previous findings, we currently observed that the fear of side effects was an important issue among non-starters. In contrast, starters were aware of the possibility of side effects, but this did not discourage them from starting the treatment. Other primary reasons that emerged in the previous studies were distrust in medication [15, 16], a low value of medication effectiveness [15, 16], and limited knowledge of osteoporosis [16]. In our study, medical advice to patients was found to be of major importance and was even identified as one of the three main themes of considerations for not starting osteoporosis treatment. Another previous study showed that fracture clinic patients reported limited understanding about osteoporosis and osteoprosis care, with ambiguity about their diagnosis, testing and treatment [21]. In our study, the purpose of the treatment was not clear for many non-starters, and many non-starters indicated to be insufficiently or ambiguously informed, whereas this was no problem for the starters. Sufficient information might also be important with respect to a low risk perception among non-starters. This observation is in line with the reduced belief compared to starters that osteoporosis is a serious disease, as observed previously [16]. In contrast to previous findings, medication costs [17] were not mentioned as primary reason for not starting bisphosphonate treatment in the current study. According to a systematic review of 24 quantitative studies, medication costs were an important factor for intentional non-initiation to any kind of medication [22]. In our study, patients did not express medication costs as a reason for not starting treatment, but this might be due to the health insurance system in the Netherlands in which most medication is reimbursed.

The currently identified considerations for non-initiation of osteoporosis treatment are very similar to previously identified considerations for non-adherence in general. Survey studies showed side effects as the most commonly reported reason to stop, but also concerns about the potential harms and motivational problems have been shown to be important [23]. A previous longitudinal qualitative study identified understanding, motivations and self-care, risk appraisal and prioritising, side effects, and decision making around medication as key themes [24]. In an overview article, the Extended Health Belief Model was used to explain medication adherence as decision making process in which perceived benefits, perceived susceptibility for and severity of fractures, concerns about or distrust in medication, medication use self-efficacy, and trust in physician are the main component [23]. The current findings fit within this framework.

In our study we explored the role of the GP in the decision about whether or not to start using osteoporosis medication. The quality of the medical consultation might be related to patient outcomes [25]. Confidence in the prescribing doctor, and trust in the healthcare system were described as important patient factors in the previous systematic review on intentional non-initiation to any kind of medication [22], and we found these factors in our study as well. From both patients' and GPs' perspective, we observed that GPs who legitimised the intention not to start treatment, or appeared to give advices hesitatingly, influenced their patients negatively. GPs who reported to have an aversion against osteoporosis treatment or preventive medicine in general, also had a negative influence on their patients. In addition, GPs who appeared to have inadequate knowledge about the current guidelines could not inform the patients properly. Although the current Dutch GP guideline for fracture prevention has been updated in 2012 and is applicable for several years now, not all GPs were aware of all treatment indications. Barriers to change, as often seen in changing health care settings, might be applicable. GP's knowledge, acceptance and beliefs about bisphosphonate indication and use may form barriers. In addition, we found that the absolute fracture risk, expressed as a percentage, was often difficult to interpret for the patient as well as for the GP, and some patients felt the percentage was not high enough to start bisphosphonate treatment. The finding that patients have difficulties interpreting fracture risk was also found in another study [26]. Furthermore, a low risk perception was expressed by several patients as well as by GPs in our study and this might be partly caused by limited information on osteoporosis discussed during the medical consultation.

A strength of our study is that we performed qualitative research into considerations for not starting bisphosphonate treatment. By performing semi-structured interviews, we could generate a detailed overview of considerations, which we could not have generated if we had used quantitative data only. Besides interviewing patients who did not start treatment, we also interviewed patients who had started, and GPs of non-starters. By doing so, we were able to explore the role of the GP in starting treatment, and to analyse whether patients who did start treatment had the same or other considerations for starting treatment. Furthermore, we were able to include patients from whom the GP had not prescribed medication during consultation, but who had an indication for treatment. These patients would have been missed if non-starters would have been identified by pharmacies.

However, because of the qualitative nature of this study, our results need to be interpreted with caution and need to be confirmed in a large and non-selective sample. The study population was a self-selected population who joined either the Dutch SOS study, or were selected via a fracture liaison service. Therefore the results might not be applicable to other populations, or patients from secondary care. What additionally might have influenced our results is that there were more patients who had experienced a fracture in the sample of starters than in the sample of non-starters. This might have led to more focus on illness awareness among the starters. On the other hand, they might have been more motivated to start medication in order to prevent a next fracture. Other limitations are the relatively large number of interviewers, and the possibility that GPs mentioned other reasons behind their reluctance to prescribe to account for their behaviour.

Previous interventions to improve medication adherence were mainly patient-focussed [27]. Our study results highlight the importance of the role of the GP in the management of intentional non-initiation of osteoporosis medication. Although patient education have been shown to only marginal improve adherence [27], combined education of GP and patient might be promising, given the current observed role of the GP in shaping the view of patients. Such an approach should be examined in future research. Firstly, GPs should have a better understanding of the current osteoporosis guidelines and treatment indication, as we observed that their knowledge was not always adequate. Secondly, GPs might contribute to a more optimal osteoporosis treatment by increasing patients' knowledge about osteoporosis and its treatment and by addressing their concerns and fears of side effects. In addition, when discussing initial fear of side effects, the GP can inform the patient that other treatment options are available, such as injectable treatment. This might help patients to make a well-informed decision about starting medication. Pharmacies might assist GPs to inform patients.

Conclusion

In conclusion, our comprehensive qualitative study examined the considerations of both osteoporosis patients and GPs concerning intentional non-initiation of bisphosphonate treatment. Most of the factors of non-initiation were comparable to the factors that play a role in non-adherence in general. New was the way patients describe that the GP had influenced their decision, either by giving the impression that they legitimized their decision, by showing doubt, or by having insufficient knowledge. It was shown that the content of medical advice of GPs to patients and their attitudes towards medication use were primary factors. Our findings suggest that primary care might be improved by increasing both GPs' and patients' knowledge as well as addressing expected barriers and discussing possible solutions, in order to increase the rate of patients who start using osteoporosis medication, and thus prevent future fractures. This suggestion needs to be further examined in interventional studies. The development of such interventions, in collaboration with patients, would be the next step.

Abbreviations
FRAX: Fracture rate assessment tool; GP: General practitioner; SOS: SALT Osteoporosis Study

Funding
The SALT Osteoporosis Study has been largely funded by Stichting Achmea Gezondheidszorg. Healthcare costs have been compensated by Achmea and VGZ Zorgverzekeraar. Additional financial support has been provided by Stichting Artsen Laboratorium en Trombosedienst. Extra funding to study medication adherence within the SALT Osteoporosis Study has been obtained after the start of the trial via unrestricted grants provided by Takeda Nederland B.V., Amgen B.V., and Teva Nederland. Funding for the evaluation of the fracture liaison service was provided by the Netherlands Organization for Health Research and Development (ZonMw). The sponsors do not have any role in the design or implementation of the study, data collection, data management, data analysis, and interpretation, or in the preparation, review, or approval of the manuscript.

Authors' contributions
Study concept and design (JH, PE, HH); obtaining funding (BZ, PE); data collection and management (MV, WH, ED, BZ, PE); warranty of infrastructure (HH), drafting the manuscript (KS, MV, WH); data analysis (KS, MV, WH, ED, BZ, PE); interpretation of data (all authors); critical revision of the manuscript for important intellectual content (all authors); study supervision (PE). All authors read and approved the final manuscript.

Competing interests
The authors declare that they have no competing interests.

Author details
[1]Department of General Practice and Elderly Care Medicine, Amsterdam Public Health research institute, Amsterdam UMC, Vrije Universiteit Amsterdam, De Boelelaan 1117, 1081 HV Amsterdam, Netherlands. [2]Stichting Artsen Laboratorium en Trombosedienst, Molenwerf 11, 1541 WR Koog aan de Zaan, Netherlands. [3]Department of Clinical Pharmacology and Pharmacy, Amsterdam Public Health research institute, Amsterdam UMC, Vrije Universiteit Amsterdam, De Boelelaan 1117, 1081 HV Amsterdam, Netherlands.

References
1. Poos M, Gommer A. Hoe vaak komt osteoporose voor en hoeveel mensen sterven eraan? RIVM: Bilthoven; 2009.
2. Hernlund E, Svedbom A, Ivergard M, Compston J, Cooper C, Stenmark J, et al. Osteoporosis in the European Union: medical management, epidemiology and economic burden. A report prepared in collaboration with the International Osteoporosis Foundation (IOF) and the European Federation of Pharmaceutical Industry Associations (EFPIA). Arch Osteoporos. 2013;8:136.
3. Abrahamsen B, van Staa T, Ariely R, Olson M, Cooper C. Excess mortality following hip fracture: a systematic epidemiological review. Osteoporos Int. 2009;20:1633–50.
4. Lotters FJ, van den Bergh JP, de Vries F, Rutten-van Molken MP. Current and future incidence and costs of osteoporosis-related fractures in the Netherlands: combining claims data with BMD measurements. Calcif Tissue Int. 2016;98:235–43.
5. Cranney A, Guyatt G, Griffith L, Wells G, Tugwell P, Rosen C. Meta-analyses of therapies for postmenopausal osteoporosis. IX: summary of meta-analyses of therapies for postmenopausal osteoporosis. Endocr Rev. 2002;23:570–8.
6. Dursun N, Dursun E, Yalcin S. Comparison of alendronate, calcitonin and calcium treatments in postmenopausal osteoporosis. Int J Clin Pract. 2001;55:505–9.
7. Wells GA, Cranney A, Peterson J, Boucher M, Shea B, Robinson V, et al. Alendronate for the primary and secondary prevention of osteoporotic fractures in postmenopausal women. Cochrane Database Syst Rev. 2008;1:CD001155.
8. Siris ES, Selby PL, Saag KG, Borgstrom F, Herings RM, Silverman SL. Impact of osteoporosis treatment adherence on fracture rates in North America and Europe. Am J Med. 2009;122(Suppl 2):3–13.
9. Ross S, Samuels E, Gairy K, Iqbal S, Badamgarav E, Siris E. A meta-analysis of osteoporotic fracture risk with medication nonadherence. Value Health. 2011;14:571–81.
10. Sharman Moser S, Yu J, Goldshtein I, Ish-Shalom S, Rouach V, Shalev V, et al. Cost and consequences of nonadherence with oral bisphosphonate therapy: findings from a real-world data analysis. Ann Pharmacother. 2016;50:262–9.
11. Vrijens B, De Geest S, Hughes DA, Przemyslaw K, Demonceau J, Ruppar T, et al. A new taxonomy for describing and defining adherence to medications. Br J Clin Pharmacol. 2012;73:691–705.
12. Hugtenburg JG, Timmers L, Elders PJ, Vervloet M, van Dijk L. Definitions, variants, and causes of nonadherence with medication: a challenge for tailored interventions. Patient Prefer Adherence. 2013;7:675–82.
13. Reynolds K, Muntner P, Cheetham TC, Harrison TN, Morisky DE, Silverman S, et al. Primary non-adherence to bisphosphonates in an integrated healthcare setting. Osteoporos Int. 2013;24:2509–17.
14. Lindsay BR, Olufade T, Bauer J, Babrowicz J, Hahn R. Patient-reported barriers to osteoporosis therapy. Arch Osteoporos. 2016;11:19.
15. Scoville EA, Ponce de Leon Lovaton P, Shah ND, Pencille LJ, Montori VM. Why do women reject bisphosphonates for osteoporosis? A videographic study. PLoS One. 2011;6:e18468.
16. Yood RA, Mazor KM, Andrade SE, Emani S, Chan W, Kahler KH. Patient decision to initiate therapy for osteoporosis: the influence of knowledge and beliefs. J Gen Intern Med. 2008;23:1815–21.
17. Yu J, Brenneman SK, Sazonov V, Modi A. Reasons for not initiating osteoporosis therapy among a managed care population. Patient Prefer Adherence. 2015;9:821–30.
18. Sabaté E. Adherence to long-term therapies. Evidence for action. Geneva: World Health Organization; 2003.
19. Charmaz K. Constructing Grounded Theory: A Practical Guide through Qualitative Analysis (1st ed.): SAGE Publications Ltd; 2006.
20. Elders PJM, Merlijn T, Swart KMA, van Hout W, van der Zwaard BC, Niemeijer C, et al. Design of the SALT osteoporosis study: a randomised pragmatic trial, to study a primary care screening and treatment program for the

prevention of fractures in women aged 65 years or older. BMC Musculoskelet Disord. 2017;18:424.

21. Sale JE, Beaton DE, Sujic R, Bogoch ER. 'If it was osteoporosis, I would have really hurt myself.' Ambiguity about osteoporosis and osteoporosis care despite a screening programme to educate fragility fracture patients. J Eval Clin Pract. 2010;16:590–6.

22. Zeber JE, Manias E, Williams AF, Hutchins D, Udezi WA, Roberts CS, et al. A systematic literature review of psychosocial and behavioral factors associated with initial medication adherence: a report of the ISPOR medication adherence & persistence special interest group. Value Health. 2013;16:891–900.

23. Schousboe JT. Adherence with medications used to treat osteoporosis: behavioral insights. Curr Osteoporos Rep. 2013;11:21–9.

24. Salter C, McDaid L, Bhattacharya D, Holland R, Marshall T, Howe A. Abandoned acid? Understanding adherence to bisphosphonate medications for the prevention of osteoporosis among older women: a qualitative longitudinal study. PLoS One. 2014;9:e83552.

25. Mead N, Bower P. Patient-centred consultations and outcomes in primary care: a review of the literature. Patient Educ Couns. 2002;48:51–61.

26. Sale JE, Gignac MA, Hawker G, Beaton D, Frankel L, Bogoch E, et al. Patients do not have a consistent understanding of high risk for future fracture: a qualitative study of patients from a post-fracture secondary prevention program. Osteoporos Int. 2016;27:65–73.

27. Hiligsmann M, Salas M, Hughes DA, Manias E, Gwadry-Sridhar FH, Linck P, et al. Interventions to improve osteoporosis medication adherence and persistence: a systematic review and literature appraisal by the ISPOR Medication Adherence & Persistence Special Interest Group. Osteoporos Int. 2013;24:2907–18.

21

Patient experiences of a lifestyle program for metabolic syndrome offered in family medicine clinics: a mixed methods study

Jennifer Klein[1], Paula Brauer[2], Dawna Royall[2], Maya Israeloff-Smith[2], Doug Klein[3]* (iD), Angelo Tremblay[4], Rupinder Dhaliwal[5], Caroline Rheaume[6], David M. Mutch[7] and Khursheed Jeejeebhoy[8]

Abstract

Background: Patient perspectives on new programs to manage metabolic syndrome (MetS) are critical to evaluate for possible implementation in the primary healthcare system. Participants' perspectives were sought for the Canadian Health Advanced by Nutrition and Graded Exercise (CHANGE) study, which enrolled 293 participants, and demonstrated 19% reversal of MetS after 1 year. The main purpose of this study was to examine participants' perceptions of their experiences with the CHANGE program, enablers and barriers to change.

Methods: A convergent parallel mixed methods design combined patients' perspectives collected by questionnaires ($n = 164$), with insights from focus groups ($n = 41$) from three sites across Canada. Qualitative data were thematically analyzed using interpretative description. Insights were organized within a socio-ecologic framework.

Results: Key aspects identified by participants included intra-individual factors (personal agency, increased time availability), inter-individual factors (trust, social aspects) and organizational factors (increased mental health support, tailored programs).

Conclusion: Results revealed participants' overall support for the CHANGE program, especially the importance of an extended program under the guidance of a family physician along with a skilled and supportive team. Team delivery of a lifestyle program in primary care or family medicine clinics is a complex intervention and use of a mixed methods design was helpful for exploring patient experiences and key issues on enablers and barriers to health behavior change.

Background

In Canada, 19% of adults have metabolic syndrome (MetS) [1, 2] exhibiting at least three of five common risk factors: high waist circumference, increased blood pressure, elevated blood glucose, elevated triglycerides and decreased high-density cholesterol levels. People with MetS have been shown to have double the annual health care costs and higher frequency of services than those without MetS [3, 4]. Progression of MetS to diabetes and heart disease can be significantly reduced by changes in diet and exercise [5–8]. Most people with MetS are treated in the primary care system.

Building on promising results from previous studies [9–11], the Canadian Health Advanced by Nutrition and Graded Exercise (CHANGE) feasibility study was completed in three diverse primary care organizations across Canada to demonstrate the possibility of achieving reversal of MetS within the Canadian primary care context. [11] This program was a practical, flexible, and personalized diet-exercise program delivered by a team of health professionals (i.e., family physician, dietitian, and exercise specialist). The CHANGE intervention was driven by the ongoing relationship that patients have with their family doctor. Key features of the program included: 1) family physician encouragement and ongoing monitoring; 2) intensive diet and exercise with individualized counseling and support by dietitians and exercise specialists each week for 3 months; followed by 3) monthly visits for the remaining part of the 1 year period. The program was successful in reversing MetS among 19% of the 293 patients and details are described elsewhere [11, 12].

* Correspondence: douglask@ualberta.ca; doug.klein@ualberta.ca
[3]Department of Family Medicine, University of Alberta, Edmonton, Canada
Full list of author information is available at the end of the article

Evaluation of patients' perspectives is particularly important for lifestyle programs, as programs vary widely and attrition can be substantial [13, 14]. Mixed methods study designs are becoming increasingly popular, being particularly helpful in identifying diverse issues and in engaging a larger cross-section of participants. The socio-ecologic framework, a theory-based framework for understanding the complex interplay of personal and environmental factors that determine behaviors, was used to organize insights at three levels: intra-individual, inter-individual, and primary care organization levels [15].

The main purpose of this study was to examine participants' perceptions of their experiences with the CHANGE program, enablers and barriers to change. Participants were from all three sites (i.e. Edmonton, Toronto and Quebec City).

Methods

A convergent parallel mixed methods design was used [16], with questionnaire and focus group data collection and analyses conducted concurrently. Results were analyzed separately and then considered together in an overall interpretation of the issues of interest. Written consent was obtained from the participants in advance of participation. Ethical approval was obtained from the University of Alberta Health Research Ethics Board.

Questionnaire
Questionnaire development
The questionnaire was a tool for assessing patients' experiences with lifestyle programs in primary care. It was developed through input from primary health care providers regarding the critical issues to be assessed for quality improvement purposes in primary care, based on a review of key indicators of primary care service quality [17]. Content validity was established through interviews with patients participating in a lifestyle program. It consisted of 21 multiple choice and 2 open-ended questions on the following dimensions as described by Wong and Haggerty [18]; access, interpersonal communication, continuity and coordination, comprehensiveness of services, trust, and patient-reported impacts of care. (See Additional file 1). The questionnaire was used as published [17], with the generic introduction modified to be specific to the CHANGE project and the entire questionnaire translated into French and Russian to meet the language needs of the participating sites.

Questionnaire administration, collection and analysis
Questionnaire administration and data collection was managed by research coordinators (RCs) from each of the three sites. Each RC had options for getting the questionnaires completed. They could complete with patients in-person or mail paper questionnaires in the

languages appropriate for their site along with pre-stamped return envelopes. The French and English paper questionnaires also included a web address to the online questionnaire so that participants could complete the questionnaire online if they wished. The online questionnaire was not translated into Russian, as the RC at the site opted to translate and complete questionnaires with participants in-person. All paper questionnaires were transcribed and downloaded into Microsoft Excel for descriptive analysis. Comments written were content analyzed for themes by one researcher (DR) and reviewed by two members of the team for consensus on theme content (PB and DR).

Focus groups
Focus group participants consisted of individuals currently participating in the CHANGE study and were recruited through a mail-out to all participants, outlining the purpose of the study. In addition, flyers were posted in the clinic, inviting people to participate in the study. Potential participants were asked to contact the researcher either by phone or email. Focus groups took place in all three cities. An experienced qualitative researcher experienced in facilitating focus groups (JK) established a relationship at the beginning of the sessions outlining the purpose of the research, her role in the project and then moderated the English sessions. The focus group in French was led by a francophone researcher (AT) who established a relationship at the beginning of the sessions with participants, outlining the purpose of the research, his role in the project and then facilitated the discussion, with input from the original facilitator (JK) who is bilingual, but had French as a second language. Open-ended questions were used to explore participant perspectives. (See Additional file 2.) Focus groups lasted approximately 1 hour each and were conducted at the participants' respective health care centre. Field notes were made after the focus groups.

Focus group analysis
Discussions were digitally recorded, transcribed and organized using NVIVO software [19], a textual database computer software program. Transcripts were analyzed by an experienced qualitative researcher (JK) using Interpretive Description, a non-categorical approach to qualitative data analysis that goes beyond description of a phenomenon to a meaningful interpretation [20]. In keeping with the general principles of interpretive description methodology, the analytic process was inductive, using constant comparative analysis to track commonalities and variations among and between participants according to the research question. Data was organized and analyzed involving coding ideas and refining themes as patterns emerged [21]. Codes were designed to capture details surrounding the experiences of participating in the

CHANGE program. These codes were then loosely organized into overarching 15 themes and subthemes (Additional file 3). These thematic patterns were identified and explored, allowing for minor adjustments in the probing questions for subsequent focus groups on issues where expansion and clarification seemed potentially fruitful. Member checking occurred at the final segment of the four focus groups to validate focus group themes; participants were provided with a summary of themes gathered to that point in the research project. Participants were asked to review and provide comments, serving as a check on the viability of the interpretations.

Availability of data and materials

The questionnaire is available in Additional file 1. Focus group questions are available in Additional file 2. Examples of themes and subthemes for focus group analysis are available in Additional file 3. Datasets used and analyzed during the current study are available from the corresponding author on request.

Results

Questionnaire

A total of 164 questionnaires were received (57 French, 107 English and 0 Russian) of 293 potential recipients (56% response rate); 76% as paper questionnaires and 24% online responses. Of the 164 responses to the survey, 27 (19.4%) respondents reversed their metabolic syndrome. This is consistent with the 19% reversal found in the entire study population (11). Therefore, the survey response reflects the population included in the larger study. Most questionnaire respondents (89%) had completed the one-year program; thus, results mostly reflect their perspectives. Numbers were inadequate to conduct subgroup analysis on the drop-outs.

Program enablers

Results of the quantitative aspects of the questionnaire and the dimension being assessed are shown in Table 1. With respect to interpersonal communication, virtually all patients (99%) felt respected and program's elements were clearly explained. Trust in the providers and their information was also very high. Participants felt they were rarely or never told different things by different providers (team functioning). While only 76% felt they were definitely involved in setting their goals, 88% felt their personal situation was taken into account when providers made recommendations. During the program, 81% felt they had received the information they needed to make changes, with 17% indicating some gaps. On a 10-point scale, 80% rated the program 8–10 regarding the importance of the lifestyle program to their health, with another 17% rating at 5–7. A notable result was the finding that 71% thought the one-year program was the

right length, while 19% found it too short. Even after 1 year, confidence in maintaining nutrition and physical activity changes was generally high, with the majority being at least moderately confident that they could maintain the diet and exercise changes (see Fig. 1).

Over 150 positive qualitative comments from the questionnaire, representing more than 80% of the comments, indicated patients felt the personalized program was motivating and had increased their awareness and knowledge of what to eat and how to exercise. Increased self-efficacy was often mentioned such as: *"They provided me with the confidence and knowledge to succeed"*. Further, patients commented that their behavior, health, and well-being had improved (e.g., *"not as susceptible to fatigue"* and *"I feel less like snacking during the day or the evening"*). Several patients noted reduced medication use or decreased blood pressure.

Program barriers

Some challenges with the program emerged. For example, 32% indicated they 'sometimes' or 'often' had problems getting to appointments due to time or cost. Only 62% felt they knew what to expect at the start of the program and 23% felt they had been involved in setting goals only to some extent.

Many participants (i.e., 49–57%) reported sometimes not trying the recommended diet or activity changes because something got in the way, while only 6–7% reported that this happened often (see Table 1). Qualitative comments denoting barriers focused on challenges maintaining the changes, such as work schedules and winter weather. Other key barriers for diet changes included the need for fast and easy food preparation, as well as the role and emphasis of food in socializing and special occasions. Others reported challenges included adhering to a specific diet pattern, *"It's hard to stick to a Mediterranean diet when you live in Alberta"*. The most common barrier to physical activity was chronic pain due to arthritis and other health issues.

When asked about services that should be added, removed or changed, a wide variety of suggestions emerged. Many participants felt the program could have been longer or more intensive with an increased frequency of meetings after the weekly phase was completed, and/or with more options for follow-up with providers or other participants. Several requested more evening and weekend appointments. Other suggestions included: encouraging participation of partners and household members, providing specialized support for mental health issues, and tailoring physical activities to participants' differing abilities, interests and pain issues.

Focus groups

There were 41 participants (15 females, 26 males) who participated in 6 focus groups across 3 clinics, each

Table 1 Responses to survey questions based on key dimensions assessed

Dimension (sub-dimension)	Question	N (%)
Access (First contact accessibility)	Able to contact a team member:	
	• Yes, definitely	125 (76%)
	• Yes, to some extent	14 (9%)
	• No, not at all	1 (1%)
	• Did not need to contact	24 (15%)
Access (Economic accessibility)	Difficulty in getting to appointments due to costs or time	
	• Never/Rarely	112 (68%)
	• Sometimes	42 (26%)
	• Often/Very often	10 (6%)
Interpersonal communication (General communication)	Knowledge of what to expect re: number of appointments, what would be learned and amount of support	
	• Yes, definitely	98 (62%)
	• Yes, to some extent	50 (32%)
	• No, not at all	10 (6%)
Interpersonal communication (General communication)	How often team members explained things clearly	
	• Always/usually	160 (98%)
	• Sometimes	2 (1%)
	• Rarely/never	1 (0.6%)
Interpersonal communication (Respectfulness)	How often team members treated with courtesy and respect	
	• Always/usually	163 (99%)
	• Sometimes	0
	• Rarely/never	1 (0.6%)
Interpersonal communication (Shared decision-making)	Involvement in setting goals	
	• Yes, definitely	122 (76%)
	• Yes, to some extent	37 (23%)
	• No, not at all	2 (1%)
Interpersonal communication (Whole-person care)	Did team members consider personal situation when making recommendations?	
	• Yes, definitely	143 (88%)
	• Yes, to some extent	19 (12%)
	• No, not at all	0
	• Don't know	1 (0.6%)
Continuity and coordination (Team functioning)	How often told different things by different providers	
	• Always/usually	7 (4%)
	• Sometimes	10 (6%)
	• Rarely/never	144 (89%)
Comprehensiveness of services (Services	How would you rate importance of this service to your health? (0 = not important at all; 10	

Table 1 Responses to survey questions based on key dimensions assessed *(Continued)*

Dimension (sub-dimension)	Question	N (%)
provided)	= extremely important)	
	• 1–4	5 (3%)
	• 5–7	28 (17%)
	• 8–10	128 (80%)
Comprehensiveness of services (Services provided)	Appropriateness of program length?	
	• Too short	31 (19%)
	• Just right	114 (71%)
	• Too long	15 (9%)
Comprehensiveness of services (Services provided)	Have the team members provided the information and support needed to make changes?	
	• Yes, definitely	132 (81%)
	• Yes, to some extent	28 (17%)
	• No, not really	2 (1%)
	• Not needed	1 (0.6%)
Trust	Comfortable sharing personal information with team?	
	• Yes, definitely	152 (93%)
	• Yes, to some extent	12 (7%)
	• No, not at all	0
Trust	Confidence in information received	
	• Yes, definitely	153 (93%)
	• Yes, to some extent	11 (7%)
	• No, not at all	0
Patient-reported impacts on care (Action on Goals)	Confidence in maintaining changes in nutrition	
	• Totally/very confident	119 (73%)
	• Moderately confident	38 (23%)
	• Little/hardly confident	7 (4%)
Patient-reported impacts on care (Action on Goals)	Confidence in maintaining changes in physical activity	
	• Totally/very confident	103 (63%)
	• Moderately confident	42 (26%)
	• Little/hardly confident	18 (11%)
Patient-reported impacts on care (Action on Goals)	Were there times when did not try nutrition changes because something got in the way?	
	• No	58 (37%)
	• Yes, sometimes	89 (57%)
	• Yes, often	10 (6%)
Patient-reported impacts on care (Action on Goals)	Were there times when did not try physical activity changes because something got in the way?	

Table 1 Responses to survey questions based on key dimensions assessed *(Continued)*

Dimension (sub-dimension)	Question	N (%)
	• No	67 (44%)
	• Yes, sometimes	75 (49%)
	• Yes, often	11 (7%)

consisting of 6–10 participants. The focus group participants reflected the larger study population, including mean age of 60 (range 45–68 years), mean BMI 32, majority Caucasian along with some participants of Asian, Russian and Arabic ethnicity.

Overall experiences
Similar to the questionnaire, focus group participants reported very positive feedback about being a part of the CHANGE program. Many shared they felt it was *"a privilege"* to be part of the program and reported the program had changed their life by educating, supporting, and implementing realistic lifestyle changes.

Program enablers
Individualized gradual approach to care. Participants emphasized the personalized and gradual approach was the biggest asset of the program and helped to differentiate it from other diets and programs previously tried as it was realistic and conceivable to adapt to individual needs. The program was reported to be *"structured, yet flexible"* enough to meet a variety of dietary, exercise, and lifestyle needs.

"It's a very structured approach to changing your diet and exercising...yet it's so flexible. The diet is about what I wanna eat and not about what somebody else is shoving down your throat." (Participant 12)

Personalities and approach of the staff. The support and enthusiasm of the staff were key factors in the adherence and success of participants. Staff reportedly created a relaxed atmosphere, never making participants feels rushed, yet *"providing gentle discipline...without being viewed as pushy"*. Many comments were made that staff were not judgmental. *"They didn't sit there and judge you, and say 'oh you shouldn't be drinking all that wine or having all that red meat...I know I was doing things wrong and I think we all know we have to make changes in our lives'"*.

Physicians as motivator and trusted mentor. Physicians played an important role in participants registering for the program. Several participants said they would not have registered independently, but did so on recommendation from their physician. Participants also spoke of adhering to the program, as they felt accountable to their physicians.

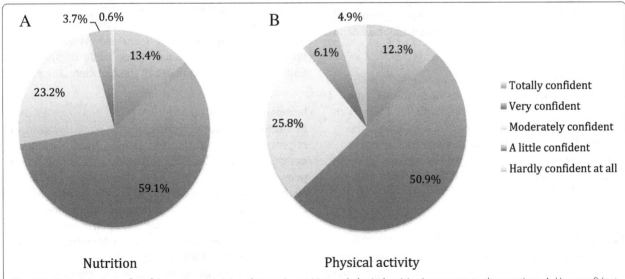

Fig. 1 Participants' ratings of confidence in maintaining changes in nutrition and physical activity. In response to the questions: A. How confident are you that you can maintain the changes in your nutrition (*n* = 164); B. How confident are you that you can maintain the changes in your physical activity (*n* = 163). *p* < 0.05 by Chi-square test

"I think if the doctor is suggesting it, that probably was one of the most powerful incentives." (Participant 27).

Frequency of meetings for the program. Surprisingly the intense weekly visits for the first 3 months were not seen as a barrier and were very well received. Not one participant felt it was too much. "*The first three month period is very good. Reinforces everything. Kind of kick starts you.*"

Accessible supervision by expert team. Participants appreciated that there were expert health professionals to guide them. Several mentioned they were apprehensive to try new lifestyle changes due to their lack of knowledge in the realms of healthy eating and exercises and/or implications of lifestyle changes on their illness or recent surgeries. Having the team involved provided confidence for them to implement the changes. Participants appreciated the open access to the dietitians and kinesiologists at all times.

Social aspect. The social aspect of the program was prominent.

"I can say coming to exercise in a group helped me because I think when you just do it by yourself or with your instructor you don't feel as much part of something that's going on, so it was always kind of neat to come to the gym and see other people that were on treadmills... That were all at different stages... that helped because I think I had felt for a long time there was no way I was ever gonna get any success out of weight loss program." (Participant 3).

Impact on significant others. Participants spoke of the impact of the program was not just individual. "*My wife got on board so that it became a family-oriented thing rather then just an individual thing*". Participants spoke of the program influencing family members and friends, which was a great motivator.

"I shared information with two colleagues. There were family members who wanted to ride with me, who wanted to exercise. It's inspiring to them. There is an impact on the family. The meals are no longer the same. There are no hamburgers and fries anymore... people around me also changed their habits. You can change the habits of 10 people through only one person." (Participant 12).

Program barriers

While participants were very positive about their experiences, several challenges were shared. These were divided into personal and program-based.

Personal. The biggest challenge was the psychological barrier to changing personal habits and maintaining self-discipline. As one participant declared, "*Controlling your diet is harder than quitting smoking*". Several participants spoke of the difficulties of maintaining their health goals when family members were not supportive. "*My biggest challenge has been trying to make the food changes with the rest of my family, who are not in the CHANGE program, and don't want to change*". Similar to the questionnaire findings, many participants shared that the lack of time to participate in exercise was challenging.

Program. There was a minimal amount of support to address mental health issues. Participants mentioned there had been a small assessment with the nutritionist, but would prefer a larger focus in this area. Offering access to a mental health professional early on in the program was deemed helpful.

"Those services take a long time to get. The assessment was done and the expectation was that your family doctor followed up on that but who do family doctors refer to? Psychologists, psychiatrists, so you're just putting another stumbling block of time and energy. Here I am on month 6, finally mentally in the game. The year's half done." (Participant 34).

In addition, several participants suggested more variety in the exercise programs and increased focus on incorporating specific health issues (e.g., arthritic knees). The program offered appointments and services only during the weekdays. Several participants requested evenings and weekend access due to conflicts with work schedules.

Discussion

Despite the questionnaire and focus group questions being framed differently, similar issues emerged from participant's responses. The focus groups elicited more reflection on intra-personal issues, while organizational issues were more prominent in the questionnaire results.

Intrapersonal level

Published literature reports the most prevalent and important barriers to lifestyle change, from participants' perspectives, are 'lack of willpower', self-discipline, and personal agency or self-efficacy, depending on the theoretical model being used [22, 23]. Lack of time (due to family, household and occupational responsibilities) is also a significant barrier that has been extensively discussed in the health behavior change literature [24–26].

In the current study, changing habits was personally challenging, but participants shared that the program mitigated some of the challenges listed above. Comments on the individualized aspects of the program, the supportive and knowledgeable personalities of the providers and the social aspects were all seen as important to promote ongoing motivation and participation.

Results from both the questionnaire and focus groups reinforced the well-known challenges with maintaining changes, even after a one-year program. While over 60% were totally or very confident to maintain both diet and physical activity changes, there was a subgroup of about 10% who were less confident in maintaining physical activity changes and 4% for dietary changes. Optimal program length for the majority of people to maintain new lifestyle habits remains controversial and has implications for program delivery costs and sustainability.

Interpersonal level

Trust has been found to be an important element to consider in patient assessment of services [27]. Focus group results highlighted the importance of the family physician as motivating the participants to change, while also acknowledging the skills and knowledge of the other providers. The role of the family physician as a trusted mentor is likely critical to the success of the program.

While the family physician plays a key role as a co-ordinator and mentor, team functioning is also known to be very important in delivery of complex interventions [28]. This was not directly assessed, as patients might not know how teams work. It was indirectly assessed in the questionnaire by asking if patients received contradictory information on diet and exercise. Most felt that different providers did not tell them different information, an issue that has been identified in some team programs [29].

People enjoyed socializing with other participants during the program. While most health counselors are trained on motivational interviewing and other counseling techniques, they may not understand the importance of, nor have been formally trained on the social benefits of the program. Since, providers in this study usually counseled one-on-one, the social aspects of the program should be further enhanced. The importance of having significant others as part of the program was mentioned both in the questionnaire comments and in the focus groups. Greater appreciation for health behavior change influencing the whole household has implications for further development of the CHANGE program.

Organizational level

Mental health is a significant factor impacting behavior change programs [30]. In both the questionnaire and focus groups, participants reported that better mental health resources and supports were needed to provide increased success in the program. Feedback from participants highlights the importance of providing focused mental health related to low mood, fears, negative perceptions of health and life changes, and lack of

motivation. Surprisingly, no studies were found that examined the impact of providing an experienced mental health worker in a similar lifestyle change program for MetS. However, the importance of providing psychological supports is reinforced in other studies [30–33].

Several comments support a need to tailor the CHANGE program to various subgroups. Many middle-aged participants were still in the workforce, so time limitation was a key barrier. Offering more evenings and weekend programming would be beneficial for this group. At the organizational level, patients often advocate for increased flexibility regarding accessing services including increased flexible clinic hours. Through the development of primary care reform, clinics are starting to address this need by hosting clinics on evenings and weekends. However, allied health services need to be expanded as well. The older adult population had more flexibility in their time, but had higher levels of social disconnectedness and perceived isolation, which are independently associated with lower levels of self-rated physical health [34]. Seniors also encounter more barriers e.g., (transportation, increased physical activity limitations). Participants with lower socioeconomic status also need to be considered as they too have increased barriers (e.g., cost of parking, public transportation, child care costs, absence from work to attend appointments) as well as low participation rates in lifestyle change programs [35, 36]. Consideration of reimbursement for out-of-pocket expenses related to participating in the program could assist with attracting more participants from this subgroup. As some cultural minorities experience a high prevalence of MetS and engage in leisure time physical activities less frequently than do adults in the rest of the population [37], developing strategies to encourage this group to participate in CHANGE would also be important. For example, targeting the program toward participants with similar cultural and linguistic backgrounds, recruiting health professionals who speak the language, and weaving components of the culture such a traditional dance and ethnic diets into the program. Further development will need to address differing issues in differing locations.

Themes from the focus groups frequently complimented the questionnaire. There were no direct contradictions in comparing the results of questionnaire and focus groups; rather different aspects emerged as important. The key role of the family physician and importance of the social aspects emerged in the focus groups, while the questionnaire confirmed the trust they had in the team. Both methods revealed trust with their health professionals, along with an individualized realistic gradual approach led to the general support for such a lengthy and intensive program. Findings that a longer and more intensive program was preferred were unexpected and needs to be further explored.

Limitations

Further validation of the questionnaire is needed including assessment of test-retest reliability and convergent and divergent validity. While we sent out the questionnaire to all participants in the study, the response rate of 56% is likely not representative. In addition, as the focus group consisted of participants self –selecting and were only offered in French or English, not Russian, there is potential for further bias. Extra concerted efforts would be needed to elicit perspectives from participants, who declined to participate in the questionnaire and focus groups, which was beyond study scope. We also have no knowledge of the needs of the wider group of people with MetS who did not agree to undertake the CHANGE intervention. Different approaches are needed to determine how to reach and promote lifestyle change among other subgroups in the population. Likely multiple strategies are needed, including web-based approaches, group programs, and programs with a stronger mental health focus. Further work is required to explore the 10% of participants who noted they were less confident in maintaining physical activity changes and 4% for dietary changes.

Conclusion

This research provides insight into patients sharing their experience of the CHANGE lifestyle program in family medicine clinics and generally confirms a large body of literature on the major enablers and barriers to lifestyle change. Overall participants' experiences were very positive especially as they emphasized the importance of participating in an individualized program led by family physicians and a skilled and supportive team. The role of the family physician as a trusted mentor is likely a key factor to the success of the program.

Due to the personalized supports, participants' confidence in maintaining the changes long term was high. Specific recommendations provided by participants (e.g., increased mental heath support, flexible hours, tailoring program to specific diseases, including families in the program) may further improve the CHANGE program and its long-term success and sustainability.

Practice implications

Implementing complex behavioral interventions such as lifestyle modification in primary care is challenging. Although intrapersonal issues (e.g., intention, self-efficacy, self-discipline) often dominate peoples' perceptions of the success of such an intervention, modifying aspects at the interpersonal (e.g., trust, team functioning) and organizational level (e.g., mental health supports, flexible

hours) can ultimately improve the effectiveness of a program. The positive participant experiences shown in our current work enhance the evidentiary basis of the CHANGE Program and supports the wide spread implementation of CHANGE in primary care. Multiple approaches may be needed to obtain future participant experiences to inform ongoing program improvements.

Abbreviations
CHANGE: Canadian Health Advanced by Nutrition and Graded Exercise; MetS: Metabolic syndrome

Funding
Metabolic Syndrome Canada is a not-for-profit charitable organization that funded the current study.

Authors' contributions
All authors contributed substantially to conception and design, or acquisition of data, or analysis and interpretation of data; drafted the article or revised it critically for important intellectual content; gave final approval of the submitted version. All authors gave final approval of the submitted version. JK contributed to acquisition and interpretation of data (focus groups), and drafted the article. PB contributed to conception and design of the study, acquisition and interpretation of quantitative data, and drafted the article. DR contributed to quantitative data collection and analysis, and article revisions. MIS contributed to data collection, translation of questionnaire and reminders, data collection and analysis. DK contributed to conception and design of the study, interpretation of the data and reviewed the article. AT contributed to the design and the development of the project, led the focus group in French, and reviewed the manuscript. RD contributed to acquisition of data, interpretation of data, and revised it critically for important intellectual content. CR contributed to the development of the project, recruitment of patients for the focus group in French and reviewed the manuscript. DMM - contributed to conception and design of the study, and reviewed the manuscript. KJ contributed to conception and design of the study and reviewed the manuscript critically for important intellectual content.

Competing interests
The authors declare that they have no competing interests.

Author details
[1]Glenrose Rehabilitation Hospital, Edmonton, Canada. [2]Department of Family Relations & Applied Nutrition, University of Guelph, Guelph, Canada. [3]Department of Family Medicine, University of Alberta, Edmonton, Canada. [4]Department of Kinesiology, Laval University, Quebec City, Canada. [5]Metabolic Syndrome Canada, Kingston, Canada. [6]Department of Family Medicine and Emergency Medicine, Laval University, Quebec City, Canada. [7]Department of Human Health & Nutritional Sciences, University of Guelph, Guelph, Canada. [8]Department of Medicine, University of Toronto, Toronto, Canada.

References
1. Riediger N, Clara I. Prevalence of metabolic syndrome in the Canadian adult population. CMAJ. 2011;183:E1127–34.
2. Rao DP, Dai S, Lagace C, Krewski D. Metabolic syndrome and chronic disease. Chronic Dis Inj Can. 2014;34:36–45.

3. Mirolla M. The cost of chronic disease in Canada. Ottawa: The Chronic Disease Prevention Alliance in Canada. 2004. http://www.gpiatlantic.org/pdf/health/chroniccanada.pdf. Accessed 26 Aug 2018.

4. Anderson G, Chronic care: making the case for ongoing care. Princeton: Robert Wood Johnson Foundation. 2010. http://www.rwjf.org/content/dam/web-assets/2010/01/chronic-care. Accessed 26 Aug 2018.

5. Knowler WC, Barrett-Connor E, Fowler SE, Hamman SF, Lachin JM, Walker EA, Nathan DM. Reduction in the incidence of type 2 diabetes with lifestyle intervention or metformin. Diabetes Prevention Program Research Group. N Engl J Med. 2002;346:393–403.

6. Gillies CL, Abrams KR, Lambert PC, Cooper NJ, Sutton AJ, Hsu RT, Khunti K. Pharmacological and lifestyle interventions to prevent or delay type 2 diabetes in people with impaired glucose tolerance: systematic review and meta-analysis. BMJ. 2007;334:299.

7. Estruch R, Ros E, Salas-Salvadó J, Covas MI, Corella D, Arós F, Gómez-Gracia E, Ruiz-Gutiérrez V, Fiol M, Lapetra J, Lamuela-Raventos RM, Serra-Majem L, Pintó X, Basora J, Muñoz MA, Sorlí JV, Martínez JA, Martínez-González MA, PREDIMED study investigators. Primary prevention of cardiovascular disease with a Mediterranean diet. N Engl J Med. 2013;368:1279–90.

8. Lindström J, Ilanne-Parikka P, Peltonen M, Aunola S, Eriksson JG, Hemiö K, Hämäläinen H, Härkönen P, Keinänen-Kiukaanniemi S, Laakso M, Louheranta A, Mannelin M, Paturi M, Sundvall J, Valle TT, Uusitupa M, Tuomilehto J. Finnish diabetes prevention study group: sustained reduction in the incidence of type 2 diabetes by lifestyle-intervention: follow-up of the Finnish diabetes prevention study. Lancet. 2006;368:1673–9.

9. Yamaoka K, Tango T. Effects of lifestyle modification on metabolic syndrome: a systematic review and meta-analysis. BMC Med. 2012;10:138.

10. Bassi N, Karagodin I, Wang S, Vassallo P, Priyanath A, Massaro E, Stone NJ. Lifestyle modification for metabolic syndrome: a systematic review. Am J Med. 2014;127(12):e1–e10.

11. Jeejeebhoy K, Dhaliwal R, Heyland D, Leung R, Day A, Brauer P, Royall D, Tremblay A, Mutch D, Pliamm L, Rhéaume C, Klein D. Family physician-led, team-based, lifestyle intervention in patients with metabolic syndrome: results of a multicentre demonstration project. CMAJ Open. 2017;5:E229–36.

12. Klein D, Jeejeebhoy K, Tremblay A, Kallio M, Rhéaume C, Humphries S, Royall D, Brauer P, Heyland D, Dhaliwal R, Mutch DM. The CHANGE program: exercise interventnionin primary care. Can Fam Physician. 2017;63:546–52.

13. Desroches S, Lapointe A, Ratté S, Gravel K, Légaré F, Turcotte S. Interventions to enhance adherence to dietary advice for preventing and managing chronic diseases in adults. Cochrane Database Syst Rev. 2013;28:CD008722. https://doi.org/10.1002/14651858.CD008722.pub2.

14. Moroshko I, Brennan I, O'Brien P. Predictors of dropout in weight loss interventions: a systematic review of the literature. Obesity Rev. 2011;12:912–34. https://doi.org/10.1111/j.1467-789X.2011.00915.x.

15. Stokols D. Translating social ecological theory into guidelines for community health promotion. AJHP. 1996;10(4):282–98.

16. Creswell JW, Clark VL. Designing and conducting mixed methods research. 2nd ed. Los Angeles: Sage Publication; 2011.

17. Brauer P, Royall D, Kaethler A, Mayhew A, Israeloff-Smith M. Development of a patient experience questionnaire to improve lifestyle services in primary care. Prim Health Care Res Dev. 2018;15:1–11. https://doi.org/10.1017/S1463423617000937. [Epub ahead of print]

18. Wong ST, Haggerty J, Measuring patient experiences in primary health care: A review and classification of items and scales used in publicly-available questionnaires. Vancouver, Centre for Health Services and Policy Research. 2013. http://www.phcris.org.au/researchevidence/item.php?id=3381&spindex=18. Accessed 26 Aug 2018.

19. NVivo qualitative data analysis Software; QSR international Pty ltd. Version 10, 2014.

20. Thorne S, Kirkham SR, MacDonald-Emes J. Interpretive description: a noncategorical qualitative alternative for developing nursing knowledge. Res Nurs Health. 1997;20:169–77.

21. Guest G. Applied thematic analysis. Thousand Oaks: Sage Publication; 2012.

22. Haberman C, Brauer P, Dwyer JJ, Edwards AM. Self-reported health behaviour change in adults: analysis of the Canadian community health survey 4.1. Chronic Dis Inj Can. 2014;34:248–55.

23. Fishbein M. An integrative model for behavioural prediction and its application to health promotion. In: DiClemente RJ, Crosby RA, Kegler MC, editors. Emerging theories in health promotion practice and research. San Francisco: Jossey-Bass; 2009.

24. Kelly S, Martin S, Kuhn I, Cowan A, Brayne C, Lafortune L. Barriers and facilitators to the uptake and maintenance of healthy behaviours by people at mid-life: a rapid systematic review. PLoS One. 2016;11:e0145074. https://doi.org/10.1371/journal.

25. Caperchione CM, Vandelanotte C, Kolt GS, Duncan M, Ellison M, George E, Mummery WK. What a man wants: understanding the challenges and motivations to physical activity participation and healthy eating in middle-aged Australian men. Am J Mens Health. 2012;6:453–61. https://doi.org/10.1177/1557988312444718.

26. Vrazel J, Saunders RP, Wilcox S. An overview and proposed framework of social-environmental influences on the physical-activity behavior of women. Am J Health Promot. 2008;23:2–12. https://doi.org/10.4278/ajhp.06070999.

27. Ozawa S, Sripad P. How do you measure trust in the health system? A systematic review of the literature. Soc Sci Med. 2013;91:10–4. https://doi.org/10.1016/j.socscimed.2013.05.005.

28. Damschroder LJ, Aron DC, Keith RE, Kirsh SR, Alexander JA, Lowery JC. Fostering implementation of health services research findings into practice: consolidated framework for advancing implementation science. Implement Sci. 2009;4:50. https://doi.org/10.1186/1748-5908-4-50.

29. Asselin J, Osunlana AM, Ogunleye AA, Sharma AM, Campbell-Scherer D. Challenges in interdisciplinary weight management in primary care: lessons learned from the 5As team study. Clin Obes. 2016;6:124–32. https://doi.org/10.1111/cob.12133.

30. Rogerson MC, Murphy BM, Bird S, Morris T. "I don't have the heart": a qualitative study of barriers to and facilitators of physical activity for people with coronary heart disease and depressive symptoms. Int J Behav Nutr Phys Act. 2012;9:140. https://doi.org/10.1186/1479-5868-9-140.

31. Følling IS, Solbjør M, Helvik AS. Previous experiences and emotional baggage as barriers to lifestyle change - a qualitative study of Norwegian healthy life Centre participants. BMC Fam Pract. 2015;16:73. https://doi.org/10.1186/s12875-015-0292-z.

32. Fagiolini A, Frank E, Scott JA, Turkin S, Kupfer DJ. Metabolic syndrome in bipolar disorder: findings from the bipolar disorder Center for Pennsylvanians. Bipolar Disord. 2005;7(5):424–30.

33. Korkiakangas EE, Alahuhta MA, Laitinen JH. Barriers to regular exercise among adults at high risk or diagnosed with type 2 diabetes: a systematic review. Health Promot Int. 2009;24(4):416–27.

34. Cornwell EY, Waite LJ. Social disconnectedness, perceived isolation and health among older adults. J Health Soc Behav. 2009;50:31–48.

35. Williamson DL, Stewart MJ, Hayward K, Letourneau N, Makwarimba E, Masuda J, Raine K, Reutter L, Rootman I, Wilson D. Low-income Canadians' experiences with health-related services: implications for health care reform. Health Policy. 2006;76:106–21.

36. Govil SR, Weidner G, Merritt-Worden T, Ornish D. Socioeconomic status and improvements in lifestyle, coronary risk factors, and quality of life: the multisite cardiac lifestyle intervention program. Am J Public Health. 2009;99:1263–70. https://doi.org/10.2105/AJPH.2007.132852.

37. Belza B, Walwick J, Shiu-Thornton S, Schwartz S, Taylor M, LoGerfo J. Older adult perspectives on physical activity and exercise: voices from multiple cultures. Prev Chronic Dis. 2004;1:A09.

Permissions

The contributors of this book come from diverse backgrounds, making this book a truly international effort. This book will bring forth new frontiers with its revolutionizing research information and detailed analysis of the nascent developments around the world.

We would like to thank all the contributing authors for lending their expertise to make the book truly unique. They have played a crucial role in the development of this book. Without their invaluable contributions this book wouldn't have been possible. They have made vital efforts to compile up to date information on the varied aspects of this subject to make this book a valuable addition to the collection of many professionals and students.

This book was conceptualized with the vision of imparting up-to-date information and advanced data in this field. To ensure the same, a matchless editorial board was set up. Every individual on the board went through rigorous rounds of assessment to prove their worth. After which they invested a large part of their time researching and compiling the most relevant data for our readers.

The editorial board has been involved in producing this book since its inception. They have spent rigorous hours researching and exploring the diverse topics which have resulted in the successful publishing of this book. They have passed on their knowledge of decades through this book. To expedite this challenging task, the publisher supported the team at every step. A small team of assistant editors was also appointed to further simplify the editing procedure and attain best results for the readers.

Apart from the editorial board, the designing team has also invested a significant amount of their time in understanding the subject and creating the most relevant covers. They scrutinized every image to scout for the most suitable representation of the subject and create an appropriate cover for the book.

The publishing team has been an ardent support to the editorial, designing and production team. Their endless efforts to recruit the best for this project, has resulted in the accomplishment of this book. They are a veteran in the field of academics and their pool of knowledge is as vast as their experience in printing. Their expertise and guidance has proved useful at every step. Their uncompromising quality standards have made this book an exceptional effort. Their encouragement from time to time has been an inspiration for everyone.

The publisher and the editorial board hope that this book will prove to be a valuable piece of knowledge for researchers, students, practitioners and scholars across the globe.

List of Contributors

Carola van Dipten, Saskia van Berkel, Wim J. C. de Grauw, Nynke D. Scherpbier-de Haan, Bouke Brongers, Karel van Spaendonck, Willem J. J. Assendelft and Marianne K. Dees
Department of Primary and Community Care, Radboud University Medical Center, HBPostal Route 117, Nijmegen, The Netherlands

Jack F. M. Wetzels
Department of Nephrology, Radboud University Medical Center, 6500 HBPostal Route 464, Nijmegen, The Netherlands

Christine P. Kowalski, Miranda Veeser and Michele Heisler
Center for Clinical Management Research (CCMR-VA), VA Ann Arbor Healthcare System, 2800 Plymouth Road Bld. 16, Ann Arbor, MI 48109, USA

Michele Heisler
Department of Internal Medicine, University of Michigan, 1500 East Medical Center Drive, Ann Arbor, MI 48109, USA

Carl de Wet and Paul Bowie
Medical Directorate, NHS Education for Scotland, Glasgow, UK

Carl de Wet, Paul Bowie and Catherine O'Donnell
General Practice & Primary Care, Institute of Health & Wellbeing, College of Medical, Veterinary and Life Science, University of Glasgow, Glasgow, Scotland

Carl de Wet
School of Medicine, Griffith University, Southport, Gold Coast, Australia

Karleen F. Giannitrapani, Thomas Day and Karl A. Lorenz
VA Palo Alto Health Care System, Center for Innovation to Implementation (Ci2i), Menlo Park, CA 94025, USA

Peter A. Glassman
VA Greater Los Angeles Health Care System, Center for the Study of Healthcare Innovation, Implementation, and Policy (CSHIIP), Los Angeles, CA 90073, USA

Peter A. Glassman
David Geffen School of Medicine, University of California, Los Angeles, 10945 Le Conte Ave, Los Angeles, CA 90024, USA

Derek Vang
VA Minneapolis Center for Chronic Disease Outcomes Research (CCDOR), 5445 Minnehaha Avenue South, Minneapolis, MN 55417, USA

Jeremiah C. McKelvey
VA Northern California Health Care System, 10535 Hospital Way, Mather, CA 95655, USA

Steven K. Dobscha
VA Portland Health Care System, Center to Improve Veteran Involvement in Care (CIVIC), 3710 SW US Veterans Hospital Rd, Portland, OR 97239, USA
Department of Psychiatry, Oregon Health and Science University, 3181 SW Sam Jackson Park RD, Portland, OR 97239, USA.

Karl A. Lorenz
Stanford Medical School, Palo Alto, CA 94305, USA
RAND Corporation, 1776 Main Street, Santa Monica, CA 90401, USA

Marie Claire Van Hout
Public Health Institute, Liverpool John Moore's University, Liverpool, UK

Marie Claire Van Hout, Des Crowley, Aoife McBride and Ide Delargy
Substance Misuse Programme, Irish College of General Practitioners, Dublin, Ireland

Nikita Roman A. Jegan, Sarah Anna Kürwitz, Lena Kathrin Kramer, Charles Christian Adarkwah, Uwe Popert and Norbert Donner-Banzhoff
Department of General Practice and Family Medicine, Philipps-University Marburg, Karl-von-Frisch-Str. 4, 35032 Marburg, Germany

Monika Heinzel-Gutenbrunner
MH Statistical Consulting, Marburg, Germany

Charles Christian Adarkwah
Department of Health Services Research, Maastricht University, Maastricht, the Netherlands

Uwe Popert
Department of General Practice, Georg-August-University, Göttingen, Germany

Christina Sandlund, Kimberly Kane and Jeanette Westman
Department of Neurobiology, Care Sciences and Society, Karolinska Institutet, Stockholm, Sweden
Academic Primary Health Care Centre, Stockholm County Council, Solnavägen 1 E, 104 31 Stockholm, Sweden

Kimberly Kane
Aging Research Center, Karolinska Institutet and Stockholm University, Stockholm, Sweden

Mirjam Ekstedt
Department of Health and Caring Sciences, Linnaeus University, Stagneliusgatan 14, SE-392 34 Kalmar, Sweden
Department of Learning, Informatics, Management and Ethics, Karolinska Institutet, Stockholm, Sweden

Concepción Violán, Albert Roso-Llorach, Quintí Foguet-Boreu, Marina Guisado-Clavero, Mariona Pons-Vigués and Enriqueta Pujol-Ribera
Institut Universitari d'Investigació en Atenció Primària Jordi Gol (IDIAP Jordi Gol), Gran Via Corts Catalanes, 587 àtic, 08007 Barcelona, Spain
Universitat Autònoma de Barcelona, Bellaterra, Cerdanyola del Vallès, Spain

Quintí Foguet-Boreu
Department of Psychiatry, Vic University Hospital, Francesc Pla el Vigatà, 1, 08500 Vic, Barcelona, Spain

Mariona Pons-Vigués and Enriqueta Pujol-Ribera
Faculty of Nursing, University of Girona, Emili Grahit, 77, 17071 Girona, Spain

Jose M. Valderas
Health Services & Policy Research Group, Academic Collaboration for Primary Care, University of Exeter Medical School, Exeter EX1 2LU, UK

J. Cárdenas-Valladolid
Dirección Técnica de Sistemas de Información, Gerencia Asistencial de Atención Primaria, Servicio Madrileño de Salud, C/ San Martín de Porres, 6, 28035 Madrid, Spain
Universidad Alfonso X el Sabio, Villanueva de la Cañada, Madrid, Spain

J. Cárdenas-Valladolid, P. Gómez-Campelo, C. de Burgos-Lunar, J. C. Abánades-Herranz and M. A. Salinero-Fort
Aging and Fragility in the Elderly Group, Hospital La Paz Institute for Health Research (IdiPAZ), Madrid, Spain

J. Cárdenas-Valladolid, A. López-de Andrés, R. Jiménez-García, P. Gómez-Campelo, C. de Burgos-Lunar, F. J. San Andrés-Rebollo, J. C. Abánades-Herranz and M. A. Salinero-Fort
MADIABETES Research Group, Madrid, Spain

A. López-de Andrés, R. Jiménez-García and C. de Burgos-Lunar
Facultad de Ciencias de la Salud, Universidad Rey Juan Carlos, Alcorcón, Madrid, Spain

M. J. de Dios-Duarte
Jefatura de Estudios del Grado en Enfermería, Universidad Alfonso X el Sabio, Villanueva de la Cañada, Madrid, Spain

P. Gómez-Campelo
Innate Immunity Group, Hospital La Paz Institute for Health Research (IdiPAZ), La Paz University Hospital, Madrid, Spain
University Centre of Health Sciences San Rafael-Nebrija, Antonio de Nebrija University, Madrid, Spain

C. de Burgos-Lunar
Dirección General de Salud Pública, Subdirección de Promoción, Prevención y Educación de la Salud, Consejería de Sanidad,Madrid, Spain
Red de Investigación en Servicios de Salud en Enfermedades Crónicas (REDISSEC), Madrid, Spain

F. J. San Andrés-Rebollo
Centro de Salud Las Calesas, Madrid, Spain

J. C. Abánades-Herranz
Centro de Salud Monóvar, Madrid, Spain

M. A. Salinero-Fort
Subdirección General de Investigación. Consejería de Sanidad, Madrid, Spain

Anna Kirstine Winthereik and Anders Bonde Jensen
Department of Oncology, Aarhus University Hospital, Noerrebrogade 44, 8000 Aarhus C, Denmark

Mette Asbjoern Neergaard
Palliative Care Team, Department of Oncology, Aarhus University Hospital, Noerrebrogade 44, 8000 Aarhus, Denmark

Peter Vedsted
Research Unit for General Practice, Department of Public Health, Aarhus University, Bartholins Allé 2, 8000 Aarhus, Denmark

Anna Kirstine Winthereik
Department of Clinical Medicine, Aarhus University, Noerrebrogade 44, 8000 Aarhus C, Denmark

Daniel Jones, Charlotte Friend and Una Macleod
Hull York Medical School, Hertford Building, University of Hull, Cottingham Road, Hull HU6 7RX, UK

Andreas Dreher
Goethe University Frankfurt, Theodor-W.-Adorno-Platz 1, 60323 Frankfurt am Main, Germany

Victoria Allgar
Faculty of Health Sciences, University of York, Heslington, York YO10 5DD, UK

Ayako Shibata
Department of Obstetrics and Gynecology, Yodogawa Christian Hospital, 1-7-50, Kunijima, Higashiyodogawa-ku, Osaka 533-0024, Japan

Makoto Kaneko
Musashikoganei Clinic, Japanese Health and Welfare Co-operative Federation, 1-15-9, Honcho, Koganei-shi, Tokyo 184-0004, Japan
Division of Clinical Epidemiology, Jikei University School of Medicine, 3-25-8, Nishishimbashi, Minato-ku, Tokyo 105-8461, Japan

Makoto Kaneko and Machiko Inoue
Department of Family and Community Medicine, Hamamatsu University School of Medicine, 1-20-1, Handayama, Higashi-ku, Hamamatsu, Shizuoka 431-3192, Japan

Ranita Hisham, Chirk Jenn Ng, Su May Liew, Pauline Siew Mei Lai, Yook Chin Chia, Ee Ming Khoo, Nik Sherina Hanafi and Sajaratulnisah Othman
Department of Primary Care Medicine, Faculty of Medicine, University of Malaya, Kuala Lumpur, Malaysia

Ping Yein Lee
Department of Family Medicine, Faculty of Medicine and Health Sciences, Universiti Putra Malaysia, UPM Serdang, Selangor, Malaysia

Khatijah Lim Abdullah
Department of Nursing Sciences, Faculty of Medicine, University of Malaya, Kuala Lumpur, Malaysia

Karuthan Chinna
Department of Social and Preventive Medicine, Julius Centre University of Malaya, University of Malaya, Kuala Lumpur, Malaysia

Yook Chin Chia
Department of Medical Sciences School of Healthcare and Medical Sciences Sunway University, Selangor, Malaysia

Aniek A. O. M. Claassen and Willemijn H. van der Laan
Department of Rheumatology, Sint Maartenskliniek, 6500, GM, Nijmegen, The Netherlands

Henk J. Schers
Department of Primary and Community Care, Radboud University Medical Center, Nijmegen, The Netherlands

Sander Koëter and Keetie C. A. L. C. Kremers-van de Hei
Department of Orthopaedic Surgery, Canisius Wilhelmina Hospital, Nijmegen, The Netherlands

Joris Botman
Stichting Gezondheidscentrum De Kroonsteen - De Vuursteen, Nijmegen, The Netherlands

Vincent J. J. F. Busch
Department of Orthopaedic Surgery, Sint Maartenskliniek, Nijmegen, The Netherlands

Wim H. C. Rijnen
Department of Orthopaedic Surgery, Radboud University Medical Center, Nijmegen, The Netherlands

Cornelia H. M. van den Ende
Department of Rheumatology, Radboud University Medical Center, Nijmegen, The Netherlands

Anja Rieckert and Andreas Sönnichsen
Institute of General Practice and Family Medicine, Faculty of Health, Witten/ Herdecke University, Alfred-Herrhausen-Str. 50, 58448 Witten, Germany

Ulrike S. Trampisch and Renate Klaaßen-Mielke
Department of Medical Informatics, Biometry and Epidemiology, Ruhr University, Universitätsstr. 105, 44789 Bochum, Germany

Eva Drewelow
Institute of General Practice, Rostock University Medical Center, Doberaner Str. 142, 18057 Rostock, Germany

Aneez Esmail
NIHR School of Primary Care Research, University of Manchester, Oxford Road 176, M13 9PL, Manchester, UK

Tim Johansson and Sophie Keller
Centre for Primary Care, NIHR School of Primary Care Research, University of Manchester, Oxford Road M13 9PL, Manchester, UK

Ilkka Kunnamo and Joonas Mäkinen
Duodecim Medical Publications Ltd., Kaivokatu 10 A, 00100 Helsinki, Finland

Giuliano Piccoliori and Anna Vögele
South Tyrolean Academy of General Practice, Wangergasse 18, 39100 Bolzano, Italy

Inbar Levkovich
The Division of Family Medicine, Department of Family Medicine, The Ruth & Bruce Rappaport Faculty of Medicine, Technion-Israel Institute of Technology, 6 Hashachaf St., Bat-Galim, 35013 Haifa, Israel

Ateret Gewirtz-Meydan and Liat Ayalon
The Louis and Gaby Weisfeld School of Social Work, Bar-Ilan University, Ramat Gan, Israel

Khaled Karkabi
Department of Family Medicine, The Ruth & Bruce Rappaport Faculty of Medicine, Technion-Israel Institute of Technology, Clalit Health Services, Western Galilee District, Haifa, Israel

Suraya Abdul-Razak, Anis Safura Ramli and Siti Fatimah Badlishah-Sham
Primary Care Medicine Discipline, Faculty of Medicine, Universiti Teknologi MARA, Selayang Campus, Jalan Prima Selayang 7, 68100 Batu Caves,Selangor, Malaysia

Suraya Abdul-Razak and Anis Safura Ramli
Institute of Pathology, Laboratory and Forensic Medicine (I-PPerForM), Universiti Teknologi MARA, Sungai Buloh Campus, Jalan Hospital, 47000 Sungai Buloh, Selangor, Malaysia

Jamaiyah Haniff
National Clinical Research Centre, Ministry of Health, Kuala Lumpur, Malaysia

Robin Lewis
Department of Nursing and Midwifery, Sheffield Hallam University, Sheffield S10 2BP, England

Shona Kelly
Department of Social Work, Social Care and Community Services, Sheffield Hallam University, Collegiate Crescent, Sheffield S10 2BP, England

Lawrence Tan and Jennifer Reath
Department of General Practice, School of Medicine, Western Sydney University, Locked Bag 1797, Penrith, NSW 2751, Australia

Gisselle Gallego
School of Medicine, University of Notre Dame, 140 Broadway, Sydney, NSW 2007, Australia

Thi Thao Cam Nguyen
Bonnyrigg Family Medical Centre, Bonnyrigg, NSW, Australia

Les Bokey
Department of Surgery, Western Sydney University, Locked Bag 1797, Penrith, NSW 2751, Australia

Karin M. A. Swart, Myrthe van Vilsteren, Wesley van Hout, Esther Draak, Babette C. van der Zwaard, Henriette E. van der Horst and Petra J. M. Elders
Department of General Practice and Elderly Care Medicine, Amsterdam Public Health research institute, Amsterdam UMC, Vrije Universiteit Amsterdam, De Boelelaan 1117, 1081 HV Amsterdam, Netherlands

Karin M. A. Swart and Myrthe van Vilsteren
Stichting Artsen Laboratorium en Trombosedienst, Molenwerf 11, 1541 WR Koog aan de Zaan, Netherlands

Jacqueline G. Hugtenburg
Department of Clinical Pharmacology and Pharmacy, Amsterdam Public Health research institute, Amsterdam UMC, Vrije Universiteit Amsterdam, De Boelelaan 1117, 1081 HV Amsterdam, Netherlands

Jennifer Klein
Glenrose Rehabilitation Hospital, Edmonton, Canada

Paula Brauer, Dawna Royall and Maya Israeloff-Smith
Department of Family Relations & Applied Nutrition, University of Guelph, Guelph, Canada

Doug Klein
Department of Family Medicine, University of Alberta, Edmonton, Canada

Angelo Tremblay
Department of Kinesiology, Laval University, Quebec City, Canada

Caroline Rheaume
Department of Family Medicine and Emergency Medicine, Laval University, Quebec City, Canada

David M. Mutch
Department of Human Health & Nutritional Sciences, University of Guelph, Guelph, Canada

Khursheed Jeejeebhoy
Department of Medicine, University of Toronto, Toronto, Canada

Index

9 781632 428776